The Self-Regulation of Health and Illness Behaviour

Over
whole
which
to att
comp
such a

Th
preser
the se
key th

• re
   sy
• cu
• he
   he
• th
• th

Partic
effecti
regula
develo
effecti

Thi
regula
practit

Linda
Auckl
of Governors Professor at Rutgers – The State University of New Jersey. He
is also a member of the Institute of Medicine of the National Academy of
Sciences.

The Self-Regulation of Health and Illness Behaviour

Edited by Linda D. Cameron and Howard Leventhal

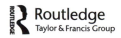
Routledge
Taylor & Francis Group

First published 2003
by Routledge
11 New Fetter Lane, London EC4P 4EE

Simultaneously published in the USA and Canada
by Routledge
29 West 35th Street, New York, NY 10001

Routledge is an imprint of the Taylor & Francis Group

©2003 Routledge

Typeset in Times by Taylor & Francis Books Ltd
Printed and bound in Great Britain by Biddles Ltd, Guildford and
King's Lynn

British Library Cataloguing in Publication Data
A catalogue record for this book is available from the British Library

Library of Congress Cataloging in Publication Data
The self-regulation of health and illness behaviour/ edited by Linda D.
Cameron and Howard Leventhal.
p. cm
Includes bibliography references and index.
1. Clinical health psychology. 2. Health behavior. 3. Sick–Psychology.
4. Self-management (Psychology). 5. Control (Psychology). 6. Goal
(Psychology). 7. Feedback (Psychology). I. Cameron, Linda D. (Linda
Diane), 1960– II. Leventhal, Howard, PhD.

R726.7 .S45 2002
613'.01'9–dc21

ISBN 0–415–29700–1 (hb)
ISBN 0–415–29701–X (pbk)

Contents

List of illustrations   viii
List of contributors   x
Acknowledgements   xiii

1   **Self-regulation, health, and illness: an overview**   1
    LINDA D. CAMERON AND HOWARD LEVENTHAL

PART I
Theoretical foundations   15

2   **Goals and confidence as self-regulatory elements underlying**
    health and illness behavior   17
    MICHAEL F. SCHEIER AND CHARLES S. CARVER

3   **The common-sense model of self-regulation of health and illness**   42
    HOWARD LEVENTHAL, IAN BRISSETTE, AND
    ELAINE A. LEVENTHAL

4   **Personality and self-regulation in health and disease:**
    toward an integrative perspective   66
    RICHARD J. CONTRADA AND ELLIOT J. COUPS

PART II
Representations of illnesses and health actions   95

5   **Representations of chronic illness**   97
    ADRIAN A. KAPTEIN, MARGREET SCHARLOO, DESIRÉE I. HELDER,
    WIM CHR. KLEIJN, INEZ M. VAN KORLAAR, AND MAAIKE WOERTMAN

6   **Representational beliefs about functional somatic syndromes**   119
    RONA MOSS-MORRIS AND WENDY WRAPSON

7   **Treatment perceptions and self-regulation**   138
    ROBERT HORNE

PART III
Emotional processes   155

8   **Anxiety, cognition, and responses to health threats**   157
    LINDA D. CAMERON

9   **Defensive denial, affect, and the self-regulation of health threats**   184
    DEBORAH J. WIEBE AND CAROLYN KORBEL

PART IV
The social and cultural context   205

10 **Carer perceptions of chronic illness**   207
    JOHN WEINMAN, MONIQUE HEIJMANS, AND MARIA JOAO
    FIGUEIRAS

11 **How gender stereotypes influence self-regulation of cardiac
    health care-seeking and adaptation**   220
    RENÉ MARTIN AND JERRY SULS

12 **Culture and illness representation**   242
    LINDA CIOFU BAUMANN

PART V
Applications and interventions   255

13 **Self-regulatory interventions for improving the management
    of chronic illness**   257
    KEITH J. PETRIE, ELIZABETH BROADBENT, AND GERALDINE
    MEECHAN

14 **Message frames and illness representations: implications for interventions to promote and sustain healthy behavior** 278
ALEXANDER J. ROTHMAN, KRISTINA M. KELLY,
ANDREW W. HERTEL, AND PETER SALOVEY

15 **Self-regulation and decision-making about cancer screening** 297
RONALD E. MYERS

16 **Self-regulation and genetic testing: theory, practical considerations, and interventions** 314
MICHAEL A. DIEFENBACH AND NATALIE HAMRICK

Index 332

Illustrations

Figures

2.1	A schematic depiction of a feedback loop	18
2.2	A hierarchy of goals	21
2.3	Two sorts of affect-generating systems and the affective dimensions we believe arise from the functioning of each	23
2.4	A flow-chart depiction of self-regulatory possibilities when obstacles to goal attainment are encountered	24
3.1	The parallel process model	46
3.2	The five domains of illness representations	50
4.1 (a)	Stress processes as mediators of personality effects on illness	71
4.1 (b)	Personality as moderator of stress-related effects on illness	72
7.1	Beliefs about HAART among consecutive HIV-positive individuals who chose either to accept or to decline the treatment	143
7.2	Treatment perceptions and the common-sense model of self-regulation	148
11.1	The influence of gender and CHD stereotypes on the interpretation of cardiac-related symptoms	225
11.2	Cardiac attributions as a function of information regarding gender and concurrent stressors	226
11.3	Levels of domestic activity undertaken by female post-MI patients and their spouses	230

Tables

4.1	Goal constructs linking personality and health-related self-regulation	88
5.1	Review of studies on illness representations and outcome in patients with asthma	103
5.2	Review of studies on illness representations and outcome in patients with chronic obstructive pulmonary disease	105
5.3	Review of studies on illness representations and outcome in patients with neurological disorders	106

5.4   Review of studies on illness perceptions and outcome
      in patients with cancer   109
5.5   Review of studies on illness representations and outcome
      in patients with cardiovascular diseases   110
6.1   Common functional somatic syndromes and their
      key characteristic symptoms   120

Contributors

Linda Ciofu Baumann, School of Nursing, University of Wisconsin-Madison, Madison, Wisconsin, USA

Ian Brissette, Institute for Health and Department of Psychology, Rutgers-The State University of New Jersey, New Brunswick, New Jersey, USA

Elizabeth Broadbent, Department of Health Psychology, The University of Auckland, Auckland, New Zealand

Linda D. Cameron, Department of Psychology, The University of Auckland, Auckland, New Zealand

Charles S. Carver, Department of Psychology, University of Miami, Miami, Florida, USA

Richard J. Contrada, Department of Psychology, Rutgers-The State University of New Jersey, Piscataway, New Jersey, USA

Elliot J. Coups, Department of Psychology, Rutgers-The State University of New Jersey, Piscataway, New Jersey, USA

Michael A. Diefenbach, Division of Population Science, Fox Chase Cancer Center, Cheltenham, Pennsylvania, USA

Maria Joao Figueiras, Instituto Piaget, Almada, Portugal

Monique Heijmans, Netherlands Institute for Health Services Research, Utrecht

Desirée I. Helder, Unit of Psychology, Leiden University Medical Centre, The Netherlands

Andrew W. Hertel, Department of Psychology, University of Minnesota, Minneapolis, Minnesota, USA

Robert Horne, Centre for Health Care Research, University of Brighton, Brighton, UK

Adrian A. Kaptein, Unit of Psychology, Leiden University Medical Centre, The Netherlands

Kristina M. Kelly, Department of Psychology, University of Minnesota, Minneapolis, Minnesota, USA

Wim Chr. Kleijn, Unit of Psychology, Leiden University Medical Centre, The Netherlands

Carolyn Korbel, Department of Psychology, University of Utah, Salt Lake City, Utah, USA

Inez M. van Korlaar, Unit of Psychology, Leiden University Medical Centre, The Netherlands

Elaine A. Leventhal, Department of Medicine, Robert Wood Johnson School of Medicine, UMDNJ, New Jersey, USA

Howard Leventhal, Institute for Health and Department of Psychology, Rutgers-The State University of New Jersey, New Brunswick, New Jersey, USA

René Martin, Department of Psychology, University of Iowa, Iowa City, Iowa, USA

Geraldine Meechan, Department of Health Psychology, The University of Auckland, Auckland, New Zealand

Rona Moss-Morris, Department of Health Psychology, The University of Auckland, Auckland, New Zealand

Ronald E. Myers, Department of Medicine, Division of Genetic and Preventive Medicine, Behavioral Epidemiology Section, Thomas Jefferson University, Philadelphia, Pennsylvania, USA

Keith J. Petrie, Department of Health Psychology, The University of Auckland, Auckland, New Zealand

Alexander J. Rothman, Department of Psychology, University of Minnesota, Minneapolis, Minnesota, USA

Peter Salovey, Department of Psychology, Yale University, New Haven, Connecticut, USA

Margreet Scharloo, Unit of Psychology, Leiden University Medical Centre, The Netherlands

Michael F. Scheier, Department of Psychology, Carnegie Mellon University, Pittsburgh, Pennsylvania, USA

Jerry Suls, Department of Psychology, University of Iowa, Iowa City, Iowa, USA

John Weinman, Guy's, Kings & St Thomas's School of Medicine, University of London, London, UK

Deborah J. Wiebe, Department of Psychology, University of Utah, Utah, USA

Maaike Woertman, Unit of Psychology, Leiden University Medical Centre, The Netherlands

Wendy Wrapson, Department of Health Psychology, The University of Auckland, Auckland, New Zealand

Acknowledgements

We would like to extend our great appreciation and thanks to the authors in this volume for their enthusiasm and efforts in generating what we believe are exciting contributions to the study of self-regulation, health, and illness. Linda would also like to thank her colleagues at The University of Auckland, and particularly Glynn Owens, Roger Booth, and Martin and Suzanne Wilkinson, for their continued support and good cheer during the preparation of this volume. Most of all, she is grateful to Paul, Michael, and Max Brown for their invaluable assistance, support, and patience. Howard would like to thank his colleagues in medicine, psychology, sociology, anthropology, and music, and his former students in these disciplines. Their ideas and efforts have greatly enriched his own understanding and approach to the study of self-regulation for the maintenance of health.

1 Self-regulation, health, and illness

An overview

Linda D. Cameron and Howard Leventhal[1]

The overall goal of this volume is to foster an integrated understanding of a self-regulation perspective of health and illness behavior. Recent years have witnessed a burgeoning interest in self-regulation within health psychology as well as in other fields, including social cognition, personality, education, and organizational psychology. We have sensed the need for a book that reviews current theory and research on self-regulation and health, not only to provide a synthesis of ideas and findings but also to orient and guide further research in this field. This volume is not designed to be a comprehensive overview of self-regulation theory and health research, but instead to provide selective reviews of principles and findings in order to familiarize readers with this area of study and stimulate new research ideas.

What is self-regulation in health and illness?

The growing popularity of self-regulation theory in psychological science has prompted the development and application of an array of self-regulation models for the study of health-related behaviors. Although there are some ambiguities and discrepancies across models regarding various principles of self-regulation, these models share some basic properties.

Virtually all models construe self-regulation as a systematic process involving conscious efforts to modulate thoughts, emotions, and behaviors in order to achieve goals within a changing environment (Zeidner *et al.*, 2000). It is a dynamic motivational system of setting goals, developing and enacting strategies to achieve those goals, appraising progress, and revising goals and strategies. Feedback loops play an integral role in these models, in which goals serve as reference values for appraising the relative success of efforts. Particularly central to this systems perspective is the principle of the TOTE (test, operate, text, exit) unit, which represents the mechanism involved in detecting and evaluating discrepancies between input (perceptions of a present state) and a reference value, generating behavior aimed at reducing the discrepancy, and appraising outcomes of that behavior in the subsequent self-regulatory cycle (Miller *et al.*, 1960).

Fundamental to many self-regulation theories is the delineation of a system of emotional processes that are integrally linked with cognitive mechanisms (Carver and Scheier, 1998; Epstein, 1994; Kuhl, 2000; Leventhal, *et al.*, 2001; Maes and Gebhardt, 2000; Miller *et al.*, 1996; Mischel and Shoda, 1999). Emotional responses are crucial elements of the motivational system – as direct responses to appraisals of goal-related progress, as experiences to be regulated, and as influences on cognitions and behaviors (see Chapter 8). Self-regulation models typically describe the parallel processing of problem-focused and emotion-focused goals, with cognitive and behavioral processes simultaneously dedicated to controlling the objective health problem and regulating emotional distress. Parallel processing of problem-focused goals and emotion-focused goals are explicitly identified, for example, by Lazarus and Folkman's (1984) stress-coping model, Maes and Gebhardt's Health Behavior Goal Model (Maes and Gebhardt, 2000), and Leventhal's Common-Sense Model (CSM; Leventhal *et al.*, 1980).

Beyond these common themes, self-regulation models diverge in their contents and processes. In the following sections, we introduce some of the primary themes that have received particular attention in self-regulation theory and research within the health domain.

Hierarchical goal structure

One important theme that receives particular emphasis in Carver and Scheier's (1998) model is the hierarchical organization of goals within the self-regulation system. Goals are arranged in a linked hierarchy whereby higher-level, more abstract goals (e.g., stay healthy) set the reference values for lower-level goals (e.g., take vitamins, keep cholesterol levels low, use sunscreen). This principle is useful for identifying the interconnectedness among various goals as well as capturing the general consistency among goals and, in turn, the coherence in actions and motivations displayed by an individual. Moreover, it provides a general framework for understanding how a particular action can serve multiple goals (see Chapter 2).

Abstract versus concrete-experiential processes

Another key theme of many self-regulation models is the distinction of abstract, conceptual processes from concrete-experiential processes (e.g., Epstein, 1994; Leventhal *et al.*, 2001). Abstract processes involve conceptual, propositional knowledge and thought whereas concrete-experiential processes incorporate imagery and perceptual-affective memories. Cognitive schemata (representations) incorporate both sorts for information; for example, one's representation of Parkinson's Disease may include knowledge that it may have some genetic basis and that it is a degenerative disease as well as vivid images of Mohammad Ali's trembling, yet controlled gestures and short, humorous verbal responses during interviews. These systems of memory and information processes have distinctive properties that differentially influence self-regulation. Conceptual-level processes tend to be more controlled and effortful, whereas concrete-experiential processes are automatic and emotionally evocative. Moreover, evidence suggests that concrete processes have a particularly strong influence on behavior (Brownlee *et al.*, 2000).

Conscious versus nonconscious regulation processes

Our general definition of self-regulation focuses specifically on conscious efforts to direct and monitor thoughts, affect, and behavior. Yet these conscious dynamics are influenced in important ways by a variety of nonconscious processes. Both abstract and concrete material may be activated below the level of awareness, and their activation can influence information processing, affective experiences, and behaviors without the individual being mindful of such influences. Nonconscious goals can also activate processes that alter conscious self-regulation dynamics. For example, motivations to protect one's self-concept or sense of safety can elicit defensive biases to process information in a manner that minimizes the threat to one's sense of well-being (see Chapter 9). Of the multitude of psychophysiological regulation processes in virtually constant operation, the vast majority occur outside of awareness – for example, neuroendocrine regulation, cardiorespiratory dynamics, and unconscious processes involved in the down-regulation or reduction of negative emotion (Kuhl, 2000). Yet these psychophysiological currents can shape conscious self-regulation dynamics through somatic experiences, affect levels, and information processing effects.

General models versus health-specific models of self-regulation

A key factor that distinguishes between different self-regulation models used in health psychology is whether it represents a general model of behavior (e.g., the Scheier and Carver model and the Lazarus and Folkman stress-coping model) or whether it applies specifically to health and illness behavior (e.g., Leventhal's CSM). Each type of model has its advantages. Health and illness are important life issues that critically influence goal selection and behavior in our daily activities. As such, general models of behavioral self-regulation must be able to account for health-related behavior. Health research generated by these models can usefully guide theoretical developments, and they can easily integrate evidence of self-regulation from other domains. In this manner, use of a general theory helps to integrate psychological science and promote cumulative knowledge about self-regulatory behavior.

4   *Linda D. Cameron and Howard Leventhal*

On the other hand, health-specific models are able to capture critical aspects of health and illness that are unique to this life domain (e.g., the primary role of symptom experiences, the survival threat posed by many illnesses, and the complexities surrounding medication use and other medical treatments). As Leventhal *et al.* note in Chapter 3, there are important characteristics of the representational contents of illnesses and treatments that must be recognized in order to sufficiently understand health and illness behaviors and experiences.

Yet these two approaches to theory and research are not inconsistent, and the field will progress most effectively if we carefully attend to how the specific models of health self-regulation map onto the more general theories of self-regulation. These theories operate at different levels of specificity, and advances at one level can serve to refine and shape understanding at the other level. Moreover, the focus of general models on self-regulatory *processes* (as opposed to *contents*) can stimulate developments concerning generic systems procedures as more content-focused theories such as the CSM can advance our understanding of the schematic contents and attributes of illness and treatment representations, and how they operate within the self-regulation system. Greater attention to the fit between general and health-specific models will ensure that theoretical developments at both levels are on the right track. Such efforts will also enhance the flow of information between the fields of social cognition, personality, and health psychology (as well as other fields) so that health psychology research can effectively inform theory development in these fields and so that the fields develop in synchrony. The advantages of such efforts are demonstrated by Contrada and Coups (Chapter 4) in their presentation of a social-cognitive perspective of self-regulation that integrates key aspects of personality theory and research with health self-regulation research.

Goals of survival and coherence

It has been suggested that humans possess two inherent, overarching goals: survival and coherence (Carver and Scheier, 1996). We may not be consciously aware of them as we go about our daily activities, but these fundamental goals are the basis from which all other goals are generated. Illness experiences can threaten both survival and a sense of coherence in one's sense of self and life goals, underscoring the critical importance of illness-related events and why adaptation to illness can present critical challenges in self-regulation. Consideration of survival and coherence goals seems crucial for understanding the cognitive, motivational, and behavioral patterns that evolve over the course of health threat experiences. In addition to Scheier and Carver's general model, health-specific models such as the CSM (see Moss-Morris *et al.*, 2002) and Myers' Preventive Health Model (see Chapter 15) identify coherence as a critical attribute of representations and goals.

Expectancies, perceived competence, and self-efficacy

Self-regulation theories vary in the extent to which they identify the role of expectancies and competence beliefs in behavioral self-regulation. Models developed by Bandura (1999), Schwartzer (1992), and Maes and Gebhardt (2000) emphasize how beliefs about one's ability to engage in a particular behavior (e.g., exercise) are crucial to the adoption of that behavior. Carver and Scheier's model delineates the importance of more general expectancies regarding potential outcomes. Other models (e.g., Leventhal's CSM) focus less explicitly on these beliefs – although ability, treatment efficacy, and expectations about disease course and treatment outcomes are seen as implicitly imbedded within illness and treatment representations. Self-efficacy and competence beliefs may be more important for complex health behaviors (e.g., exercise and dietary changes), yet less important for a substantial proportion of illness behaviors. For example, there may be relatively little variation in perceptions of one's ability to take oral medication or to seek medical care for serious symptoms (practical access issues notwithstanding).

The role of the self in self-regulation

Self-regulation theories of health and illness behavior generally tend to focus on the psychological dynamics that are specific to selected episodes and illness experiences. Yet there is increasing recognition of the need to connect these self-regulation dynamics with the more general self-system (Contrada and Ashmore, 1999). The self has been defined as a multi-faceted knowledge structure within which a web of self-representations and identities are connected with multiple sets of scripts and strategies for achieving related goals (Cantor and Kihlstrom, 1987). Illness challenges the integrity of the self, and managing illness requires the regulation of critical aspects of the self – in particular, emotional states and physical states. Social cognition theorists are making gains in clarifying the connections between self-constructs (e.g., self-efficacy and self-guides) and self-regulation, and Contrada and Coups (Chapter 4) identify a number of connections between these constructs and health-related self-regulation. As Kuhl (2000) notes, cognitive representations of goals and activities cannot energize behavior until they have personal meaning – that is, until they connect with the self. Once these connections are made, then cognitive representations of goals and activities may be translated into specific behavioral routines that can become dissociated from personal meaning over time. Scheier and Carver (Chapter 2) and Leventhal *et al.* (Chapter 3) discuss how the personal meaning of health-related goals and activities influence behavior, and how appraisals of health status and health-related activities shape the self-concept. Moreover, motivations to protect the self can bias health-related construals and cognitions, as discussed by Wiebe and Korbel (Chapter 9); the extent to which these effects can lead to the development of serious functional somatic syndromes is addressed by Moss-Morris and Wrapson (Chapter 6).

Self-regulation within the social and cultural systems

Although self-regulation theories tend to focus on internal processes and mechanisms, they must take into account that these processes occur in a sociocultural context and that knowledge structures of illnesses, health, and treatment methods reflect experiences within the family, neighborhood, community, and society at large (Jackson *et al.*, 2000). Moreover, social and economic resources constrain or permit health-related behavior and critically influence cognitive and affective experiences when dealing with health threats. Indeed, sociocultural factors affect virtually every component of the self-regulation system: definitions of the self, construals of illness, development of desires and goals, identification of strategies for coping, reference values for appraising progress, and even emotional responses and use of emotion regulation strategies. Self-regulation theory offers a framework with which to systematically examine the interactions between persons and contexts – that is, how self-regulation is linked with social relationships and the cultural environment (see Chapter 12).

Health and illness self-regulation occurs within dynamic social contexts, and illness management is often a shared task involving family members and significant friends. As social experiences involving the sharing of ideas, treatment procedures, and emotional regulation with others, illness behavior is best understood within the social context and by considering the congruence and incongruence of self-regulation systems among those involved (see Chapters 10 and 11).

Are these models different from other models popular in the health domain?

The term 'self-regulation' has been used so widely in recent years that there is some speculation as to whether self-regulation models are really that different from other models of health and illness behavior – indeed, whether most health-related behavior models *are* self-regulation models. Yet although a model may include some combination of cognitive processes, affective factors, and behavioral goals, it is not a self-regulation model unless it sufficiently captures the dynamic elements of feedback, motivation, and goal pursuit. Comprehensive comparisons of self-regulation models with other health/illness behavior models exist, and the reader is directed to these extensive treatments of this issue (Brownlee *et al.*, 2000; Maes and Gebhardt, 2000; Leventhal *et al.*, 2001). We briefly identify key attributes of two categories of health behavior models that characterize their similarities with and, more importantly, their distinctiveness from self-regulation models.

Subjective utility models such as the Health Belief Model (Becker, 1974), the theory of reasoned action (Ajzen and Fishbein, 1980), and the more recent theory of planned behavior (Ajzen, 1991) all consider the individual as a rational decision-maker who weighs up his or her attitudes and values when evaluating the overall utility of the behavior in question. As Maes (2000) notes, these conceptual processes represent an initial, rudimentary phase of self-regulation: the phase of setting behavioral goals. However, these models fail to capture several important aspects of behavioral self-regulation: they do not incorporate emotional processes; they view behavioral decisions as static events rather than as dynamic processes that change over time; and they fail to delineate feedback processes for appraising progress toward or away from goal states. In this volume, Rothman *et al.* (Chapter 14) and Myers (Chapter 15) integrate aspects of subjective utility models into self-regulatory perspectives of health persuasion and decision-making. This approach is needed in order to meld the many insights provided by these models with current self-regulation perspectives.

Stage theories of health behavior represent another category of health behavior change. Models such as the transtheoretical model (Prochaska and DiClemente, 1984), the precaution adoption process (Weinstein, 1988), and the health action process approach (Schwartzer, 1992) have in common the identification of distinct phases in the process of selecting, adopting, and maintaining a change in behavior. Although these models attend to the dynamic nature of behavior over time, they (to varying degrees) are less successful in delineating the roles of emotional processes in influencing behavior, the nature of the psychological processes within the stages, and the influence of the social and environmental context on behavior change throughout the stages. In particular, the reliance of the transtheoretical model on defining all beliefs, attitudes, emotional experiences, and social factors as 'pros' and 'cons' obscures the complexities of the cognitive, affective, and social processes influencing behavior.

A focus on Leventhal's CSM and the Scheier and Carver model of self-regulation

The authors in the present volume focus to a great extent on the CSM and the Scheier and Carver self-regulation model, although other self-regulation models are also discussed. We take this focus because we believe there is much to be gained in health psychology theory and research by highlighting these two theories. First, they complement each other in many ways. For example, the CSM has developed primarily to explain health and illness behavior and gives particular attention to schematic contents, whereas Scheier and Carver's model has developed as a more general theory of behavior and elaborates on process. Second, both theories have been particularly successful in stimulating research and empirical advances in health psychology (and, in the case of the Scheier and Carver model, in social and personality psychology). This volume highlights the extent to which these theoretical perspectives can be integrated. Their joint consideration can facilitate the process of identifying gaps in these models and, in turn, ways to refine and develop these frameworks.

Intervening in self-regulation

As an applied discipline, one of the primary goals of health psychology is to develop interventions for promoting health and quality of life. Effective interventions will be those that promote successful self-regulation – that is, adaptive problem-focused strategies and emotion regulation, both of which are essential for achieving the goals of survival and coherence.

Self-regulation models can be useful as templates for evaluating existing interventions. By appraising interventions and evidence regarding their outcomes from a self-regulatory perspective, we can better understand why they succeed and why they fail. Moreover, we may have a better understanding of the conditions under which they are likely to succeed or fail, and which individuals are most likely to benefit and when (see Chapter 13). More proactively, self-regulation models can serve as theoretical frameworks for designing new interventions. To date, few interventions have been designed specifically on the basis of self-regulation models (e.g., Petrie *et al.*, 2002), but the initial efforts are encouraging and we strongly believe that interventions guided by self-regulation theory will most effectively foster health and well-being. These interventions will, by their very nature, require much more tailoring, flexibility, and complexity than have interventions based on more simplistic theoretical models. Yet the modest success of many existing psychosocial interventions suggests that this more sophisticated approach is necessary.

Self-regulation interventions are likely to be of particular relevance in the growing number of conditions requiring informed decision-making as opposed to unquestioning acceptance of a treatment or behavior. Advances in medical technology are leading consumers into gray areas of treatment choices, in which available medical assessments and procedures are of unknown utility. In these conditions, it is critical that consumers make informed decisions about whether to undergo these procedures or not. Cancer screening (see Chapter 15) and genetic testing (see Chapter 16) are two areas in which there is an increasing demand for interventions aimed at fostering effective decision-making.

We have been enlightened by the insights regarding a self-regulation approach to behavioral interventions offered by the authors in this volume. We would like to supplement their suggestions with a few of our own comments on intervention design from a self-regulatory perspective. First, we agree that interventions need to be tailored to the individual's belief system and personal context. In doing so, interventions should assist individuals in identifying realistic and feasible behavior goals, using techniques for enabling the individual to develop a coherent system of beliefs (illness and treatment representations) that support and motivate the behaviors needed to achieve these goals. This belief system must integrate the concrete experiences of the disease (e.g., symptoms and functional status) in a manner that is congruent with goal-relevant behavior. When possible, these concrete experiences should be used as motivational cues for desired behavior. For example, cardiac patients could be taught that one way to restore energy is to identify feelings of lethargy as cues to eat a healthy meal or to take a walk. Interventions also need to identify ways to make 'quiet periods salient'. Many illnesses and illness-risk conditions involve lengthy periods when the individual is symptom-free or else experiences stable levels of symptomatology (e.g., prolonged fatigue and weakness). Symptoms are salient motivators of protective action, and acute, changing symptoms are more alarming and motivating than vague, unchanging symptoms (thereby reflecting a fundamental psychological principle: stimulus change triggers attention/awareness whereas stimulus constancy does not). Interventions must use methods for attracting attention to health-protective efforts and activating motivation to engage in those efforts during the quiet times. Interventions also must carefully attend to emotion regulation needs, as failure to effectively process and resolve distress can derail illness self-regulation and undermine health and well-being (see Chapter 8). Finally, interventions must be sensitive to the changing dynamics of behavior over time and the need for feedback on how well individuals are doing in their self-regulation efforts. Monitoring and feedback are critical to motivating sustained behavior.

Outline of the book

This volume is organized into five parts. Part I is devoted to reviewing the theoretical foundations of self-regulation, and the chapters in this section present three different, yet largely complementary theoretical orientations to self-regulation in health and illness. Scheier and Carver (Chapter 2) provide an overview of their general self-regulatory model and its application to understanding illness-related behavior. They consider the particular relevance of confidence and doubt in relation to coping with health threats, and the challenges of deciding whether to maintain or let go of important life goals when illness or aging makes them difficult to achieve. As they note, these issues highlight the importance of maintaining hope and engagement in goals that provide a sense of purpose when dealing with the adversities of illness. Leventhal *et al.* (Chapter 3) continue the section with a presentation of the CSM, describing its development over the past decades. They discuss the need for models that delineate the contents of representations in order to fully understand illness self-regulation, the interactive links of illness self-regulation with the self-system, and changes in self-regulation strategies associated with aging. Next, Contrada and Coups (Chapter 4) address the important role of personality in understanding self-regulation in health and illness. In addition to providing an overview of key constructs that link personality to health and illness, they describe the merits of a social-cognitive perspective for understanding personality influences in health self-regulation and note important implications for statistical and methodological approaches for further research in these intersecting areas.

Part II reviews empirical developments in the role of illness representations in determining health behaviors and outcomes. Significant advances in illness representations research have taken place in the last decade, with substantial contributions from researchers in the United Kingdom, Europe, and New Zealand; the majority of these efforts have been guided by the CSM. Kaptein *et al.* (Chapter 5) review empirical findings on relationships between illness beliefs and outcomes for five major chronic illnesses, noting some emerging patterns and trends within and across illness domains and identifying issues for further research. Illness representations take on a particularly intriguing nature when dealing with functional somatic syndromes. These conditions, for which there is generally little or no evidence of primary biological pathology, are particularly mysterious to patients, and their common-sense representations of these syndromes bear some interesting similarities. Moss-Morris and Wrapson (Chapter 6) review this literature, noting how the CSM provides a useful framework for identifying cognitive, emotional, behavioral, and personality (self-concept) factors that contribute to the development and perpetuation of these syndromes. Horne (Chapter 7) focuses on representations of medical treatments, detailing his model and reviewing supportive research. As his work demonstrates, further developments in our understanding of treatment representations will significantly enhance the breadth and depth of self-regulation theory.

Part III focuses on the emotional processes influencing the self-regulation of health-related behaviors. Emotional processes are a key feature of self-regulation models, and recent years have witnessed considerable advances in research on how affective experiences influence cognitive processing and decision-making. Anxiety and fear are pervasive features of critical illness experiences, and Cameron (Chapter 8) reviews the processes by which anxiety arousal can shape information processing and coping behaviors during these experiences. Wiebe and Korbel (Chapter 9) focus on the influential role of defensive biases in affect regulation when confronted with health threats. Moreover, they identify how defensive biases link with the self-system. In both of these chapters, the authors suggest that anxiety arousal and anxiety-induced defensive biases can play adaptive roles in self-regulation during health threats. For example, anxiety activation motivates protective attentional and behavioral efforts, and defensive biases can serve to regulate distress in order to maintain optimal levels of motivation and attention to danger control.

The chapters in Part IV explore interpersonal and cultural influences on self-regulatory behavior and health outcomes. Weinman and colleagues (Chapter 10) begin with a discussion of how partners' and caregivers' beliefs about a patient's illness can shape the patient's coping behaviors and outcomes. The research presented in this chapter underscores the important point that illnesses are social experiences. Not only do illnesses affect the lives of others, but the course of illness can be significantly shaped by the illness beliefs held by others. Martin and Suls (Chapter 11) further address the social context of illness experiences. They describe how social stereotypes are connected with illness representations, and how cognitive heuristics and processes responsible for stereotyped responses are integrated into illness self-regulation. The authors draw on the stereotyping and gender literatures in articulating these connections, and their work demonstrates the utility of these linkages in exploring the role of social stereotypes in the management of illness. Finally, Baumann (Chapter 12) provides a cultural perspective of illness representations, reviewing methodologies for exploring variations in illness construals across cultures and identifying key ways in which culture shapes illness beliefs and behaviors.

Part V focuses on the practical applications of self-regulation theory and, in particular, its utility in designing health care interventions. Petrie *et al.* (Chapter 13) review interventions for chronic illness patients that are based on self-regulatory principles, and they describe a recent self-regulation intervention aimed at instilling adaptive illness representations in myocardial infarction patients. Rothman *et al.* (Chapter 14) review empirical developments, guided by the Prospect Theory of decision-making, in framing messages to effectively promote health-protective behaviors. They propose an empirical approach for addressing the dynamic nature of these behavior representations, noting that changes in these representations over repeated use of the behavior will require coordinated changes in the message frames in order for them to be persuasive. The final two chapters address the increasing need to promote informed decision-making in situations where the health behavior in question is of uncertain utility. Myers (Chapter 15) considers cancer-screening decisions and describes the Preventive Health Model, a self-regulation theory that integrates key factors relating to screening use. He then discusses how self-regulation approaches to cancer screening can integrate decision-making tools such as Analytic Hierarchical Processing techniques. These techniques can foster informed decision-making for situations such as prostate cancer tests, in which the test's benefits are unclear and its use should be based on personal values and choice. In a similar vein, Diefenbach and Hamrick (Chapter 16) take a self-regulatory perspective on genetic testing, noting the applicability of the theory in understanding the dynamics surrounding genetic-testing decisions and outlining a self-regulation intervention for fostering informed decisions. These last three chapters identify important ways in which self-regulation theory can be advanced to integrate key aspects of decision-making theories.

We complete this volume with a respect for the substantial foundations that have been laid and the proliferation of advances made in understanding the self-regulation of health and illness behavior. We appreciate the complementary perspectives offered by our international team of authors, and we hope that this volume serves to integrate empirical advances in health self-regulation and stimulate further syntheses in theory and research across nations. We look forward with optimism to these future developments.

Note

1   Correspondence concerning this chapter should be addressed to Linda D. Cameron, Department of Psychology (Tamaki Campus), The University of Auckland, Private Bag 92019, Auckland, New Zealand. E-mail: l.cameron@auckland.ac.nz

References

Ajzen, I. (1991) 'The theory of planned behavior,' *Organizational Behavior and Human Decision Processes* **50**: 179–211.

Ajzen, I. and Fishbein, M. (1980) *Understanding Attitudes and Predicting Social Behavior*, Englewood Cliffs, NJ: Prentice-Hall.

Bandura, A. (1986) *Social Foundations of Thought and Action : A Social Cognitive Theory*, Englewood Cliffs, NJ: Prentice-Hall.

—— (1999) 'Social-cognitive theory of personality,' in L.A. Pervin and O.P. John (eds) *Handbook of Personality: Theory and Research*, 2nd edn, New York: Guilford, pp. 154–196.

Becker, M.H. (1974) 'The health belief model and personal health behaviors,' *Health Education Monographs* **2**: 376–423.

Brownlee, S., Leventhal, H. and Leventhal, E.A. (2000) 'Regulation, self-regulation, and construction of the self in the maintenance of physical health,' in M. Boekaerts, P.R. Pintrich and M. Zeidner (eds) *Handbook of Self-Regulation*, San Diego, CA: Academic Press, pp. 369–416.

Cantor, N. and Kihlstrom, J.F. (1987) *Personality and Social Intelligence*, Englewood Cliffs, NJ: Prentice-Hall.

Carver, C.S. and Scheier, M.F. (1996) *Perspectives on Personality*, 3rd edn, Boston, MA: Allyn and Bacon.

—— (1998) *On the Self-Regulation of Behavior*, New York: Cambridge University Press.

Contrada, R.J. and Ashmore, R.D. (eds) (1999) *Self and Social Identity Vol. 2: Self, Social Identity, and Physical Health*, New York: Oxford University Press.

Epstein, S. (1994) 'Integration of the cognitive and the psychodynamic unconscious,' *American Psychologist* **49**: 709–724.

Jackson, T., Mackenzie, J. and Hobfoll, S.E. (2000) 'Communal aspects of self-regulation,' in M. Boekaerts, P.R. Pintrich and M. Zeidner (eds) *Handbook of Self-Regulation*, New York: Academic Press, pp. 275–300.

Kuhl, J. (2000) 'A functional-design approach to motivation and self-regulation: the dynamics of personality systems and interactions,' in M. Boekaerts, P.R. Pintrich and M. Zeidner (eds) *Handbook of Self-Regulation*, San Diego, CA: Academic Press, pp. 111–169.

Lazarus, R.S. and Folkman, S. (1984) *Stress, Appraisal, and Coping*, New York: Springer.

Leventhal, H., Leventhal, E.A. and Cameron, L. (2001) 'Representations, procedures, and affect in illness self-regulation: a perceptual-cognitive model,' in A. Baum, T.A. Revenson and J.E. Singer (eds) *Handbook of Health Psychology*, Mahwah, NJ: Lawrence Erlbaum Associates, pp. 19–47.

Leventhal, H., Meyer, D. and Nerenz, D.R. (1980) 'The common sense representation of illness danger,' in S. Rachman (ed.) *Contributions to Medical Psychology*, vol. 2, New York: Pergamon Press, pp 7–30.

Maes, S. and Gebhardt, W. (2000) 'Self-regulation and health behavior: the health behavior goal model,' in M. Boekaerts, P.R. Pintrich and M. Zeidner (eds) *Handbook of Self-Regulation*, San Diego, CA: Academic Press, pp. 343–368.

Maes, S., Leventhal, H. and De Ridder, D. (1996) 'Coping with chronic disease,' in N. Endler and M. Zeidner (eds) *Handbook of Coping*, New York: Wiley.

Miller, G., Galanter, E. and Pribram, K. (1960) *Plans and the Structure of Behavior*, New York: Henry Holt & Co.

Miller, S.M., Shoda, Y. and Hurley, K. (1996) 'Applying cognitive-social theory to health-protective behavior: breast self-examination in cancer screening,' *Psychological Bulletin* **118**: 70–94.

Mischel, W. and Shoda, Y. (1999) 'Integrating dispositions and processing dynamics within a unified theory of personality: the cognitive-affective personality system,' in L.A. Pervin and O.P. John (eds) *Handbook of Personality: Theory and Research*, 2nd edn, New York: Guilford, pp. 197–218.

Moss-Morris, R., Weinman, J., Petrie, K.J., Horne, R., Cameron, L.D. and Buick, D. (2002) 'The Revised Illness Perception Questionnaire (IPQ-R),' *Psychology and Health* **17**: 1–16.

Petrie, K.J., Cameron, L.D., Ellis, C., Buick, D. and Weinman, J. (2002) 'Changing illness perceptions following myocardial infarction: an early intervention randomized controlled trial,' *Psychosomatic Medicine* **64**: 580–586.

Prochaska, J. and DiClemente, C. (1984) *The Transtheoretical Approach: Crossing the Traditional Boundaries of Therapy*, Homewood, IL: Dow Jones-Irwin.

Schwartzer, R. (ed.) (1992) *Self-Efficacy: Thought Control of Action*, Washington: Hemisphere.

Weinstein, N.D. (1988) 'The precaution adoption process,' *Health Psychology* **7**: 355–386.

Zeidner, M., Boekaerts, M. and Pintrich, P.R. (2000) 'Self-regulation: directions and challenges for future research,' in M. Boekaerts, P.R. Pintrich and M. Zeidner (eds) *Handbook of Self-Regulation*, San Diego, CA: Academic Press, pp. 750–768.

Part I

Theoretical foundations

2 Goals and confidence as self-regulatory elements underlying health and illness behavior

Michael F. Scheier and Charles S. Carver[1]

The purpose of this chapter is to discuss some of the ways in which self-regulatory models of behavior relate to today's understanding of health and illness. Although self-regulatory models have been around for a number of years in social and personality psychology, the systematic application of those models to health and disease is of more recent origin. As a result, many health psychologists are still becoming aware of the nature of self-regulatory models and how they relate to some of the phenomena that health psychologists seek to understand.

We think it useful to begin this chapter by describing a set of orienting assumptions and principles embedded in models of self-regulation, placing the heaviest emphasis on our own approach. Then we turn to issues that self-regulatory models raise with respect to health and illness behaviors. One set of issues has to do with the importance of maintaining confidence when illness episodes and health threats are encountered. A second set of issues has to do with a tension that arises between holding on to and letting go of important values and goals as those values and goals are threatened by disease processes or by deterioration in biological functioning associated with normal aging. A final set of issues has to do with the implications of self-regulatory models for understanding why some types of interventions might work better for some types of patients than others.

A model of behavioral self-regulation

Goals and feedback processes

For the past two and a half decades, our research has been guided by a particular model of behavioral self-regulation (Carver and Scheier, 1981, 1990, 1998). Central to our view is the notion that people live life by identifying goals and behaving in ways aimed at attaining these goals. The idea that goals form an important part of human behavior is shared with a variety of contemporary personality theorists (e.g., Austin and Vancouver, 1996; Bandura, 1997; Cantor and Kihlstrom, 1987; Carver and Scheier, 1998; Elliott and Dweck, 1988; Emmons, 1986; Higgins, 1987, 1996; Klinger, 1975;

Little, 1989; Markus and Nurius, 1986; Miller and Read, 1987; Pervin, 1982, 1989). Common to all these views is the belief that goals energize and direct activities (Pervin, 1982). All these views also convey the sense that understanding a person means understanding the person's goals – that goals give meaning and purpose to people's lives (Baumeister, 1989; Scheier and Carver, 2001).

People's goals would not be very interesting if they were not somehow linked to their actions. But how exactly are goals and action linked? For us, goals serve as reference values for feedback processes. A feedback loop consists of four elements in a particular organization (cf. Miller *et al.* 1960). The elements are an input function, a reference value, a comparator, and an output function (see Figure 2.1).

An input function is a sensor that brings in information about the current state of affairs. It can be thought of as perception. The reference value provides information about what is intended or desired, thereby providing the target around which the system regulates. In the kinds of feedback loops we will be discussing, reference values are roughly equivalent to goals. The comparator is a device that makes comparisons between input and reference value, yielding one of two outcomes: either the values being compared are noticeably different from one another or they are not. Following the comparison is an output function. For present purposes, output is behavior, though sometimes the behavior is internal.

The nature of the output varies, depending on whether the loop under consideration is discrepancy *reducing* or discrepancy *enlarging*. In a discrepancy reducing feedback loop, the output is aimed at diminishing differences

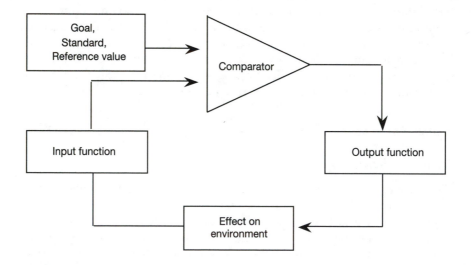

Figure 2.1 A schematic depiction of a feedback loop

between input and reference value. In human behavior, discrepancy reduction (matching of input to reference value) is reflected in attempts to approach desired goals. For example, a health conscious person who has the goal of consuming 1800 calories per day will adjust caloric intake upward or downward, in order to minimize discrepancies between what is actually consumed and what is intended to be consumed each day.

In a discrepancy enlarging feedback loop, the output increases differences between input and reference value. Thus, the reference value is one to avoid rather than one to approach. It may be simplest to think of such values as 'anti-goals.' An example from the health domain would be the case of a person whose goal is to avoid any symptoms of illness, or to never visit a physician's office.

Regardless of whether the feedback loop is discrepancy enlarging or discrepancy reducing, feedback is essential to the system's functioning. Without feedback, comparisons cannot be made, and evaluation of the effects of one's self-regulatory actions would not be possible. Research from health psychology suggests that informational feedback matters so much that people will seek it out and rely on it *even when it doesn't tell them anything*, and even when relying on it creates *problems* for their health. Under such circumstances, the feedback loop governing behavior continues to operate, continues to sense, compare, and guide behavior, but it does so in a manner that is counter-productive.

Several studies that illustrate this point examine the behavior of people being treated for hypertension (Baumann and Leventhal, 1985; Meyer *et al.*, 1985). People with hypertension have no reliable symptoms. Yet most people who enter treatment for hypertension quickly come to believe that they *can* isolate a symptom of it. Indeed, the longer they're in treatment, the more likely they are to think they can tell when their blood pressure is up. More than 90 per cent of those in treatment for more than three months claim to be able to tell (Meyer *et al.*, 1985). Patients then use the symptoms to make medical decisions. Most importantly, they use the symptoms to tell them whether to take their medication, or whether to remain in treatment.

This example illustrates how much people need and rely on feedback to guide behavior. If the people with hypertension perceive a discrepancy between present state (symptom) and standard (no symptoms), they act in a way they think will reduce the discrepancy (take their medication). They are using feedback, just as the self-regulation approach suggests people do all the time. The problem is that the input channel is providing faulty information.

Hierarchical organization among goals

The distinction made above between approach goals and avoidance goals is one way in which goals differ. Another way goals differ is in the level of abstraction (for broader treatment of this issue, see Carver and Scheier, 1998). For example, a man might have the goal, at a high level of abstraction, of being healthy. He may also have the goal, at a lower level of abstraction, of going to the gym to work out on a daily basis. The first goal is to be a particular kind of *person*, the second concerns completing particular kinds of *action*. You can also imagine goals even more concrete than the latter one, such as the goal of completing thirty minutes on a treadmill. Such goals are closer to specifications of individual acts than was the second goal mentioned, which was more a summary statement about the overriding intent that provides the organizational focus for a set of action patterns.

These examples of concrete goals link directly to the example of an abstract goal, helping to illustrate the idea that goals can be connected hierarchically. In 1973, William Powers argued that behavior occurs via a hierarchical organization of discrepancy reducing feedback loops. Inasmuch as such loops imply goals, his argument assumed a hierarchical model of goals (see also Vallacher and Wegner's (1985, 1987) theory of action identification). Powers reasoned that the output of a high-level system consists of resetting reference values at the next lower level. To put it differently, higher-order systems 'behave' by providing goals to the systems just below them. In this manner, there is a 'cascade' of control from higher-order, more abstract loops to lower-order, more concrete loops, as the constituents of the higher-order goal are embodied in more and more specific aspects of action (cf. Leventhal *et al.*, 1980; Leventhal and Carr, 2001; Leventhal *et al.*, 2001).

Figure 2.2 shows a simple portrayal of Power's hierarchy. This diagram omits the loops of feedback processes, using lines to indicate only the links among goal values. Terms on the left side of the figure provide the labels that Powers (1973) used to identify the top levels of control in the specific hierarchy that he proposed. The lines imply that moving toward a particular lower goal contributes to the attainment of a higher goal (or even to several at once). Multiple lines to a given goal indicates that several lower-level action qualities can contribute to its attainment. The figure can also be read in the opposite direction, as indicating that a given higher-order goal specifies more concrete goals at the next lower level. As indicated previously, there are goals to 'be' a particular way and goals to 'do' certain things (and at lower levels, goals to create physical movement). Goals of 'being' particular ways are attained by 'doing' particular actions.

Hierarchical models have also been an important aspect of theory within the domain of health psychology. For several decades, Leventhal has been studying the common-sense models of illness that people hold (Leventhal *et al.*, 1980; Leventhal and Carr, 2001; Leventhal *et al.*, 2001). Common-sense models of illness reflect the ways in which people represent illnesses to themselves. Illness representations are thought to have five different attributes: an identity (involving a disease label and symptoms); a timeline (e.g., time to onset, time to cure or recovery, time to death); a cause (e.g., genetic versus environmental); controllability; and consequences (see, e.g., Lau and Hartman, 1983; Leventhal *et al.*, 1980).

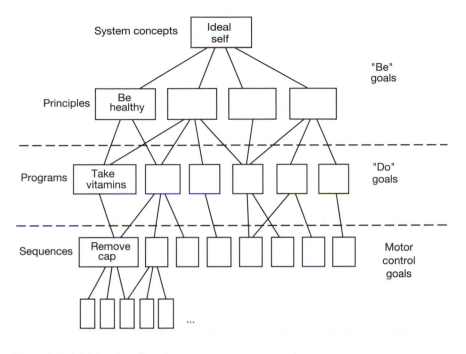

Figure 2.2 A hierarchy of goals

Source: Adapted from Carver and Scheier (1998).

What is important for present purposes is that each of these attributes is thought to be represented in two ways (Leventhal and Carr, 2001). That is, illness attributes are represented both at an abstract, cognitive level and at a more concrete, perceptual level (Meyer *et al.*, 1985). As an example, consider illness identity. At a concrete level, illnesses are identified by a collection of discrete symptoms and bodily cues. At a more abstract level, these collections of symptoms give rise to an illness label. A scratchy throat, cough, fever, and stuffy nose is identified as a cold; the combination of shortness of breath accompanied by extreme pain radiating down the left arm is identified as a heart attack. It is possible to construe these two levels of illness representation as existing within a simple hierarchy of feedback control (Leventhal and Carr, 2001). At the higher level, people regulate their activities so as to avoid the recognition that they have a particular illness. They do this by managing and regulating their lower-level symptoms upon which the illness label depends.

The notion of hierarchicality as we have described it has implications for several issues in conceptualizing behavior (see Carver and Scheier, 1998, 1999b). Most notably for present purposes, goals vary in importance. That is, the higher in the organization, the more tied to the sense of self are the goals. Thus, goals at higher levels tend to be more important than those at lower levels. At the same time, two goals at a lower level are not necessarily equivalent in importance. There are two ways for importance to accrue to a lower goal. First, a lower goal that is more central to attaining a valued abstract goal is more important than one that is less central to attaining the abstract goal. Second, a lower goal that contributes to attaining several higher level goals at once is more important than one that contributes to attaining only one such goal (see also Carver and Scheier, 1999b).

Affect

The model described up to this point addresses the control of action, but there is more to be considered. People also experience feelings during their actions. We have suggested that feelings arise via the operation of a second feedback process (for details, see Carver and Scheier, 1990, 1998, 1999b). One way to characterize what this second feedback system does is to say that it is checking on how well the behavior system is doing at carrying out its job. For discrepancy reducing behavioral loops, the perceptual input for the affect-creating loop is a representation of the *rate of discrepancy reduction in the action system over time* (we consider discrepancy enlarging loops shortly).

We do not believe that the rate of discrepancy reduction creates affect by itself, because a given rate of progress has different affective conse-quences under different circumstances. As in any feedback system, this input is compared against a reference value (cf. Frijda, 1986, 1988): an acceptable or desired rate of behavioral discrepancy reduction. We believe that the result of the comparison process at the heart of this loop (the error signal from the comparator) manifests itself phenomenologically in two ways. The first is as a hazy and nonverbal sense of confidence or doubt. The second is as affect – a sense of positivity or negativity. Several studies have yielded evidence that tends to support this view of the source of affect (e.g., Brunstein, 1993; Guy and Lord, 1998; Hsee and Abelson, 1991; Lawrence *et al.*, in press; for a more thorough discussion, see Carver and Scheier, 1998).

The view we just described rests on the idea that positive feelings arise when an action system is doing well at *doing what it's organized to do*. Approach systems are organized to reduce discrepancies. When approach systems are making good progress toward desired goals, positive affect is experienced. When satisfactory progress is not being made, affect turns more negative. We see no obvious reason why the same principle should not also apply to systems organized to increase discrepancies. Thus, if avoidance systems are doing well at what they are organized to do – distancing the person from anti-goals – positive affect should result. If they are doing poorly at what they are organized to do, the affective experience should be negative.

This much seems the same for both types of systems. On the other hand, we do see a difference in the specific affects that are involved (Carver, 2001; Carver and Scheier, 1998). For both approach and avoidance systems there is a positive pole and a negative pole, but the positives are not quite the same, and neither are the negatives (see Figure 2.3). Our view of this difference derives partly from the insights of Higgins and colleagues (Higgins 1987, 1996). Following his lead, we suggest that the affect dimension relating to discrepancy reducing loops (in its purest form) runs from depression to elation. Discrepancy reducing systems are presumed to yield sadness or depression when progress is below standard, and happiness or elation when progress is above standard. The affect dimension that relates to discrepancy enlarging loops (in its purest form) runs from anxiety to relief or contentment. Discrepancy enlarging systems are presumed to yield anxiety when progress is below standard, and relief or contentment when progress is above standard.

Confidence and doubt

The preceding account of the experience of affect suggested that one mechanism yields two subjective read-outs: affect, and a hazy sense of confidence versus doubt. We believe that the affect and expectancies that get generated 'on-line' as behavior unfolds are intertwined. As affect becomes more negative, doubt tends to increase; as affect becomes more positive, hopefulness, confidence, and favorable expectations also rise. Thus, what we have said

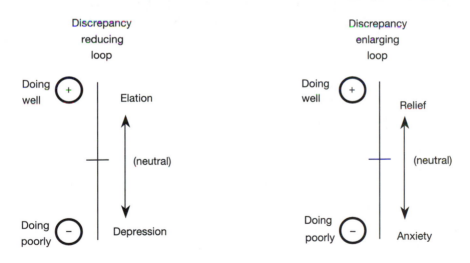

Figure 2.3 Two sorts of affect-generating systems and the affective dimensions we believe arise from the functioning of each

Source: Carver and Scheier (1998); © Cambridge University Press, reprinted with permission.

about affect applies equally well to the vague sense of confidence versus doubt that also emerges in parallel with ongoing action, as rate of progress falls above or below a desired level.

The on-line sense of confidence and doubt does not operate in a vacuum, though. Having one's efforts at goal attainment disrupted by adversity can yield distress emotions and doubtful feelings. But sometimes those immediate reactions are blended with, colored, or overridden by other information. We have suggested that when people experience adversity in trying to move toward goals, they periodically interrupt their effort and assess in a more deliberative way the likelihood of success (e.g., Carver and Scheier, 1981, 1990, 1998). In effect, people suspend the behavioral stream, step outside of it, and judge what outcome is likely (see Figure 2.4). In doing so, people presumably use memories of prior outcomes in similar situations, thoughts about alternative approaches to the problem, and thoughts about other resources they might bring to bear (cf. Lazarus, 1966; MacNair and Elliott, 1992). They may also use social comparison information (e.g., Wills, 1981; Wood, 1989; Wood *et al.*, 1985) and attributional analyses of prior events (Abramson *et al.*, 1978; Peterson and Seligman, 1984; Pittman and Pittman, 1980; Wong and Weiner, 1981).

How do these thoughts influence the expectancies that result? In some cases, people retrieve chronic expectancies from memory. As such, the information already *is* the person's expectancies: summaries of products of previous behavior. For example, a person with a long history of receiving adverse information from medical tests may find himself automatically expecting the worst from a newly conducted test.

In other cases, people think more expansively about how the situation might be changed. For such possibilities to influence expectancies, their

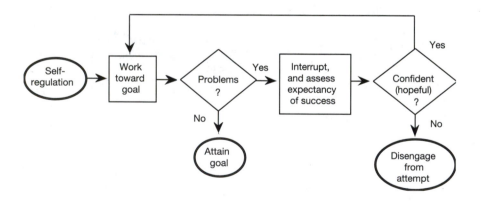

Figure 2.4 A flow-chart depiction of self-regulatory possibilities when obstacles to goal attainment are encountered

Source: Adapted from Carver and Scheier (1981).

consequences must be evaluated. This can be done by playing them through mentally as behavioral scenarios (cf. Taylor and Pham, 1996). For example, a cancer patient considering a new therapy may play through a scenario of undergoing the therapy, experiencing limited side effects, and having an improvement in health. She may derive from that scenario a sense of confidence. Effective mental scenarios emphasize explicit processes needed for reaching a goal, the concrete steps that must be enacted in order to get there (Taylor *et al.*, 1998; see also Cameron and Nicholls, 1998). Simply imagining the goal as having been attained is not enough to facilitate self-regulatory activities, and can even be detrimental (Oettingen, 1996).

Efforts and giving up

Expectancies – whether generated on-line or through further processing – have an important influence on behavior (see Figure 2.4). If expectations are favorable enough, the person renews effort. If doubts are strong enough, there is an impetus to disengage from effort, and even from the goal itself. We have argued that these two classes of reactions form a 'watershed' or bifurcation (Carver and Scheier, 1981, 1998, 1999b); that is, one set of responses involves continued efforts at movement forward, while the other set consists of disengagement and quitting (see also Klinger, 1975; Kukla, 1972; Wortman and Brehm, 1975).

The fact that hierarchically arranged goals vary in specificity – from very abstract to very concrete and specific – suggests that expectancies can also vary in the same way (Armor and Taylor, 1998; Carver and Scheier, 1998). To put it more concretely, a cancer patient can be confident or doubtful about regaining health and recovering from cancer, about finishing one more day of chemotherapy, or about lifting her arm.

Which of these sorts of expectancies matter? Probably all of them. Expectancy-based theories often hold that behavior is predicted best when the specificity of the expectancy matches that of the behavior. Sometimes it is argued that prediction is best when taking into account several levels of specificity. But many outcomes in life have multiple causes, people often face situations they have never experienced before, and situations unfold and change over time. It has been suggested that in circumstances such as these, generalized expectations are particularly useful in predicting behavior and emotions (Scheier and Carver, 1985).

What exactly are generalized expectancies? They are expectancies that pertain to very diverse outcomes. In terms of the hierarchy presented earlier, they bear on both abstract and concrete goals. Similarly, they pertain not just to one kind of goal but to many kinds of goals. Thus, people who are generally optimistic are those who believe that they will attain not just one higher-order goal, but all of the higher-order goals that their goal hierarchies contain, along with all of the subgoals to which those higher-order goals are linked.

Issues in the self-regulation of health and illness behaviors

The model of self-regulation presented in the preceding pages was meant to capture the structure and processes underlying 'behavior in general.' That is, it was meant to provide a generic model of motivated action. The model was not specifically designed with health behaviors and illness episodes in mind. On the other hand, we believe that the model can readily be applied to phenomena of interest within the health domain (for a more thorough treatment of this topic, see Scheier and Carver, in press).

Take, for example, the question of illness and disease. How might one understand the experience of illness and disease vis-à-vis the principles in the model? In our view, illness episodes are no different from a host of other adversities that a person might encounter on the way to goal attainment. They function in a manner similar to what are labeled in Figure 2.4 as 'problems,' indirectly undermining people's confidence in achieving the collection of their ongoing life goals. Of course, the onset of a disease or an illness episode also directly threatens the desire to be healthy and stay alive (valued goals in their own right).

What about active attempts on the part of the person to stay healthy and to engage in health-promoting activities? Here again the application of the model seems straightforward. Being healthy reflects a particular higher-order goal. Presumably, higher-order goals imply organizations of hierarchically arranged lower-order goals that allow the higher-order goals to be realized (recall Figure 2.2). Thus, someone whose goal is to be healthy might achieve this by engaging in a program of regular exercise, avoiding fatty foods, taking vitamins, and drinking wine in moderate amounts. Even lower-level goals might specify the pattern of muscle movements that underlie these health-related actions. From this perspective, health-promoting behavior thus reflects the operation of a hierarchically arranged series of interconnected feedback loops.

In sum, we believe that the self-regulatory framework provides a useful heuristic by which health and illness behaviors might be viewed. By providing a theoretical superstructure, self-regulatory models help to identify central variables and processes for study. At the same time, those same models raise important issues about the nature of a person's self-regulatory activities, and what it is about those activities that may predispose a person to favorable or unfavorable health-related outcomes. In the sections that follow, we explore some of the issues raised by the self-regulatory model described in the preceding sections.

The importance of positive expectations

An important theme in our discussion of self-regulatory activities was that expectations play a pivotal role in responses to adversity. When people expect positive outcomes, even when things are difficult, they should experience less negative emotion and more positive emotion. When people are more pessimistic, they should experience a stronger bias toward negative feelings (Carver and Scheier, 1998; Scheier and Carver, 1992). These differences play themselves out in the various ways in which people respond to illness threats.

The expectancies we have been most interested in are general feelings of optimism and pessimism. A simple characterization of the literature on dispositional optimism is that optimists experience less distress and greater positive affect than do more pessimistic people. To illustrate this, we briefly describe a portion of the literature relating optimism to surgical treatment for coronary artery disease (for more comprehensive reviews involving other diseases and illnesses, see Carver and Scheier, 1999a, or Scheier *et al.*, 2001).

One early study examined men undergoing and recovering from coronary artery bypass surgery (Scheier *et al.*, 1989). Prior to surgery, optimists reported lower levels of hostility and depression than did pessimists. A week after surgery, optimists reported feeling more relief and happiness, greater satisfaction with their medical care, and greater satisfaction with the emotional support they had received from friends. Six months after surgery, optimists reported a higher quality of life than did pessimists. In a follow-up of the same patients five years after surgery (cited in Scheier and Carver, 1992), optimists continued to experience greater subjective well-being and general quality of life compared to pessimists. All these differences remained significant when medical factors were statistically controlled for. We should also note, however, that quality of life was only assessed post-surgically in this study, so it is difficult to determine whether post-surgical differences in quality of life between optimists and pessimists were due to changes in life quality over time or due to differences that were also apparent at the beginning of the study.

Another study on optimism and quality of life after coronary artery bypass surgery (Fitzgerald *et al.*, 1993) assessed participants one month prior to surgery and eight months later. Analysis revealed that optimism was negatively related to pre-surgical distress. Furthermore, controlling for pre-surgical life satisfaction, optimism was positively related to post-surgical life satisfaction. Further analysis revealed that the general sense of optimism appeared to operate on feelings of life satisfaction through a more focused sense of confidence about the surgery. That is, the general sense of optimism about life seems to have been funneled into a specific kind of optimism regarding the surgery, and from there to satisfaction with life. All of the effects involving optimism reported by Fitzgerald *et al.* (1993) were found to be independent of disease severity.

Similar salutary effects of optimism have been observed in a group of women undergoing coronary artery bypass surgery (King *et al.*, 1998). At all assessment points, optimism demonstrated significant adaptive relationships with positive mood, negative mood, and satisfaction with life. More importantly, optimism assessed at one week was associated with more positive mood and less negative mood at one month, independent of initial levels of positive and negative mood.

These findings concern psychological adjustment following diagnosis and treatment of heart disease. Other data link optimism to physical health outcomes as well. Scheier *et al.* (1999), for example, recently reported findings from another sample of bypass patients that bear on a medical problem that sometimes arises after bypass surgery: the need for rehospitalization due to infection from the surgery or to complications from the underlying disease. Scheier *et al.* (1999) found that optimists were significantly less likely to be rehospitalized, controlling for medical variables and other personality measures.

Another research group (Leedham *et al.*, 1995) has explored the effects of positive expectations on experiences surrounding heart transplant surgery (this study did not examine dispositional optimism per se, but variables conceptually linked to optimism). Positive expectations assessed at an earlier stage related to a higher quality of life being assessed at a later stage, even among patients who had health setbacks. Importantly, patient confidence predicted better adherence to the postoperative medical regimen (reflecting engagement), and strongly predicted nurses' ratings of patients' physical health at six months after surgery. There was also a tendency for positive expectations to predict longer delays before the development of infection (which is a near-universal side effect of heart transplantation).

Taken together, these various findings strongly suggest that a generalized optimistic orientation to life helps to promote better adaptation to the stress associated with being diagnosed and treated for a major, potentially life-threatening illness. The findings suggest that optimism may also enhance physical well-being.

When to persist, when to give up

Positive expectations play an important role in the self-regulation of action. Confidence fosters persistence and perseverance. A person who gives up easily whenever difficulty is encountered will not accomplish much in life. Positive expectations regarding ultimate outcomes can help a student work through a series of bad examination grades to go on to master the course material at hand. Positive expectations can also help a woman undergoing chemotherapy to persist in attaining important life goals even in the face of significant treatment-induced side effects.

Perseverance is clearly important in a great many activities. However, this is only part of the story. An equally important role is played by processes that are precisely the *opposite* of those just described. A critical role in life is also played by doubt and disengagement – by giving up (Carver and Scheier, 1998, in press; Wrosch *et al.*, in press).

Giving up has a bad reputation in Western thought. 'Winners never quit and quitters never win' is the credo of American sports and business alike. And even patients suffering from terminal diseases are admonished to 'never give up hope.' However, there are occasions when one has to quit. No one goes through life without confronting an insoluble problem at some stage, and eventually everyone has to die, due to the progression of a disease, the gradual failure of critical organ systems associated with normal aging – from something. People also have accidents, compromising aspects of their physical functioning, which render certain future activities impossible. Disengagement turns out to be a necessity – a natural and indispensable aspect of effective self-regulation (Klinger, 1975).

Sometimes disengagement involves scaling back in order to work toward a less ambitious goal in the same domain as the abandoned goal. People in effect *trade the threatened goal for a less demanding one*. This is a kind of limited disengagement. They have given up on the first goal at the same time as adopting a lesser one. This limited disengagement has an important positive consequence, however: by doing so, people remain engaged in the domain they had wanted to quit (or felt the need to quit). By scaling back (giving up in a small way), they keep trying to move ahead (thus *not* giving up in a larger way).

An illustration of limited disengagement comes from research on couples in which one partner was ill and was dying from AIDS (Moskowitz *et al.*, 1996). Some healthy subjects had as their goal the aim of overcoming their partners' illness and continuing their active lives together. As the illness progressed, however, and it became apparent that this goal would not be met, the healthy partners often scaled back their aspirations. Now, for example, the goal was to do more limited activities during the course of a day. Choosing a goal that is more limited and manageable ensures that it will be possible to move toward it. The result was that despite adversity, the person experienced more positive feelings than would have otherwise have been the case, and thus remained engaged behaviorally with efforts to move forward with this aspect of life.

We believe this principle of scaling back – partial disengagement without completely abandoning the goal domain – is a very important one. By keeping the person engaged in goal pursuits in particular domains, it keeps the person engaged with life. It is easy to envision how the ability to scale back goals as needed can assist a person in adjusting to the progression of a disease, or to the gradual erosion of behavioral and biological resources associated with normal aging.

Sometimes disengagement involves scaling back to a less ambitious goal in the same domain as the abandoned goal. Other times the disengagement is more radical. Rather than scale back, people disengage from the unattainable goal completely and substitute an attainable alternative. If one path is blocked, people need to be able to jump to another one. Consider a cancer patient who has great personal investment in family ties. If chemotherapy destroys the ability to have children, positive family experiences can be obtained in other ways (cf. Clark *et al.*, 1991). If long-term career ambitions are threatened by a potentially fatal illness, the person might reprioritize various aspects of his or her life and spend less time working and more time in close relationships.

Of course, recognizing that goal disengagement can be beneficial says nothing about the ease with which people can actually disengage. It is clear that people often have a hard time giving up on unattainable goals, even when they realize that goal disengagement may be the most adaptive response they can make. What makes goal disengagement difficult? A key reason stems from the idea that goals are hierarchically organized. Recall that goals are more central to the self as one moves to higher levels. Recall also that some lower-order goals connect to only a few higher ones, where other lower-order goals connect to many higher ones. Some lower goals connect intimately to higher ones, other lower goals connect only weakly to higher ones. There also are, of course, individual differences in the organization.

Presumably, disengaging from higher-order goals is always hard. Disengaging from a high-order goal means giving up a core element of the self, which is not done lightly (Greenwald, 1980). Less obvious is the fact that disengagement from a concrete goal is also hard if the concrete goal is closely linked to a higher-order goal. Under such circumstances, giving up on a lower-order goal means more than simply abandoning the concrete behavior. It also means creating a problem for the higher-order goals to which the lower goal is linked. As a result, disengagement from the concrete goal is difficult.

It should be apparent from the preceding discussion that a critical question in life concerns when to stay engaged with and when to dissolve a goal commitment (cf. Pyszczynski and Greenberg, 1992). On the one hand, giving up (at some level, at least) is a necessity. It is part of self-regulation. If people are ever to turn away from efforts at achieving unattainable goals, if they are ever to back out of blind alleys, they must be able to disengage, to give up and to start again somewhere else.

The importance of disengagement is obvious when considering such concrete goals, but it is also important with regard to some higher-level ones. A vast literature attests to the importance of moving on with life after the loss of close relationships, even if the moving on does not imply a complete putting aside of the old (e.g., Cleiren, 1993; Orbuch, 1992; Stroebe *et al.*, 1993). Being stuck in the past instead of moving on has been found to create problems for people who have experienced a variety of life traumas (Holman and Silver, 1998). For example, paraplegia currently has no remedy. A person who loses the use of his legs and focuses only on regaining the ability to walk may expend extensive resources in a futile effort to do so.

We would argue that giving up is an adaptive response *when it leads to the taking up of other goals*, whether these goals represent substitutes for the lost one or simply new goals in a different domain. By providing for the pursuit of alternate goals, giving up creates an opportunity to re-engage and move ahead again (Carver and Scheier, 1998; Scheier and Carver, 2001). In such cases, giving up serves the broader function of keeping the person engaged with life. This appears to apply to values that extend fairly deeply into the sense of self. People need multiple paths to such values (cf. Linville, 1985, 1987; Showers and Ryff, 1996; Wicklund and Gollwitzer, 1982). If one path is blocked, people need to be able to move to another.

It seems likely that substituting a new path for an obstructed one is made easier by having clearly identified values at the more abstract level. For example, consider the case of a highly competitive athlete who loses his mobility. A person in this situation who understands that his core desire is to *compete* can more readily recognize that there are many ways to satisfy that desire than can someone who is less clear about the nature of the core desire. Similarly, it seems likely that a person who already recognizes the multiple paths that exist to a given goal will be better prepared to move between these paths as necessary.

In any case, it appears that the ability to adopt a new goal, or to take a new path toward an existing goal, is an important part of remaining goal-engaged. What happens if there is no alternative to take up? In such circumstances, disengagement from an unattainable goal cannot be accompanied by a shift of focus. This is the worst situation: nothing to pursue, nothing to take the place of the unattainable (cf. Moskowitz *et al.*, 1996).

There is reason to believe that this situation is implicated in suicide (Beck *et al.*, 1985). There is even reason to suspect that it may be implicated in premature death from natural causes (Carver and Scheier, 1998, Chapter 18). That is, popular wisdom holds that people (and other animals) can die from a loss of the 'will to live.' The folklore of many cultures also contains the idea that people can die from hexes and curses. Such voodoo deaths have been documented often enough to suggest that the phenomenon is in fact real (see, e.g., Cannon, 1942). What causes it? Apparently, it is not a matter of making up one's mind to die, but rather a matter of coming to believe that one is bound to die (cf. Cannon, 1942), that survival is impossible. Under such circumstances, it makes little sense to remain engaged in the activities of living, so people just give up. Dying in these cases can thus be construed as resulting from the failure to keep living.

We have recently collected data that speak directly to the psychological benefits of disengagement and re-engagement. In an initial study, we examined relations between goal disengagement, goal re-engagement, and subjective well-being in college students (Wrosch *et al.*, 2001, Study 1). We expected that the transition to a university setting might require students to abandon at least some of the life goals that were previously being pursued, as well as restructure the life goals governing current and future behavior. The results showed that the participants' capacities to reduce effort and to relinquish commitment to blocked goals were related to low levels of perceived stress and intrusive thoughts and high levels of self-mastery. In addition, the capacity to pursue alternative goals was significantly related to high levels of self-mastery and purpose in life and to low levels of perceived stress and intrusive thoughts. Finally, among participants who had not identified alternative goals to pursue, those who reported being unable to disengage from unattainable goals showed particularly high levels of perceived stress and low levels of self-mastery.

In a second study, we examined whether goal disengagement becomes even more important when people face extremely challenging life circumstances. To study this hypothesis, we assessed goal disengagement, goal re-engagement, and negative affect in twenty parents of children with cancer and twenty-five parents of healthy children (Wrosch *et al.*, 2001, Study 2). We reasoned that the diagnosis of a life-threatening disease in their own children might force parents to give up some important life goals (e.g., giving up career goals to spend more time with their children). Thus, we expected an inverse correlation to emerge in the data between disengagement and negative affect, particularly among parents of children with cancer. Consistent with these expectations, the study results showed that high levels of both goal disengagement and goal re-engagement predicted low levels of negative affect (specifically depression), particularly among parents whose children were diagnosed with cancer. Unfortunately, the small sample size in this study prevented us from assessing the interactive effects of goal disengagement and goal re-engagement.

A final data set that has been recently collected examined the experience and management of life regrets among college students (Wrosch and Scheier, 2002a). We asked the participants to report their most severe commission regrets (i.e., regrets over things they had done). They also reported the amount of negative affect and intrusive thoughts they experienced with respect to the regret. In addition, we asked the participants to report whether the negative consequences of the regrettable behavior could in fact be undone. Finally, to obtain a measure of disengagement, we asked the participants to report whether they were putting forth effort and whether they were committed toward undoing the negative consequences of the regrettable behavior.

We expected that high levels of disengagement would be related to lower levels of negative affect and intrusive thoughts, but only among people who perceived low opportunities to undo the negative consequences of their regrets. That is what we found. Among participants who perceived little opportunity to undo their regrets, those who could disengage more easily reported less negative affect and intrusive thoughts. In contrast, disengagement was unrelated to negative affect and intrusive thoughts in participants who perceived opportunities to undo the negative consequences of their regrettable behaviors. The results from this study, in conjunction with the results already described, clearly suggest that disengagement and re-engagement can be associated with positive states of psychological well-being.

Disengagement may also have physical health benefits. Wrosch and Scheier (2002b) have recently collected data on life regrets, depression, and physical symptoms in a sample of older adults. Their study showed that the intensity of the regrets that older participants reported was positively related to the amount of depressive symptomatology and physical symptomatology (e.g., constipation and skin problems) that was reported. More importantly, the associations between intensity of life regrets, depressive symptoms, and physical symptoms were significant only among those who had failed to disengage from the attempt to undo their life regrets. The results from this study thus lend support to the idea that the inability to disengage from unattainable goals can adversely affect physical well-being, at least in older adults.

Psychosocial interventions and disease severity: targeting hope versus purpose

We have chosen to ground our discussion of goal-directed activities within a self-regulatory framework. Although we have not mentioned it thus far, aspects of our self-regulatory model belong to a broad family of expectancy-value theories of motivation. That is, in the view that we have presented, two factors are important in keeping the person involved in goal-directed pursuits. One is the person's ability to identify goals that are valued. People do not take up goals that do not matter to them, and if they did, they would not persist with them for very long when things got difficult. Valued goals provide a purpose for living.

The second important factor is the sensed attainability of the goal. If a goal seems unattainable at the outset, effortful behavior will never even begin. If people continually fail to make progress toward the goals that they have committed themselves to, they will begin to withdraw effort and start to perceive those goals as out of reach. In contrast, hope enables one to hold on to valued goals, to remain engaged in the process of goal striving, and to stay committed to the attempt to move forward.

These general themes have been emphasized by generations of expectancy-value models of motivation (Atkinson, 1964; Feather, 1982; Shah and Higgins, 1997; Vroom, 1964). In such models, if engagement of effort is to occur, then there must be a goal that matters enough for a person to try and reach it (value), and that person must have sufficient confidence about its eventual attainment (expectancy). Thus, the view we have taken on behavior is one instantiation of this larger class of models.

Most expectancy-value theories afford hope (positive expectations) and purpose (valued goals) equal status. Both are required in order for goal-directed action to be sustained. On the other hand, one can imagine a situation in which one of these might be harder to maintain or more important to maintain than the other. Similarly, there might be certain kinds of people who are more vulnerable to the erosion of hope, and others who are more vulnerable to the erosion of purpose.

Elsewhere (Scheier and Carver, 2001), we have discussed how hope and purpose might be differentially affected by the stage or severity of a disease with which a person has been diagnosed. Consider, for example, two cancer patients, one at an early stage of the disease and one at a later stage. Realistically, the early-stage cancer patient has a better prognosis. Since the disease was caught quickly, medical treatment should be more effective and the odds of cancer-free survival should be higher. Given the enhanced odds of dealing effectively with the disease, the cancer should pose less a threat to ongoing life tasks, and consequently be less likely to permanently disrupt long-term life projects. For this type of person, maintaining hope and positive expectations may be paramount. Given the patient's life situation, there may be little objective need to abandon or re-evaluate ongoing life goals.

The situation for someone with a disease at an advanced stage may be quite different. For this person, ongoing life goals may in fact be objectively threatened. While we think it is important for even this type of person to begin the treatment process with a positive orientation, and to maintain that orientation as long as possible, should the treatment begin to falter and the prognosis become less favorable, maintaining a sense of purpose may become the more critical factor. Someone in this situation may begin to sense that life-long ambitions may go unrealized. As the hope of attaining these long-term goals begins to wane, it is important that the patient find purpose in life elsewhere, either in scaled-back versions of the threatened longer-term goals or in alternative, shorter-term substitute goals. Thus, as the ability to maintain hope fades, it becomes more important to find renewed purpose (about which hope is more realistic).

These considerations suggest that it may be important to take the patients' stage of disease into account when planning psychosocial interventions. What is important for the early-stage patient is the maintenance of hope. What is important for the late-stage patient is the maintenance of purpose. Perhaps different interventions are differentially effective in promoting hope versus purpose.

Several studies of interventions among cancer patients may provide useful illustrations of this idea. For example, Helgeson *et al.* (1999) studied early-stage breast cancer patients and found that an educational intervention enhanced their emotional adjustment. Antoni *et al.* (2001) also studied early-stage breast cancer patients and found that a cognitive-behavioral stress management intervention reduced the prevalence of depressive symptoms. It is noteworthy that both of these interventions were aimed at providing patients with tools to use when dealing with their illness. The educational groups in the Helgeson *et al.* study provided patients with certain kinds of illness information and coping techniques. The stress management groups in the Antoni *et al.* study provided patients with a variety of skills to use in dealing with whatever stressors they were confronting. It seems likely that these interventions helped the patients to maintain the hope of coping well with the effects of the illness. Consistent with this, patients in the Antoni *et al.* study even reported slight increases in their overall levels of optimism.

In contrast to these two studies, Spiegel *et al.* (1981) looked at metastatic breast cancer patients and found that a social support intervention enhanced both psychological adjustment and survival time (Spiegel *et al.*, 1989), although the effect on survival has been difficult to replicate (see, e.g., Cunningham *et al.*, 1998; Goodwin *et al.*, 2001). It seems likely that the later-stage patients studied by Spiegel *et al.* were experiencing vulnerability with respect to the erosion of the sense of purpose in their lives. Given the context (i.e., discussions of end-of-life issues), it also seems likely that the activities that occurred within the groups helped the patients to maintain their sense of purpose, and perhaps even to identify different but positively valued goals for what remained of their lives. Indeed, in discussing mechanisms underlying their findings, Spiegel *et al.* (1981) were struck by how important the group members had become for each other, and how the act of caring for each other had provided group members with an important reason for living. In the authors' words, 'being of help to others, even at the very end of life, helped to imbue members with a vital sense of meaningfulness' (Spiegel *et al.*, 1981: 532). Thus, for the individual members the group offered an important sense of purpose.

We believe that it may be important to think more generally about what needs different patients might have, and especially about how those needs might vary as a function of the patients' stage of disease. We have couched the discussion here in terms of stages of the cancer experience, but similar reasoning should apply across different diseases. Someone who has just been diagnosed with the early stages of congestive heart failure (or renal disease, or any other kind of potentially life-threatening disease) may have quite different needs from someone whose congestive heart failure (or renal disease, or any other kind of disease) is about to place significant restrictions on physical and social activities. As diseases progress from early to late stages, there may in fact be an accompanying shift in what is most important, hardest, and beneficial for the patient to do – maintain hope versus maintain purpose. Interventions might increase in effectiveness if they explicitly take these differential needs into account.

Concluding comment

We began this chapter by laying out some of the principles and processes that self-regulatory models embody, and then used those principles and processes to identify a set of issues that might be important to consider when thinking about disease outcomes and health and illness behaviors. In so doing, we made a case that positive expectations play a central role in determining one's psychological and physical response to disease, and that disengagement processes may at times be as likely as persistence to lead to greater well-being. We also suggested that patients at different stages of an illness may have quite different needs in terms of the importance of hope and purpose, and that interventions might be optimized if these issues were taken into account. We have long held that self-regulatory models provide a useful heuristic enabling one to better understand the nature of goal-directed activities, regardless of the particular domain of behavior in which those goal-directed activities are taking place. We hope the comments offered here will help convince others of the value of self-regulatory principles in understanding the kinds of behaviors involved in maintaining health and dealing with illness.

Note

1   Preparation of this chapter was facilitated by support from the National Cancer Institute (grants CA64710, CA64711, CA78995, and CA84944) and the National Heart, Lung, and Blood Institute (grants HL65111 and HL65112). Correspondence should be addressed to Michael F. Scheier, Department of Psychology, Carnegie Mellon University, Pittsburgh, PA 15213, USA. E-mail: scheier@cmu.edu

References

Abramson, L.Y., Seligman, M.E.P. and Teasdale, J.D. (1978) 'Learned helplessness in humans: critique and reformulation,' *Journal of Abnormal Psychology* **87**: 49–74.

Antoni, M.H., Lehman, J.M., Klibourn, K.M., Boyers, A.E., Culver, J.L., Alferi, S.M., Yount, S.E., McGregor, B.A., Arena, P.L., Harris, S.D., Price, A.A. and Carver, C.S. (2001) 'Cognitive-behavioral stress management intervention decreases the prevalence of depression and enhances benefit finding among women under treatment for early-stage breast cancer,' *Health Psychology* **20**: 20–32.

Armor, D.A. and Taylor, S.E. (1998) 'Situated optimism: specific outcome expectancies and self-regulation,' in M. Zanna (ed.) *Advances in Experimental Social Psychology*, vol. 29, San Diego: Academic Press, pp. 309–379.

Aspinwall, L.G. and Taylor, S.E. (1992) 'Modeling cognitive adaptation: a longitudinal investigation of the impact of individual differences and coping on college adjustment and performance,' *Journal of Personality and Social Psychology* **61**: 755–765.

Atkinson, J.W. (1964) *An Introduction to Motivation*, Princeton, NJ: Van Nostrand.

Austin, J.T. and Vancouver, J.B. (1996) 'Goal constructs in psychology: Structure, process, and content,' *Psychological Bulletin* **120**: 338–375.

Bandura, A. (1997) *Self-Efficacy: The Exercise of Control*, New York: W.H. Freeman.

Baumann, L.J. and Leventhal, H. (1985) ' "I can tell when my blood pressure is up, can't I?" ' *Health Psychologist* **4**: 203–218.

Baumeister, R.F. (1989) 'The problem of life's meaning,' in D.M. Buss and N. Cantor (eds) *Personality Psychology: Recent Trends and Emerging Directions*, New York: Springer-Verlag, pp. 138–148.

Beck, A.T., Steer, R.A., Kovacs, M. and Garrison, B. (1985) 'Hopelessness and eventual suicide: a 10-year prospective study of patients hospitalized with suicidal ideation,' *American Journal of Psychiatry* **142**: 559–563.

Brunstein, J.C. (1993) 'Personal goals and subjective well-being: a longitudinal study,' *Journal of Personality and Social Psychology* **65**: 1061–1070.

Cameron, L.D. and Nicholls, G. (1998) 'Expression of stressful experiences through writing: effects of a self-regulation manipulation for pessimists and optimists,' *Health Psychology* **17**: 84–92.

Cannon, E.B. (1942) ' "Voodoo" death,' *American Anthropologist* **44**: 169–181.

Cantor, N. and Kihlstrom, J.F. (1987) *Personality and Social Intelligence*, Englewood Cliffs, NJ: Prentice-Hall.

Carver, C.S. (2001) 'Affect and the functional bases of behavior: on the dimensional structure of affective experience,' *Personality and Social Psychology Review* **5**: 345–356.

Carver, C.S. and Scheier, M.F. (1981) *Attention and Self-Regulation: A Control-Theory Approach to Human Behavior*, New York: Springer Verlag.

—— (1990) 'Origins and functions of positive and negative affect: a control-process view,' *Psychological Review* **97**: 19–35.

—— (1998) *On the Self-Regulation of Behavior*, New York: Cambridge University Press.

—— (1999a) 'Optimism,' in C. R. Snyder (ed.) *Coping: The Psychology of What Works*, New York: Oxford University Press, pp. 182–204.

—— (1999b) 'Themes and issues in the self-regulation of behavior,' in R.S. Wyer, Jr. (ed.) *Advances in Social Cognition*, vol. 12, Mahwah, NJ: Lawrence Erlbaum Associates, pp. 1–105.

—— (in press) 'Three human strengths,' in L.G. Aspinwall and U.M. Staudinger (eds) *A Psychology of Human Strengths: Perspectives On an Emerging Field*, Washington, DC: American Psychological Association.

Clark, L.F., Henry, S.M. and Taylor, D.M. (1991) 'Cognitive examination of motivation for childbearing as a factor in adjustment to infertility,' in A.L. Stanton and C. Dunkel-Schetter (eds) *Infertility: Perspectives from Stress and Coping Research*, New York: Plenum, pp. 157–180.

Cleiren, M. (1993) *Bereavement and Adaptation: A Comparative Study of the Aftermath of Death*, Washington, DC: Hemisphere.

Cunningham, A.J., Edmonds, C.V., Jenkins, G.P., Pollack, H., Lockwood, G.A. and Warr, D.A. (1998) 'A randomized controlled trial of the effects of group psychological therapy on the survival of women with metastatic breast cancer,' *Psychooncology* **7**: 508–517.

Elliott, E.S. and Dweck, C.S. (1988) 'Goals: an approach to motivation and achievement,' *Journal of Personality and Social Psychology* **54**: 5–12.

Emmons, R.A. (1986) 'Personal strivings: an approach to personality and subjective well being,' *Journal of Personality and Social Psychology* **51**: 1058–1068.

Feather, N.T. (ed.) (1982) *Expectations and Actions: Expectancy-Value Models in Psychology*, Hillsdale, NJ: Lawrence Erlbaum Associates.

Fitzgerald, T.E., Tennen, H., Affleck, G. and Pransky, G.S. (1993) 'The relative importance of dispositional optimism and control appraisals in quality of life after coronary artery bypass surgery,' *Journal of Behavioral Medicine* **16**: 25–43.

Frijda, N.H. (1986) *The Emotions*, Cambridge: Cambridge University Press.

—— (1988) 'The laws of emotion,' *American Psychologist* **43**: 349–358.

Goodwin, P.J., Leszcz, M., Ennis, M., Koopmans, J., Vincent, L., Guther, H., Drysdale, E., Hundleby, M., Chochinov, H.M., Navarro, M., Speca, M., Masterson, J., Dohan, L., Sela, R., Warren, B., Paterson, A., Pritchard, K.I., Arnold, A., Doll, R., O'Reilly, S.E., Quirt, G., Hood, N. and Hunter, J. (2001) 'The effect of group psychosocial support on survival in metastatic breast cancer,' *New England Journal of Medicine* **345**: 1719–1726.

Greenwald, A.G. (1980) 'The totalitarian ego: fabrication and revision of personal history,' *American Psychologist* **35**: 603–618.

Guy, J.L. and Lord, R.G. (1998) 'The effects of perceived velocity on job satisfaction: an expansion of current theory,' paper presented at the 10th Annual Conference of the American Psychological Society, Washington, DC.

Helgeson, V.S., Cohen, S., Schulz, R. and Yasko, J. (1999) 'Education and peer discussion group interventions and adjustment to breast cancer,' *Archives of General Psychiatry* **56**: 340–347.

Higgins, E.T. (1987) 'Self-discrepancy: a theory relating self and affect,' *Psychological Review* **94**: 319–340.

—— (1996) 'Ideals, oughts, and regulatory focus: affect and motivation from distinct pains and pleasures,' in P.M. Gollwitzer and J.A. Bargh (eds) *The Psychology of Action: Linking Cognition and Motivation to Behavior*, New York: Guilford, pp. 91–114.

Holman, E.A. and Silver, R.C. (1998) 'Getting "stuck" in the past: temporal orientation and coping with trauma,' *Journal of Personality and Social Psychology* **74**: 1146–1163.

Hsee, C.K. and Abelson, R.P. (1991) 'Velocity relation: satisfaction as a function of the first derivative of outcome over time,' *Journal of Personality and Social Psychology* **60**: 341–347.

King, K.B., Rowe, M.A., Kimble, L.P. and Zerwic, J.J. (1998) 'Optimism, coping, and long-term recovery from coronary artery bypass in women,' *Research in Nursing and Health* **21**: 15–26.

Klinger, E. (1975) 'Consequences of commitment to and disengagement from incentives,' *Psychological Review* **82**: 1–25.

Kukla, A. (1972) 'Foundations of an attributional theory of performance,' *Psychological Review* **79**: 454–470.

Lau, R.R. and Hartman, K.A. (1983) 'Common sense representations of common illnesses,' *Health Psychology* **2**: 167–185.

Lawrence, J.W., Carver, C.S. and Scheier, M.F. (in press) 'Velocity toward goal attainment in immediate experience as a determinant of affect,' *Journal of Applied Social Psychology*.

Lazarus, R.S. (1966) *Psychological Stress and the Coping Process*, New York: McGraw-Hill.

Leedham, B., Meyerowitz, B.E., Muirhead, J. and Frist, W.H. (1995) 'Positive expectations predict health after heart transplantation,' *Health Psychology* **14**: 74–79.

Leventhal, H. and Carr, S. (2001) 'Speculations on the relationship of behavioral theory to psychosocial research on cancer,' in A. Baum and B.L. Andersen (eds) *Psychosocial Interventions for Cancer*, Washington, DC: American Psychological Association, pp. 375–400.

Leventhal, H., Leventhal, E.A. and Cameron, L. (2001) 'Representations, procedures and affect in illness self-regulation: a perceptual-cognitive model,' in A. Baum, T. Revenson and J.E. Singer (eds) *Handbook of Health Psychology*, Hillsdale, NJ: Lawrence Erlbaum Associates, pp. 19–47.

Leventhal, H., Meyer, D. and Nerenz, D. (1980) 'The common sense representation of illness danger,' in S. Rachman (ed.) *Medical Psychology*, vol. 2, New York: Permagon Press, pp. 7–30.

Linville, P. (1985) 'Self-complexity and affective extremity: don't put all of your eggs in one cognitive basket,' *Social Cognition* **3**: 94–120.

—— (1987) 'Self-complexity as a cognitive buffer against stress-related illness and depression,' *Journal of Personality and Social Psychology* **52**: 663–676.

Little, B.R. (1989) 'Personal projects analysis: trivial pursuits, magnificent obsessions, and the search for coherence,' in D.M. Buss and N. Cantor (eds) *Personality Psychology: Recent Trends and Emerging Directions*, New York: Springer-Verlag, pp. 15–31.

MacNair, R.R. and Elliott, T.R. (1992) 'Self-perceived problem-solving ability, stress appraisal, and coping over time,' *Journal of Research in Personality* **26**: 150–164.

Markus, H. and Nurius, P. (1986) 'Possible selves,' *American Psychologist* **41**: 954–969.

Meyer, D., Leventhal, H. and Gutmann, M. (1985) 'Common-sense models of illness: the example of hypertension,' *Health Psychology* **4**: 115–135.

Miller, G.A., Galanter, E. and Pribram, K.H. (1960) *Plans and the Structure of Behavior*, New York: Holt, Rinehart and Winston.

Miller, L.C. and Read, S.J. (1987) 'Why am I telling you this? Self-disclosure in a goal-based model of personality,' in V.J. Derlega and J. Berg (eds) *Self-Disclosure: Theory, Research, and Therapy*, New York: Plenum, pp. 35–58.

Moskowitz, J.T., Folkman, S., Collette, L. and Vittinghoff, E. (1996) 'Coping and mood during AIDS-related caregiving and bereavement,' *Annals of Behavioral Medicine* **18**: 49–57.

Oettingen, G. (1996) 'Positive fantasy and motivation,' in P. M. Gollwitzer and J.A. Bargh (eds) *The Psychology of Action: Linking Cognition and Motivation to Behavior*, New York: Guilford Press, pp. 219–235.

Orbuch, T.L. (ed.) (1992) *Close Relationship Loss: Theoretical Approaches*, New York: Springer-Verlag.

Pervin, L.A. (1982) 'The stasis and flow of behavior: toward a theory of goals,' in M.M. Page and R. Dienstbier (eds) *Nebraska Symposium on Motivation*, vol. 30, Lincoln: University of Nebraska Press, pp. 1–53.

—— (ed.) (1989) *Goal Concepts in Personality and Social Psychology*, Hillsdale, NJ: Lawrence Erlbaum Associates.

Peterson, C. and Seligman, M.E.P. (1984) 'Causal explanations as a risk factor for depression: theory and evidence,' *Psychological Review* **91**: 347–374.

Pittman, T.S. and Pittman, N.L. (1980) 'Deprivation of control and the attribution process,' *Journal of Personality and Social Psychology* **39**: 377–389.

Powers, W.T. (1973) *Behavior: The Control of Perception*, Chicago: Aldine.

Pyszczynski, T. and Greenberg, J. (1992) *Hanging On and Letting Go: Understanding the Onset, Progression, and Remission of Depression*, New York: Springer-Verlag.

Scheier, M.F. and Carver, C.S. (1985) 'Optimism, coping and health: assessment and implications of generalized outcome expectancies,' *Health Psychology* **4**: 219–247.

—— (1992) 'Effects of optimism on psychological and physical well-being: theoretical overview and empirical update,' *Cognitive Therapy and Research* **16**: 201–228.

—— (2001) 'Adapting to cancer: the importance of hope and purpose,' in A. Baum and B.L. Andersen (eds) *Psychosocial Interventions for Cancer*, Washington, DC: American Psychological Association, pp. 15–36.

—— (in press) 'Self-regulatory processes and responses to health threats: effects of optimism on well-being,' in J. Suls and K.A. Wallston (eds) *Social Psychological Foundations of Health*, Oxford: Blackwell Publishers.

Scheier, M.F., Carver, C.S. and Bridges, M.W. (2001) 'Optimism, pessimism, and psychological well-being,' in E.C. Chang (ed.) *Optimism and Pessimism: Implications for Theory, Research, and Practice*, Washington, DC: American Psychological Association, pp. 189–216.

Scheier, M.F., Matthews, K.A., Owens, J.F., Magovern, G.J., Lefebvre, R.C., Abbott, R.A. and Carver, C.S. (1989) 'Dispositional optimism and recovery from coronary artery bypass surgery: the beneficial effects on physical and psychological well-being,' *Journal of Personality and Social Psychology* **57**: 1024–1040.

Scheier, M.F., Matthews, K.A., Owens, J.F., Schulz, R., Bridges, M.W., Magovern, G.J., Sr. and Carver, C.S. (1999) 'Optimism and rehospitalization following coronary artery bypass graft surgery,' *Archives of Internal Medicine* **159**: 829–835.

Shah, J. and Higgins, E.T. (1997) 'Expectancy X value effects: regulatory focus as determinant of magnitude *and* direction,' *Journal of Personality and Social Psychology* **73**: 447–458.

Showers, C.J. and Ryff, C.D. (1996) 'Self-differentiation and well being in a life transition,' *Personality and Social Psychology Bulletin* **22**: 448–460.

Spiegel, D., Bloom, J.R. and Yalom, I. (1981) 'Group support for patients with metastatic cancer,' *Archives of General Psychiatry* **38**: 527–533.

Spiegel, D., Bloom, J.R., Kraemer, H.C. and Gottheil, E. (1989) 'Effect of psychosocial treatment on survival of patients with metastatic breast cancer,' *Lancet* **2**: 888–891.

Stroebe, M.S., Stroebe, W. and Hansson, R.O. (eds) (1993) *Handbook of Bereavement: Theory, Research, and Intervention*, Cambridge: Cambridge University Press.

Taylor, S.E. and Pham, L.B. (1996) 'Mental stimulation, motivation, and action,' in P.M. Gollwitzer and J.A. Bargh (eds) *The Psychology of Action: Linking Cognition and Motivation to Behavior*, New York: Guilford, pp. 219–235.

Taylor, S.E., Pham, L.B., Rivkin, I.D. and Armor, D.A. (1998) 'Harnessing the imagination: mental simulation, self-regulation, and coping,' *American Psychologist* **53**: 429–439.

Vallacher, R.R. and Wegner, D.M. (1985) *A Theory of Action Identification*, Hillsdale, NJ: Lawrence Erlbaum Associates.

—— (1987) 'What do people think they're doing? Action identification and human behavior,' *Psychological Review* **94**: 3–15.

Vroom, V.H. (1964) *Work and Motivation*, New York: Wiley.

Wicklund, R.A. and Gollwitzer, P.M. (1982) *Symbolic Self-Completion*, Hillsdale, NJ: Lawrence Erlbaum Associates.

Wills, T.A. (1981) 'Downward comparison principles in social psychology,' *Psychological Bulletin* **90**: 245–271.

Wong, P.T.P. and Weiner, B. (1981) 'When people ask "why" questions, and the heuristics of attributional search,' *Journal of Personality and Social Psychology* **40**: 650–663.

Wood, J.V. (1989) 'Theory and research concerning social comparisons of personal attributes,' *Psychological Bulletin* **106**: 231–248.

Wood, J.V., Taylor, S.E. and Lichtman, R.R. (1985) 'Social comparison in adjustment to breast cancer,' *Journal of Personality and Social Psychology* **49**: 1169–1183.

Wortman, C.B. and Brehm, J.W. (1975) 'Responses to uncontrollable outcomes: an integration of reactance theory and the learned helplessness model,' in L.

Berkowitz (ed.) *Advances in Experimental Social Psychology*, vol. 8, New York: Academic Press, pp. 277–336.

Wrosch, C. and Scheier, M.F. (2002a) 'Disengagement and regrets,' unpublished manuscript.

—— (2002b) 'Giving-up on life regrets: beneficial effects on well-being and health in older adults,' unpublished manuscript.

Wrosch, C., Scheier, M.F., Carver, C.S. and Schulz, R. (in press) 'The importance of goal disengagement in adaptive self-regulation: when giving up is beneficial,' *Self and Identity*.

Wrosch, C., Scheier, M.F., Miller, G.E., Carver, C.S. and Schulz, R. (2001) 'Goal disengagement, goal re-engagement, and subjective well-being: the benefits of giving up unattainable goals,' unpublished manuscript.

Zeidner, M. and Hammer, A.L. (1992) 'Coping with missile attack: resources, strategies, and outcomes,' *Journal of Personality* **60**: 709–746.

3 The common-sense model of self-regulation of health and illness

Howard Leventhal, Ian Brissette, and Elaine A. Leventhal [1]

The past decade has been witness to an unprecedented growth in research on self-regulation. For example, of the 2,700-plus chapters, dissertations, and journal articles containing the keyword 'self-regulation' archived in PsychINFO, a well-used social science citation index, over 1,800 have been published since 1990 alone. It is not entirely clear whether this trend is due to a shift in the Zeitgeist or a change in semantics. Though we suspect that both are involved, the Zeitgeist in Western, industrialized nations is the likely driving force. The focus on the consumer, individual choice, and populist movements that emphasize individual and community empowerment create a context congenial to self-regulation models. These models represent efforts at maintaining a sense of individual autonomy in the face of technological changes and monopolistic, corporate conglomerates that are actually shrinking the individual's options. Whereas the exact reason for the proliferation of self-regulation models is not clear, what is clear is that an increasing number of researchers and practitioners in the fields of health and social science are adopting concepts and principles from self-regulation theory to explain human behavior and promote behavior change in different contexts (see Boekaerts *et al.* (2000) for a discussion of applications in areas other than health).

The overall goal of this chapter is to present our perspective on the nature of self-regulation as it applies to the enactment of health and illness behaviors. We begin by defining self-regulation. Then we provide a brief historical overview of the factors leading to the development of the common-sense model (CSM) of self-regulation. We describe the assumptions and features of the CSM and review the empirical and theoretical work that contributed to its development. In the process, we discuss how the CSM differs from existing frameworks of self-regulation (e.g., see Scheier and Carver, this volume, Chapter 2) and from theories of the factors governing the enactment of health behaviors (Ajzen and Fishbein, 1980; Becker, 1974; Rogers, 1983; Rosenstock, 1974).

History and the current status of the common-sense of self-regulation

Conceptualizing self-regulation as regulation of the self-system

Much of human cognition and behavior is characterized as inherently purposeful, directed to achieve goals and to reduce and remove obstacles to those goals (Anderson, 1983; Newell, 1980). The term 'problem solving' is often used to refer to the processes involved in purposeful action: identifying goals, representing one's current state relative to these goals, selecting and enacting strategies to achieve the goals and to remove any obstacles, and determining the utility of implemented strategies. Many of our daily activities can be characterized as forms of problem solving, assuming that we apply the phrase to a broad range of actions rather than a narrow set of highly complex, consciously generated executive functions. Activities such as getting up in the morning and making coffee and navigating one's car through traffic jams, through to managing daily work tasks and working social plans into a busy routine, involve goal setting, comparing present and imagined future states to goals, and selecting and generating plans for goal attainment. The essential elements of problem solving have been represented in self-regulation frameworks using different labels. Goals are represented by reference values; the representation of one's current state by an input function; the selection and implementation of strategies to achieve goals, reduce barriers to goals, and move closer to goals, by an output function; and the process of evaluating whether or not implemented strategies are successful in achieving, moving closer to, and reducing barriers to goals, by a comparator (Carver and Scheier, 1981; Powers, 1973).

Some have argued that any system capable of individual problem solving can be considered to be capable of self-regulation (Powers, 1973). This approach to self-regulation is based on the principles of cybernetic control theory and posits a simple feedback loop or TOTE (test, operate, test, exit) unit governs the actions of self-regulating systems (Miller *et al.*, 1960). The self-regulating system *tests* its current status against a reference value, *operates* to produce output that alters the input so it is closer to the reference value, and *tests* input against the reference value again, repeating this process until a satisfactory degree of concordance between the input and reference is met and the system ceases to produce an output (*exit*).

The TOTE mechanism provides a generic model for conceptualizing feedback systems; it can be applied to physical as well as biological systems. It does not, however, tell us what is being regulated and how regulation is achieved. These 'details' are critically important for understanding the behavior of biological systems, including the efforts of human beings to protect and maintain health and to avoid and control illness. As we view it, the CSM provides a framework and specific variables that begin to specify some of these details. Problem solving is the management of the physical self and the subjective feelings of the self (Brownlee *et al.*, 2000). The term self-regulating refers not only to the fact that the system can operate to achieve identified goals, but to the fact that what is being regulated is the physical machinery and functional resources of the self. The goals for self-regulation are the concrete, perceptual experiences, the physical sensations or symptoms, moods and emotions, and feelings of vigor and competence generated by the biological and psychological self. The specific procedures and strategies chosen for regulation are defined by the properties of the threat to health, and the resources available to the individual and the social context and culture. Within the context of the CSM, self-regulation is both a description of the property of the system and a label connoting what is being regulated. This emphasis on content is one of the features that distinguishes the CSM from alternative frameworks, and in our view leads it to be more suitable for studying self-regulation as it pertains to health. The addition of content has two effects: first, it allows for more specific hypotheses; second, it introduces new structural and functional mechanisms into the self-regulation system.

Fundamental features of the common-sense model of self-regulation: historical development

A very brief review of the origins of the CSM will help to contrast it with other models of health behavior; for example, the health belief model and models of coping. Our review differs from prior ones as its emphasis is on the origins of the substantive features of the common-sense self-regulation system.

The CSM is an extension of the parallel processing model, a model designed to account for the findings of studies of fear-arousing communications focused on health behaviors (Leventhal, 1970). The first studies were based upon the Fear-Drive model which assumed that fear was a motivational state and that actions or procedures that reduced or eliminated fear were reinforced or learned (Dollard and Miller, 1950). The studies presented low and high fear messages about specific health threats (e.g., tetanus, lung cancer) by varying the language (technical and impersonal versus graphic and personal) and photographs (black and white and benign versus color images of tracheotomy wounds) describing the health threat, though presenting otherwise identical information (see Leventhal, 2000 for a review). In three studies, two on the threat of tetanus (Leventhal *et al.*, 1966; Leventhal *et al.*, 1965) and one on cigarette smoking (Leventhal *et al.*, 1967), some of the participants were randomly assigned to conditions where they were encouraged to develop specific action plans for coping with the threat. For example, the tetanus studies participants were asked to review their daily schedules and find the time when their class changes would bring them near the medical center where tetanus shots were available. The Fear-Drive model predicted that when the strategies were paired with a high as opposed to a low fear message, participants would develop more favorable attitudes about the strategies for avoiding the threat presented and be more likely to enact them (Leventhal and Singer, 1966).

The data from these studies were consistent with high fear messages being more effective than low fear messages in changing attitudes in the direction advocated in the communication. The effects of fear on attitudes, however, proved short-lived (lasting from 24 to 48 hours; Leventhal and Niles, 1965). Moreover, and more detrimental to the Fear-Drive model, high fear messages were no more effective than low fear messages in generating adherence to recommended health promoting actions. Thus, whether the messages were high or low in fear content, they succeeded in generating action if they were combined with an action plan. The combination of a low or high threat message and an action plan produced substantial increments in tetanus vaccination (Leventhal *et al.*, 1966; Leventhal *et al.*, 1965), and significant reductions in cigarette smoking (Leventhal *et al.*, 1967). These behavioral effects were both significant in size and durable, emerging days and weeks after exposure to the threat message, well after message-generated fear states had decayed (Leventhal and Niles, 1965).

Taken together, the absence of the interaction of fear level and action plans and the results of studies varying factors hypothesized to facilitate fear reduction and learning (Dabbs and Leventhal, 1966; Leventhal and Singer, 1966; Leventhal and Watts, 1966) proved to be fatal to the Fear-Drive model. The absence of an interaction of fear and action plans should not, however, be interpreted to mean that these two key factors had completely independent effects on behavior. By consulting the 'off design' conditions (when subjects were presented only with action plan messages), it was clear that there was a fundamental dependency between the two types of information. Namely, no subject exposed to an action plan asked for a tetanus inoculation in the absence of exposure to a threat message. Thus, although the effects of action plans were 'independent' of the level of fear, they affected behavior only in the presence of a fear message. Recent studies confirm that plans to implement goal-directed action have large effects on the performance of health behaviors as diverse as breast self-examination, cervical cancer screening, and vitamin supplement use (Gollwitzer and Oettingen, 1998; Orbel and Sheeran, 2002).

These data led to the development of the parallel process model (Leventhal, 1970). This model posited that health threats generate both emotional states of fear and distress and a corresponding need for procedures to manage these emotions (fear control) as well as a cognitive representation of the threat and a corresponding need for procedures for managing these threats (danger control). *Fear control* and *danger control* referred to the parallel actions that were undertaken and appraised for their efficacy in reducing the negative emotions evoked by health threats (fear control) and reducing the threats themselves (danger control; see also Lazarus and Launier, 1978). A diagram of the parallel process model is depicted in Figure 3.1. The

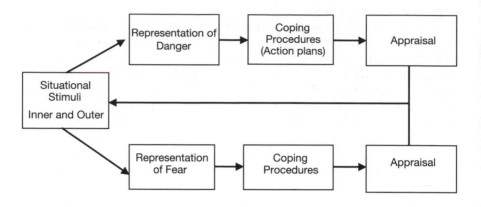

Figure 3.1 The parallel process model

model proposed that somatic stimuli and information about health threats are processed as perceived representations of danger and as emotional experience. Action plans are the activities that are undertaken to reduce fear and danger. Individuals are depicted as actively appraising the efficacy of these action plans and incorporating this information into their representations.

The parallel process model proposed that a cognitive representation of the health threat was a necessary condition for danger control. This representation established the goals for danger control, the specific procedures and strategies for control, the criteria for appraising success, and the ongoing perceptions of response efficacy. Though the combination of a threat message and an action plan succeeded in generating the motivation which led to the performance of specific procedures for controlling danger (e.g., take a tetanus shot; quit smoking), it was not clear which features of the message were essential for generating this motivation.

Self-regulation in navigating noxious medical treatments

If fear per se is not the source of motivation for health-promoting action, what aspect or specific content of the message is responsible for activating plans of action? Neither our early studies (Leventhal, 1970) nor more recent ones have answered this critical question (Witte and Allen, 2000).[2] In fact, we did not know whether the motivational effect was due to specific content or to how the content was structured. Four types of data strongly suggested, however, that the critical source for the motivational effects of illness representations, and indeed of fear itself, was the individual's concrete, perceptual experience and how that experience was interpreted! The first source of evidence came from the fear studies themselves: action planning involved concretizing future actions, imagining the time and place to initiate specific acts. The second source was from the findings of the first health belief model studies: they showed that perceived risk was best assessed by accessing visual images of the self as either healthy or sick, and the observation of others infected with flu (Rosenstock *et al.*, 1960); responses to Likert or probability scales did not predict behavior. The third source was the observations of patients during medical procedures indicating that concrete, somatic stimuli created fear states that interfered with patients' effective participation in the procedure. Finally, anthropological data indicated that people develop representations of health threats when left to their own devices (Whiting and Child, 1953). The lay health-threat theories that they developed were typically symptom-based and motivated the performance of health practices to reduce the perceived dangers. It was also clear that these lay representations of health dangers often had little correspondence to Western medical models.

The focus on perception led us to undertake a series of studies to evaluate the hypothesis that perceptual experience of somatic sensations could either stimulate fear or lead to effective self-management (danger control) depending upon how the sensations were interpreted. The studies were conducted with patients about to undergo a noxious medical procedure such as an endoscopy (Johnson and Leventhal, 1974) or a post-surgical colonoscopy (Johnson, 1975). The sensations experienced during these procedures could elicit fear and powerful avoidance reactions if they were interpreted and experienced as signs of impending danger. In contrast, these identical sensations could stimulate appropriate behaviors if they were perceived as cues for well-defined, participatory responses. The prototypical study varied two factors: sensory information and specific coping instructions. The sensory information used to prepare patients for an endoscopy first described and then provided benign interpretations of specific somatic sensations that would be felt during the examination (e.g., they inflate your stomach with air and you will feel as if you had eaten a large meal). Examples of specific coping instructions included suggestions as to how to breath when the throat is being swabbed with anesthetic and how to make swallowing motions when the endoscopy tube is introduced into the gullet.

The results showed that sensory information and coping plans had independent effects in reducing emotional reactions (e.g., gagging) and enhanced instrumental behaviors for managing the immediate situation (e.g., controlling the rate of swallowing the endoscope). It was clear that information that prepared an individual to expect specific sensory cues and provided benign views of these cues could shift the response from fearful avoidance to self-regulated problem solving. The results reinforced the notion that health threats were represented on at least two levels: semantically as abstract knowledge, and perceptually as concrete experience. Moreover, they suggested that these two representational levels were interactive (see also

Epstein, 1994). Somatic sensations could elicit fear by means of bottom-up influence and activate beliefs that one was in danger. Abstract information about the meaning of these physical sensations could short-circuit the perception of danger and the experience of fear by exerting a top-down influence (defining the symptoms as benign and manageable). Action plans reduced distress by linking sensory information to specific responses that allowed the patient to participate in and exert control over the noxious examination. Action plans and sensory information allowed patients to experience the somatic sensations during examination as predictable, controllable and benign by-products of a novel and noxious medical examination.

That fear is a product of the interaction of abstract and concrete levels of processing was clear from a study of cancer-worry conducted by Easterling and Leventhal (1989). Questionnaires featuring items on worrying about cancer, daily mood (anxious or depressed), symptom reports (non-cancer symptoms such as fatigue, headaches), and a question asking, 'What do you think the chances are that you will get cancer?' were completed by 54 women who had been successfully treated for cancer and by 81 women who had no history of cancer. The 81 women in the control group were either friends of the ex-patients or women who did not know the ex-patients. In both groups, cancer-worry was greater for women who felt the chances were great that they would get cancer, but only if they experienced (non-cancer) symptoms. Women who felt that their chances of recurrence were great were not worried if they did not have symptoms. Similarly, women who had symptoms did not worry if they did not feel they would get cancer. Worry required both factors, symptoms and a belief that one could get cancer. The pattern was identical within the two groups, but the women who had been treated for breast cancer reported higher levels of cancer-worry than the women lacking a history of breast cancer. The two groups did not differ in daily anxious mood, suggesting that the worry was specific to the threat of cancer. The finding that the experience of somatic symptoms would activate a cognitive label, and that providing a cognitive label could influence the interpretation of somatic sensations was consistent with Schachter and Singer's (1962) proposal that emotions are a product of physiological arousal and cognitive interpretation. The similarity of findings does not require, however, that one accept the Schacter–Singer model as a complete and adequate account of emotional processes (Leventhal, 1984).

Representations: content and rules/heuristics for construction

Content: identity as a core domain

We suspected and soon found that the joining of abstract cognition (feelings of vulnerability) to concrete experience (general symptoms) was important not only for the experience of emotion, but for the identity of illness threats.

Interviews with patients suffering from hypertension (Meyer *et al.*, 1985) indicated that 45 out of 50 patients who had been in continuing treatment for hypertension believed that their symptoms (e.g., flushed face, headache, shakiness) indicated when their blood pressure was elevated. Moreover, they used their medication as prescribed if they perceived that it controlled their symptoms; they were non-compliant (and experiencing poor blood-pressure control) if the medication was perceived not to control their symptoms. Notably, 40 out of these same 50 patients agreed that 'People cannot tell when their blood pressure is up.' Thus, while they agreed that others were ignorant of their blood pressure, the core, or identity, of their personal representation of hypertension, was a combination of symptoms and a label. Studies across a variety of illness conditions, ranging from mundane, everyday illnesses (Lau and Hartman, 1983) to life-threatening conditions such as cancer (Nerenz *et al.*, 1982), find that this combination of symptoms and label lies at the heart of illness representations.

Five content domains

Common sense suggested, and subsequent investigations validated, that symptoms represented only one type of perceptual information associated with the experience of a health condition, and that the label represented only a small portion of its semantic information. The other domains of illness representations were identified by methods ranging from open-ended interviews that elicited qualitative data on participants' understanding and management of conditions such as the common cold (Lau, Bernard, and Hartmann, 1989; Lau and Hartmann, 1983), hypertension (Bauman and Leventhal, 1985; Meyer *et al.*, 1985), and pulmonary disease (Lacroix *et al.*, 1991), to quantitative approaches such as multidimensional scaling and factor analysis that assessed the structure underlying representations of health conditions (Bishop, 1991; Bishop and Converse, 1986). For example, Penrod's (1980) application of multidimensional scaling to disease labels and symptoms identified three additional domains: consequences (severity), timelines (duration), and cause. A combination of methods were used by Bishop (1991): open-ended to obtain descriptions of symptom experiences, and quantitative to classify these descriptions. When participants were asked to indicate what else would be experienced by individuals describing specific sets of symptoms, 90 per cent of their responses could be classified as relating to one of five categories: identity, cause, timeline, consequences, and cure.

The empirical data was congruent with the two, basic propositions that underlie the self-regulation model: first, that people act as common-sense scientists when constructing representations of illness threats; and, second, that these representations generate goals for self-management and suggest procedures for goal attainment and criteria for evaluating response efficacy. The information or knowledge about disease threats within each of the five domains consisted of factors such as symptoms and names (identity), expected duration or expected age of onset (timeline), severity of pain and impact on life functions (consequences), infection or genes (internal and external causes), and whether the disease was perceived as preventable, curable, or controllable (controllability). Each of these domains contains specific types of semantic and perceptual information about an illness threat and each variable in a domain is both abstract and concrete. For example, our causal concept of contagion includes the concept of germs and the perception of contact with an infected person (Nemeroff and Rozin, 1994). Timelines, meanwhile, are represented abstractly ('This viral flu will last for two to three weeks') and experientially ('It seems as if this cold has lasted as long as this house!'). Time is often concretized by spatial representations (Boroditsky and Ramscar, 2002).

Heuristics / Rules for evaluating illness indicators

Figure 3.2 depicts the five content domains of illness representations: identity, timeline, cause, consequences, and control. The information represented within each of these domains is represented in both abstract (semantic) and concrete (perceptual or experiential) form. A number of rules or heuristics have been identified as being involved in converting stimuli into representations. These heuristics are used in the ongoing interpretation of the stimuli generated by an illness and efforts to control it. The result is an increasingly elaborate representation of the illness threat. The *symmetry* rule refers to the pressure to connect abstract experience with labels. Our hypertension patients and cancer patients linked labels to symptoms (Easterling and

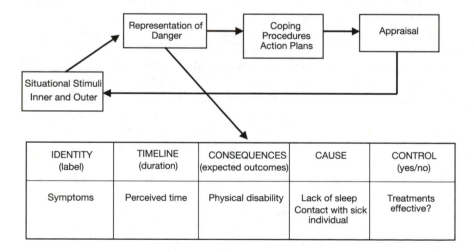

Figure 3.2 The five domains of illness representations

Leventhal, 1989; Meyer *et al.*, 1985). Moreover, subjects in laboratory studies reported symptoms when told that their blood pressure was very high (Bauman *et al.*, 1989). The connection is bi-directional and symmetrical, as labels seek symptoms and symptoms seek labels. Symmetry, by anchoring abstractions to perceptual experience, provides depth to the representation.

As new information is integrated with existing schematic structures, representations develop breadth; their content can expand from one or two domains to all five. Information can be generated by disease-related biological changes that create new symptoms and behavioral dysfunctions, by the observation of these changes in others, and by input from various media. Representations are shaped and reshaped by the success or failure of specific procedures for preventing, moderating, and curing disease processes. How such information is processed, and its meaning and the conclusions drawn from it, will reflect the questions or heuristics the individual uses for evaluating its implications. Data are available on four such rules, in addition to that of symmetry: the stress-illness rule, the age-illness rule, the prevalence rule (Croyle and Jemmott, 1991), and the duration rule (Mora *et al.*, 2002). The first two rules question whether symptoms or functional changes reflect an underlying disease process (illness) or a non-disease process (in particular, age-related changes or temporary changes due to work or interpersonally induced emotional stress). The prevalence and duration rules address the potential severity or seriousness of a symptom or risk indicator. The question implicit in each of these heuristics leads to specific procedures for evaluating and enriching the representation.

Stress-illness appraisals appear to involve an evaluation of one's ongoing reaction to environmental events. This evaluation of one's stress level can be explicit (e.g., elicited by instructions to review the events of the day on which a set of symptoms first appear) or implicit (e.g., if the day on which they appear happens to be a high- versus a low-stress day). Whether explicit or not, if the events of the day are stressful, symptoms are more likely to be interpreted as signs of stress rather than as indicators of illness (Baumann *et al.*, 1989). At least two conditions limit the application of the stress-illness heuristic: the nature of the symptoms and the duration of the stressor. Stress interpretations are most likely when symptoms are psychophysiological (e.g., fatigue, aching, headache) and have low specificity as indicators of disease. In addition, when stressors are relatively chronic, they can be seen as causes of illness, and medical care will be sought even for ambiguous symptoms of low specificity (Cameron *et al.*, 1995). The stress-illness heuristic is not applied mindlessly: it has limiting conditions (see Cameron, this volume, Chapter 8). Common sense also suggests that the duration and failure of a stress symptom to respond to treatment (e.g., the headache that does not respond to aspirin) will raise questions about a benign, stress interpretation and activate social communication and care seeking. Indeed, duration is one of the most powerful predictors of care seeking (Mora *et al.*, 2002), and can be considered a heuristic or rule for judging symptom seriousness. And whereas symptom duration implies seriousness, perceptions that a symptom or condition is prevalent among others can reduce inferences of its severity (Croyle and Jemmott, 1991).

It is conceivable that heuristics may differ with regard to the point at which they are most likely to be applied. For example, symmetry, stress-illness and age-illness rules seem especially valuable for deciding that one is or is not ill, whereas the prevalence rule seems to serve as an indicator of disease severity and to affect the decision to call for care. The duration rule, on the other hand, might be equally likely to function for both decisions – that is, that one is ill and in need of medical care. Studies examining the duration of appraisal delay (the time from noticing symptoms to the decision that one is ill) and illness delays (the time from deciding one is ill to calling for care), have not examined this issue (E. Leventhal *et al.*, 1993; E. Leventhal *et al.*, 1995). Hopefully, these questions will be addressed in future studies.

Coping procedures and action plans

Illness representations set the stage for coping; they guide the selection of procedures to eliminate and control potential or ongoing illness threats. The procedures for managing illness threats are legion, ranging from the use of dietary supplements and other 'natural' products, through over-the-counter medications, to treatments prescribed by physicians, non-traditional practitioners, family members, friends, and acquaintances. Nowadays, personal recommendations can be made both face-to-face and over the Internet (Berland *et al.*, 2001; Rice and Katz, 2001).

Anthropological studies provide dramatic examples of the way in which representations shape self-regulation coping procedures (Chrisman, 1977; Heurtin-Roberts and Reisin, 1992; Kleinman, 1980; Pachter, 1993; Simons, 1993). For example, parents of babies suffering from 'molera caida,' the folk name for the fallen fontanelle that is a symptom of dehydration, will apply pressure to the roof of the mouth or suck and draw up the fontanelle in efforts to cure the disease and prevent infant death. Similar mechanical/geographical principles are common in everyday life in Western cultures; the choice of procedure often reflects concrete-perceptual relationships between symptoms and procedures. We apply cold compresses to the head to ease headaches and salves to skin irritations, we imbibe home remedies for stomach upset, and billions of dollars are spent (Consumer Reports, 2000) on vast quantities of vitamins, herbal 'medications' and other alternative products (Cassileth, 1998; Eisenberg *et al.*, 1998). Cold compresses and salves seem irrelevant as cures for stomach upsets, and although we take pills to cure headaches, intuition suggests they are less relevant for curing skin rashes. Each procedure seems of special value for dealing with specific disorders and their symptoms; the linkages are not random.

Given the expected match between representations and procedures, it follows that the features of procedures can also be classified in the five domains. Procedures have identities with labels and symptomatic side effects, timelines, causal routes of action, consequences (expected outcomes including both somatic and non-somatic side effects), and control expectations regarding particular symptoms and diseases. For example, food supplements and diet selection can be perceived as useful ways of preventing and controlling cancer (the consequence) by strengthening immune function (the causal route). In addition, many traditional, well-validated medications such as analgesics and anti-depressants are perceived to have consequences or 'side effects,' including harm to the body, weakening of the immune system, and risk of addiction (Horne, 1997; see also this volume, Chapter 7). As with illness representations, individuals' representations of procedures also have abstract and experiential components. In terms of a medication's timeline, for example, a medication can have an expected timeline ('I should feel better in a week'), an actual timeline ('The patient should begin to feel better in about four weeks'), and an experiential timeline ('It feels like it is taking forever for this medication to work'). Taking account of the bi-level nature of these representations can be useful in understanding individuals' adherence to their pharmacological and behavioral regimens.

Procedures specify both a class of actions (e.g., use an analgesic) and a specific choice (e.g., ibuprofren); action plans specify the time and place for the initial and subsequent steps required for act completion. Once the representation and procedures are linked to an action plan, the self-regulation system is complete and coherent (Horowitz *et al.*, in review). From the perspective of the individual, coherence can be expressed as an '*if-then*' question (Brownlee *et al.*, 2000). That is, if I am suffering from a stress headache (identity) due to a bad day at work (cause; timeline), then taking two aspirins (procedure) should eliminate the pain (consequences; control) in 20 to 30 minutes (time frame for consequences).

Moderators and mediators of self-regulation

Coherent self-regulation systems (systems in which representations have set goals and defined procedures for goal attainment, and which lead to specific action plans) are generated in contexts of the self and the social system. The *if-then* questions that generate a self-regulation system refer to self-knowledge and social factors when drawing conclusions about a pathogen. For example, deciding if a symptom reflects illness or age requires reference to the self and what it means to be old (what symptoms or signs are indicators of aging). The *if-then* question that is raised and answered reflects the properties of the self. Hooker and Kaus (1994) have examined future, health-relevant identities, but relatively little work has been done examining the interaction of the self-system and illness representations. Heidrich *et al.*'s (1994) analysis of the factors affecting emotional distress in breast cancer patients suggests that the self-system (discrepancies between current and hoped-for self) mediates the effects of factors such as chronic timelines on elevations of emotional distress. It is unclear, however, whether or not the statistical notion of mediation provides the appropriate interpretation as to how self-discrepancies relate to the variables of chronic timelines and physical dysfunction that are central to these women's representations of breast cancer.

Self-regulation strategies

Elderly patients regularly express their strategies for self-regulation in clinical encounters with their geriatric physician (Leventhal and Crouch, 1997). These strategies appear to be linked to self-identities. For example, many elderly patients express concerns about taking medication as they perceive their bodies as unusually sensitive. Beliefs that one possesses a 'sensitive soma' have been related to concerns about medication (Horne, 1997), and this self-construal encourages a strategy of minimizing contact with medication.

Conservation, a self-management strategy designed to protect the age-related decline in somatic resources and to avoid risk from pathogenic processes, appears to be at the core of the rapid seeking of medical advice and health care by elderly patients (Leventhal and Crouch, 1997). In comparison to individuals aged 45-55 (the middle-aged) those over 65 years of age are swifter to appraise symptoms as signs of illness, and use medical care when symptoms are perceived as potentially serious (Leventhal *et al.*, 1995; Leventhal *et al.*, 1993). The elderly and middle-aged are equally swift to use care when symptoms are clearly serious. Minimizing delay avoids prolonged worry and the depletion of energy, and it reduces the risk of developing an advanced and incurable disease. Conservation is not always beneficial, however. When serious health problems disrupt ongoing activities, then conservation (unlike optimism, social support, and social demands) will detract from finding replacements and re-engaging with life activities (Duke *et al.*, 2002; see also Scheier and Carver, this volume, Chapter 2). A contrasting strategy, a commitment to *vigor through use*, encourages the use of exercise and herbal supplements as an alternative approach to self-maintenance (Carr, 2000). Whether the effects of a specific strategy will be beneficial or harmful depends upon the representation guiding its use and their relationship to the individual's biological status.

The social context

It is a gross misconception to think of self-regulation as a process carried out in solitude or to think of the individual as an isolated problem-solving machine. Self-regulation is dependent on the input and expertise of others. The research literature on social isolation and social integration suggests that the presence of others may be a necessary condition for the successful self-regulation of both physical health (Berkman and Syme, 1979; House *et al.*, 1988; Lynch, 1979) and psychological health (Jaco, 1954; Thoits, 1983). At any specific instance and over the individual's developmental history, every component of the self-regulation system will be shaped and reshaped by the social environment.

The case of a newborn child provides an illustration of the inherently social nature of self-regulation. Infants lack the capacity to be direct agents for their well-being. However, they possess instincts and skills that allow them to achieve the goals necessary to insure their survival. Babies are equipped with organ systems that signal hunger, with lungs and vocal cords to propel their screams to their mothers' attentive ears, and with reflexes to seek out and draw milk from their mothers' breasts. Infants regulate their emotions and physical selves (they self-regulate) by virtue of their ability to evoke and extract needed resources from their social environments. Conceptualizing and assessing the effects of such early experiences on later-life representations of threats to health, strategies for self-management, and patterns marshaling social resources, will be a major research challenge.

Self-regulation is also a social process for adults, and the CSM reveals both the importance and complexity of cultural and social factors for self-regulation in adult behavior. The contribution of the social system is immediately apparent when we consider how people engage in the diagnosis and management of symptoms. Individuals turn to medical practitioners for diagnosis and treatment when they experience somatic changes that are novel, vague, and/or of unexpected duration (Mora *et al.*, 2002). Expert input is critical as the perceptual input provided by the body is often vague and diffuse. In most cases, it is only through formal consultation with an expert that a cluster of symptoms becomes an identifiable illness. Here, the 'expert' other determines the nature of the dysfunction responsible for generating symptoms and suggests an appropriate intervention.

Though the use of medical care provides what may be the clearest example of social input, it is usually not the first social input for self-regulation. Data suggest that consultation with a family member and/or friend precedes the formal use of medical care for virtually every care seeker (Cameron *et al.*, 1993; Suls *et al.*, 1997). People use others to determine whether or not they need to seek care, to get 'permission' to do so, and to find partners for care seeking (Zola, 1966). The social network provides a convoy of ongoing contacts throughout the care-seeking and treatment process (Pescosolido, 1992) to determine whether one's experiences are normal, or to predict how one should expect to feel; self-regulation is inherently social (Buunk and Gibbons, 1997). The nature of the target of the social comparison is likely to differ depending on whether the individual is interested in evaluating an existing belief or predicting how one is going to feel (Suls *et al.*, 2000). Social contacts, however, often fail to lead to appropriate self-management. Indeed, other persons may encourage the individual's preference to manage the symptoms alone because these others distrust or dislike the health-care delivery system (Suls and Goodkin, 1994). Several studies have also found that individuals in strong social networks are more likely to delay seeking medical intervention (Berkanovic *et al.*, 1981; Granovetter, 1978; Liu and Duff, 1972). Failures to seek care and delays in seeking care may be serious, as many ignored symptoms could benefit from medical attention (Suls *et al.*, 1997).

Social information can have powerful effects on behavior even when it does not come from medical experts or intimate and trusted social contacts. For example, patients who spend time with and observe patients who are further along the treatment trajectory gain significant information that helps to clarify expectations about their future experiences and provides either reassurance (Kulik and Mahler, 1987) or doubt. Individuals often select targets for social comparison in order to make themselves feel better rather than obtaining an accurate conception of their own state of affairs (Perloff and Fetzer, 1986; Taylor, 1983). Whereas in the context of adaptation to a chronic illness this tendency can promote well-being (e.g., Helgeson *et al.*, 1999), in the context of promoting preventive health behaviors it represents a barrier that can lead to overly optimistic appraisals about individual risk. When assessing their personal risk of contracting HIV, for example, individuals can compare themselves to peers who are more promiscuous than they are. Or when assessing their risk for lung cancer, young smokers can justify that they are not at risk because of the age differences that exist between them and the typical lung cancer patients. Whereas theoretical and empirical work point to the importance of social comparisons in self-regulation, the goals of comparison (e.g., self-appraisal, anticipating future outcomes, acquiring skills, etc.) and the point in time at which these goals emerge have yet to be articulated. The CSM provides a basis for doing so (Leventhal *et al.*, 1997).

Although the individual, and therefore the self-regulation system, is embedded in a social context, except under unusual circumstances (e.g., under surgical anesthesia), the individual is the nexus for the intake and use of social information. Individuals attend to some and ignore other inputs from their social network, decide when to solicit care from other people, and choose whether or not to act on the medical advice and guidance they receive. The self remains the primary agent of self-regulation; more importantly, the process of self-regulation makes use of subjective information, symptoms, and emotional states that are not directly available to observing others. In fact, past work demonstrates that individuals hold different views about their health and the nature of their health conditions than do their family members (Clipp and George, 1992; Hatchett *et al.*, 1997; Peyrot *et al.*, 1988) and the health professionals with whom they consult (Eichenberger and Rossler, 2000; Maddox and Douglass, 1973). In such circumstances, individuals seem to reject input from social sources by virtue of it being inconsistent with personal experience. Social influence and input alter self-regulation, but they do not define it entirely.

Other frameworks for understanding self-regulation as it pertains to health behavior do not adequately address the social nature of self-regulation. The TOTE framework implies that the social environment may operate as a disturbance that may alter the self-system's efforts to change its behavior to align itself more closely with its goal state. However, it does not account for other means by which social relationships can influence self-regulation. Social relationships can serve to set the reference values that individuals strive to achieve. For example, doctors can instruct patients about the appropriate levels for their cholesterol, weight, and blood pressure. Or a model depicted in a commercial for a fitness center may establish a reference value. Social relationships can also influence the selection and implementation of coping strategies to manage health conditions through both direct and indirect means (Brissette *et al.*, 2002; Thoits, 1986). Family members and medical practitioners can offer instruction to individuals regarding how they can alter their behaviors so as to move themselves toward reference states (Lewis and Rook, 1999). Moreover, the actions of family members and peers can serve as models to follow. Finally, social relationships can provide the input that initiates the comparison of the self against the reference value. For example, a family member's remark that one does not look well may initiate a process of self-analysis and trigger important self-care that may not have occurred without the availability of social input.

Attitudinal models of the performance of health behaviors, such as the theory of reasoned action (TRA; Ajzen and Fishbein, 1980) and the theory of planned behavior (TBP; Ajzen, 1991), are less comprehensive in evaluating the contribution of social relationships to self-management. For example, both the TRA and the TPB postulate that positive evaluations of a recommended action from significant others creates a norm encouraging the performance of that action. The concept of social norms fails to capture, however, the role of the social environment in the acquisition of skills, the effectiveness of observations of others in reducing distress (Kulik and Mahler, 1987), and the many ways in which the social environment can shape the representations of health threats and associated strategies for threat control.

The influence of social and cultural factors on self-regulation is depicted in the CSM (Brownlee *et al.*, 2000; Leventhal *et al.*, 1998); that is, social and cultural factors are depicted as shaping individuals' representations of their health conditions. Leventhal and colleagues (Leventhal *et al.*, 1998) identified two ways in which social and cultural factors influence individuals' illness representations: first, they contended that culture provides the linguistic labels for differentiating and categorizing the array of events that constitute illness; second, they argued that specific social contacts can influence the interpretation of somatic information and the acquisition of specific procedures for self-management. Studies of self-care and the use of social comparison in adapting to health threats point to the prominent role other people play in shaping each of the five domains of illness representation. Identifying the processes by which this occurs and how social input from different sources (family, physicians, peers) can improve individual self-regulation continues to be a priority.

Future directions: process, schemata, and the self

The complexity of the self-regulation system, the possible variables within each of the five domains describing the representation of health threats and procedures for threat management, and the multiplicity of appraisals arising from the combination of these factors, may seem daunting even to the experienced investigator, let alone the investigator in training. Whether we like it or not, social-biological systems are complex; the enormous number of possible interactions among their many parts pose a challenge to our theoretical ingenuity and methodological skills. Fortunately, a limited number of simple rules can generate interesting predictions about the operation of the system, its interaction with the self, and some of the likely patterns underlying the self-regulation process.

Process rules, illness schemata, and representations of the self

What simple rules can we use for the analysis of the complex processes involved in the creation of representations, their bi-directional relationship to procedures for self-management, and the criteria for appraising response efficacy? At the heart of the CSM is the proposition that representations are generated and shaped by the experience of disease biology. The pain, nausea, rashes, disruptions of cognitive and physical function, fatigue, and mood changes evoked by disease make powerful and, at times, dominating contributions to the illness representation. And the greater the magnitude and rapidity of change of these somatic indicators, the greater their contribution to the representation of a health threat. Similarly, procedures that produce large, rapid, and sustained decrements in these indicators will be greatly valued and contribute to the interpretation or identity of the representation. What are the implications of these 'psychophysics' of illness cognition?

Illness schemata

Evidence suggests an initial division between schemata for acute, cyclic, and chronic illnesses. Although most (but not all) acute conditions are caused by external pathogens and are unlikely to be life threatening, all are time-limited. Chronic illnesses, by contrast, are permanent and embedded in the very fabric of the self. Cyclic conditions involve a series of episodes that may be predictable (as is the case for seasonal allergies) or unpredictable (as may be the case for episodes of asthma or congestive heart failure). Whether an illness is represented in one or the other of these three classes is more likely to reflect the individual's experience with the disease and the communications from medical authorities, family members, and other patients rather than the actual biology of the disease. For example, although asthma is a chronic condition, the sudden onset of its attack leads many asthmatics to self-regulate as though the disease is episodic. They consequently use preventive medication only when severely symptomatic. Even patients with advanced, life-threatening disease may be slow to make the transition from acute or cyclic to chronic. Many patients first entering treatment for hypertension (Meyer *et al.*, 1985) or chemotherapy for metastatic breast cancer perceive their illnesses as time-limited and curable (Leventhal *et al.*, 1986). It is clearly more attractive to represent either of these chronic conditions as a mundane, non-life-threatening illness that is treatable and non-recurrent. The biology and treatments encourage an acute model: hypertension is asymptomatic, and cancer patients are exposed to noxious chemotherapy (the intensity of which can be borne if one hopes and feels that it promises a cure).

Self-system and self-regulation

Our discussion of the self focused on generic, trait-like features of the self – that is, identities (such as sensitive soma) and strategies for self-management (such as conservation and vigor through use). These factors ignore specific features of self-representation that may shape and interact with the representation of health threats. For example, self-perceptions include specific factors such as the timeline of the self (age and expected longevity), factors associated with disease causation such as the self-assessment of health, and the individual's perception of the vigor of her immune system. These specific features of the self can be expected to interact with the representation of specific diseases and to play a role in generating perceptions of vulnerability and the availability of motivation for self-protective action. For example, when asked to guess the age at which women are most likely to fall ill with breast cancer, the majority of responses fall within a ten-year interval of 45-55 years of age. The actual modal range for breast cancer occurrence, however, is 70-75 years of age (Ries et al., 2002). Does this perception account for the gradual decline in the annual use of mammography that seems to begin at 70 years of age and older? Do people take more liberties with exposure to cancer-causing agents if they perceive themselves as having a strong immune system? These and other similar questions have not been addressed.

Interventions, schemata and self-regulation

In our judgment, the future health of the CSM depends upon its success in generating conceptually clear interventions that prove effective in enhancing behaviors for reducing disease risk and improving the management of chronic illness. We believe that interventions, including mass media programs, will best succeed when their contents are informed by the representations of specific illnesses and procedures for their control. As suggested by Petrie and colleagues' successful intervention in recovery from myocardial infarction (Petrie *et al.*, 2002), it is likely that initial efforts will be individualized and conducted in clinical settings (see Petrie *et al.*, this volume, Chapter 13). We believe, however, that both the content and the processes uncovered in studies of common-sense reasoning and health-related behavior will prove effective in developing campaigns for informing large segments of the population that resonate for those who possess the motivation and skills for effective self-regulation. Ongoing studies will provide evidence for or against this judgment.

Notes

1   Correspondence should be addressed to Howard Leventhal, Institute for Health, Health Care Policy and Aging Research, Rutgers – The State University of New Jersey, 30 College Avenue, New Brunswick, NJ 08901-1293. E-mail: hleventhal@ihhcpar.rutgers.edu
2   Meta-analyses of more recent studies show a consistent, if small advantage of high relative to low fear messages for behavioral change ($r's$ = 0.10 to 0.15) and a larger effect size for attitude change and behavioral intentions (Witte and Allen, 2000).

References

Ajzen, I. (1991) 'The theory of planned behavior,' *Organizational Behavior and Human Decision Processes* **50**: 179–211.
Ajzen, I. and Fishbein, M. (1980) *Understanding Attitudes and Predicting Social Behavior*, Englewood Cliffs, NJ: Prentice-Hall.
Anderson, J.A. (1983) *The Architecture of Cognition*, Cambridge, MA: Harvard University Press.
Baumann, L.J. and Leventhal, H. (1985) 'I can tell when my blood pressure is up, can't I?' *Health Psychology* **4**: 203–218.
Baumann, L.J., Cameron, L.D., Zimmerman, R. and Leventhal, H. (1989) 'Illness representations and matching labels with symptoms,' *Health Psychology* **8**: 449–470.
Becker, M.H. (1974) 'The health belief model and personal health behaviours,' *Health Education Monographs* **2**: 376–423.
Berkanovic, E., Telesky, C. and Reeder, S. (1981) 'Structural and social psychological factors in the decision to seek medical care for symptoms,' *Medical Care* **19**: 693–709.
Berkman, L.F. and Syme, S.L. (1979) 'Social networks, host resistance, and mortality: a nine-year follow-up study of Alameda county residents,' *American Journal of Epidemiology* **109**: 186–204.
Berland, G.K., Elliot, M.N., Morales, L.S., Algazy, J.I., Kravitz, R.L., Broder, M.S., Kanouse, D.E., Munoz, J.A., Puyol. J., Lara, M., Watkins, K.E., Yang, H. and McGlynn, E.A. (2001) 'Health information on the Internet: accessibility, quality, and readability in English and Spanish,' *Journal of American Medical Association* **285**: 2612–2621.

Bishop, G.D. (1991) 'Understanding the understanding of illness: Lay disease representations,' in J.A. Skelton and R.T. Croyle (eds) *Mental Representation in Health and Illness*, New York: Springer-Verlag, pp. 32–59.

Bishop, G.D. and Converse, S.A. (1986) 'Illness representations: a prototype approach,' *Health Psychology* **5**: 95–114.

Boekaerts, M., Pintrich, P.R. and Zeidner, M. (eds) (2000) *Handbook of Self-Regulation*, San Diego, CA: Academic Press.

Boroditsky, L. and Ramscar, M. (2002) 'The roles of body and mind in abstract thought,' *Psychological Science* **13**: 185–189.

Brissette, I., Scheier, M.F. and Carver, C.S. (2002) 'The role of optimism in social network development, coping and psychological adjustment during a life transition,' *Journal of Personality and Social Psychology* **82**: 102–111.

Brownlee, S., Leventhal, H. and Leventhal, E.A. (2000) 'Regulation, self-regulation and regulation of the self in maintaining physical health,' in M. Boekaerts, P.R. Pintrich and M. Zeidner (eds) *Handbook of Self-Regulation*, San Diego, CA: Academic Press, pp. 369–416.

Buunk, B. and Gibbons, F.X. (1997) *Social Comparisons, Health, and Coping*, Hillsdale, NJ: Lawrence Erlbaum Associates.

Cameron, L.D., Leventhal, E.A. and Leventhal, H. (1993) 'Symptom representations and affect as determinants of care seeking in a community dwelling adult sample population,' *Health Psychology* **12**: 171–179.

—— (1995) 'Seeking medical care in response to symptoms and life stress,' *Psychosomatic Medicine* **57**: 37–47.

Carver, C.S. and Scheier, M.F. (1981) *Attention and Self-Regulation: A Control-Theory Approach to Human Behavior*, New York: Springer-Verlag.

Carr, S. (2000) 'Self-regulation strategies and the use of exercise and herbal supplements,' unpublished MA thesis, Rutgers University.

Cassileth, B.R. (1998) *The Alternative Medicine Handbook: The Complete Reference Guide to Alternative and Complementary Therapies*, New York: W.W. Norton.

Chrisman, N.J. (1977) 'The health seeking process: an approach to the natural history of illness,' *Culture, Medicine, and Psychiatry* **1**: 351–177.

Clipp, E.C. and George, L.K. (1992) 'Patients with cancer and their spouse caregivers,' *Cancer* **69**: 1074–1079.

Consumer Reports (2000) 'The mainstreaming of alternative medicine,' May, 17–25.

Croyle, R.T. and Jemmott, J.B. III (1991) 'Psychological reactions to risk factor testing,' in J.A. Skelton and R.T. Croyle (eds) *Mental Representation in Health and Illness*, New York: Springer-Verlag, pp. 85–107.

Dabbs, J.M., Jr. and Leventhal, H. (1966) 'Effects of varying the recommendations in a fear-arousing communication,' *Journal of Personality and Social Psychology* **4**: 525–531.

Dollard, J. and Miller, N.E. (1950) *Personality and Psychotherapy*, New York: McGraw-Hill.

Duke, J., Brownlee, S., Leventhal, E.A. and Leventhal, H. (2002) 'Giving up and replacing activities in response to illness,' *Journal of Gerontology: Psychological Sciences,* **57**: 367–376.

Easterling, D. and Leventhal, H. (1989) 'The contribution of concrete cognition to emotion: neutral symptoms as elicitors of worry about cancer,' *Journal of Applied Psychology* **74**: 787–796.

Eichenberger, A. and Rossler, W. (2000) 'Comparison of self-ratings and therapist ratings of outpatients' psychological status,' *Journal of Nervous and Mental Disease* **188**: 297–300.

Eisenberg, D.M., Davis, R.B., Ettner, S.L., Appel, S., Wilkey, S., Van Rompay, M. and Kessler, R.C. (1998) 'Trends in alternative medicine use in the United States, 1990–1997: results of a follow-up national survey,' *Journal of the American Medical Association* **280**: 1569–75.

Epstein, S. (1994) 'Integration of the cognitive and the psychodynamic unconscious,' *American Psychologist* **49**: 709–724.

Gollwitzer, P.M. and Oettingen, G. (1998) 'The emergence and implementation of health goals,' *Psychology and Health* **13**: 687–715.

Granovetter, M.S. (1978) 'The strength of weak ties,' *American Journal of Sociology* **31**: 1360–1369.

Hatchett, L., Friend, R., Symister, P. and Wadhwa, N. (1997) 'Interpersonal expectations, social support and adjustment to chronic illness,' *Journal of Personality and Social Support* **73**: 560–673.

Heidrich, S.M., Forsthoff, C.A. and Ward, S.E. (1994) 'Psychological adjustment in adults with cancer: the self as mediator,' *Health Psychology* **13**: 346–353.

Helgeson, V., Cohen, S., Schulz, R. and Yasko, J. (1999) 'Education and peer discussion group interventions and adjustment to breast cancer,' *Archives of General Psychiatry* **56**: 340–347.

Heurtin-Roberts, S. and Reisin, E. (1992) 'The relation of culturally influenced lay models of hypertension to compliance with treatment,' *American Journal of Hypertension* **5**: 787–792.

Hooker, K. and Kaus, C. (1994) 'Health-related possible selves in young and middles adulthood,' *Psychology and Aging* **9**: 126–133.

Horne, R. (1997) 'Representations of medication and treatment: advances in theory and measurement,' in K.J. Petrie and J.A. Weinman (eds) *Perceptions of Health and Illness*, Amsterdam: Harwood Academic, pp. 155–188.

Horowitz, C.R., Rein, S.B. and Leventhal, H. (in review) 'Challenges to effective self-management of heart failure: a grounded theory approach.'

House, J.S., Landis, K.R. and Umberson, D. (1988) 'Social relationships and health,' *Science* **241**: 540–545.

Jaco, E. (1954) 'The social isolation hypothesis and schizophrenia,' *American Sociological Review* **19**: 567–577.

Jemmott, J.B., Ditto, P.H. and Croyle, R.T. (1986) 'Judging health status: effects of perceived prevalence and personal relevance,' *Journal of Personality and Social Psychology* **50**: 899–905.

Johnson, J.E. (1975) 'Stress reduction through sensation information,' in I.L. Sarason and C.D. Spielberger (eds) *Stress and Anxiety*, Washington, DC: Hemisphere Publishing, pp. 361–373.

Johnson, J.E. and Leventhal, H. (1974) 'The effects of accurate expectations and behavioral instructions on reactions during a noxious medical examination,' *Journal of Personality and Social Psychology* **29**: 710–718.

Kleinman, A. (1980) *Patients and Healers in the Context of Culture: An Exploration of the Borderland Between Anthropology, Medicine, and Psychiatry*, Los Angeles: University of California Press.

Kulik, J.A. and Mahler, H.I.M. (1987) 'Effects of preoperative roommate assignment on preoperative anxiety and recovery from coronary-bypass surgery,' *Health Psychology* 6: 525–543.

Lacroix, J.M., Martin, B., Avendano, M. and Goldstein, R. (1991) 'Symptom schemata in chronic respiratory patients,' *Health Psychology* 10: 268–273.

Lau, R.R. and Hartman, K.A. (1983) 'Common sense representations of common illnesses,' *Health Psychology* 2: 167–185.

Lau, R.R., Bernard, T.M. and Hartman, K.R. (1989) 'Further explorations of common sense representations of common illnesses,' *Health Psychology* 8: 195–219.

Lazarus, R.S. and Launier, R. (1978) 'Stress related transactions between person and environment,' in L.A. Pervin and M. Lewis (eds) *Perspectives in Interactional Psychology*, New York: Plenum, pp. 287–327.

Leventhal, E.A. and Crouch, M. (1997) 'Are there differences in perceptions of illness across the lifespan?' in K.J. Petrie and J.A. Weinman (eds) *Perceptions of Health and Illness*, Amsterdam: Harwood Academic, pp. 77–102.

Leventhal, E.A., Easterling, D.V., Leventhal, H. and Cameron, L.D. (1995) 'Conservation of energy, uncertainty reduction, and swift utilization of medical care among the elderly: study II,' *Medical Care* 33: 988–1000.

Leventhal, E.A., Leventhal, H., Schaefer, P. and Easterling, D.V. (1993) 'Conservation of energy, uncertainty reduction, and swift utilization of medical care among the elderly,' *Journal of Gerontology* 48: 78–86.

Leventhal, H. (1970) 'Findings and theory in the study of fear communications,' *Advances in Experimental Social Psychology* 5: 119–186.

—— (1984) 'A perceptual-motor theory emotion,' in L. Berkowitz (ed.) *Advances in Experimental Social Psychology*, Orlando, FL: Academic Press, pp.117–182.

Leventhal, H. and Niles, P. (1965) 'Persistence of influence for varying durations of exposure to threat stimuli,' *Psychological Reports* 16: 223–233.

Leventhal, H. and Singer, R.P. (1966) 'Affect arousal and positioning of recommendations in persuasive communications,' *Journal of Personality and Social Psychology* 4: 137–146.

Leventhal, H. and Watts, J.C. (1966) 'Sources of resistance to fear-arousing communications on smoking and lung cancer,' *Journal of Personality* 34: 155–175.

Leventhal, H., Hudson, S. and Robitaille, C. (1997) 'Social comparison and health: a process model,' in B. Buunk and F.X. Gibbons (eds) *Health, Coping and Well Being: Perspectives From Social Comparison Theory*, Hillsdale, NJ: Lawrence Erlbaum Associates, pp. 411–432.

Leventhal, H., Jones, S. and Trembly, G. (1966) 'Sex differences in attitude and behavior change under conditions of fear and specific instructions,' *Journal of Experimental Social Psychology* 2: 387–399.

Leventhal, H., Leventhal, E.A. and Contrada, R.J. (1998) 'Self-regulation, health, and behavior: a perceptual-cognitive approach,' *Psychology and Health* 13: 717–733.

Leventhal, H., Singer, R. and Jones, S. (1965) 'Effects of fear and specificity of recommendations upon attitudes and behaviour,' *Journal of Personality and Social Psychology* 2: 20–29.

Leventhal, H., Watts, J. C. and Pagano, F. (1967) 'Effects of fear and instructions on how to cope with danger,' *Journal of Personality and Social Psychology* **6**: 313–321.

Leventhal, H., Easterling, D.V., Coons, H.L., Luchterhand, C.M. and Love, R.R. (1986) 'Adaptation to chemotherapy treatments,' in B.L. Andersen (ed.) *Women with Cancer: Psychological Perspectives*, New York: Springer Verlag, pp. 172–203.

Lewis, M.A. and Rook, K.S. (1999) 'Social control in personal relationships: impact on health behaviors and psychological distress,' *Health Psychology* **18**: 63–71.

Liu, W.T. and Duff, R.W. (1972) 'The strength in weak ties,' *Public Opinion Quarterly* **42**: 361–367.

Lynch, J.J. (1979) *The Broken Heart*, New York: Basic Books.

Maddox, G.L. and Douglass, E.B. (1973) 'Self-assessment of health: a longitudinal study of elderly subjects,' *Journal of Health and Social Behavior* **14**: 87–93.

Meyer, D., Leventhal, H. and Guttman, M. (1985) 'Common-sense models of illness: the example of hypertension,' *Health Psychology* **4**: 115–135.

Miller, G., Galanter, E. and Pribram, K. (1960) *Plans and the Structure of Behavior*, New York: Henry Holt & Co.

Mora, P., Robitaille, C., Leventhal, H., Swigar, M. and Leventhal, E.A. (2002) 'Trait negative affect relates to prior weak symptoms, but not to reports of illness episodes, illness symptoms and care seeking,' *Psychosomatic Medicine* **64**: 436–449.

Nemeroff, C. and Rozin, P. (1994) 'The contagion concept in adult thinking in the United States: transmission of germs and of interpersonal influence,' *Ethos* **22**: 158–186.

Nerenz, D.R., Leventhal H. and Love, R.R. (1982) 'Factors contributing to emotional distress during cancer chemotherapy,' *Cancer* **50**: 1020–1027.

Newell, A. (1980) 'Reasoning, problem-solving, and decision processes: the problem space as a fundamental category,' in R. Nickerson (ed.) *Attention and Performance*, vol. 8, Hillsdale, NJ: Lawrence Erlbaum Associates.

Orbell, S. and Sheeran, P. (2002) 'Changing health behaviours: the role of implementation intentions,' in D. Rutter and L. Quine (eds) *Changing Health Behaviour: Intervention and Research with Social Cognition Models*, Buckingham, UK: Open University Press, pp. 123–137.

Pachter, L.M. (1993) 'Latino folk illnesses: methodological considerations,' *Medical Anthropology* **15**: 103–108.

Penrod, S. (1980) 'Cognitive models of symptoms and diseases,' paper presented at the Annual Meeting of the American Psychological Association.

Perloff, L.S. and Fetzer, B.K. (1986) 'Self-other judgments and perceived vulnerability to victimization,' *Journal of Personality and Social Psychology* **50**: 502–510.

Pescosolido, B.A. (1992) 'Beyond rationale choice: the social dynamics of how people seek help,' *American Journal of Sociology* **97**: 1096–1138.

Petrie, K.J., Cameron, L.D., Ellis, C., Buick, D. and Weinman, J. (2002) 'Changing illness perceptions following myocardial infarction: an early intervention randomized controlled trial,' *Psychosomatic Medicine* **64**: 580–586.

Peyrot, M., McMurry, J.F. and Hedges, R. (1988) 'Marital adjustment to adult diabetes: interpersonal congruence and spouse satisfaction,' *Journal of Marriage and the Family* **50**: 363–376.

Powers, W.T. (1973) *Behaviour: The Control of Perception*, Chicago: Adline.

Rice, R.E. and Katz, J.E. (2001) *The Internet and Health Communication*, Thousand Oaks, CA: Sage Publications.

Ries, L.A.G., Eisner, M.P., Kosary, C.L., Hankey, B.F., Miller, B.A., Clegg, L. and Edwards, B.K. (eds) (2002) *SEER Cancer Statistics Review, 1973–1999, National Cancer Institute*, Bethesda, MD, http://seer.cancer.gov/csr/1973_1999/.

Rogers, R.W. (1983) 'Cognitive and physiological processes in fear appeals and attitude: a revised theory of protection motivation,' *Social Psychophysiology: A Sourcebook*, New York: Guilford, pp. 153–176.

Rosenstock, I.M. (1974) 'The health belief model and preventative health behavior,' *Health Education Monographs* **2**: 354–386.

Rosenstock, I.M., Hochbaum, G.M. and Leventhal, H. (1960) *The Impact of Asian Influenza on Community Life: A Study of Five Cities*, Publication No. 766, Washington, DC: US Department of Health, Education, and Welfare, the Public Health Service.

Schachter, S. and Singer, J.E. (1962) 'Cognitive, social, and physiological determinants of emotional state,' *Psychological Review* **69**: 379–399.

Simons, R.C. (1993) 'A simple defense of Western biomedical explanatory schemata,' *Medical Anthropology* **15**: 201–208.

Suls J. and Goodkin, F. (1994) 'Medical gossip and rumor: their role in the lay referral system,' in R.F. Goodman and A. Ben-Zeev (eds) *Good Gossip*, Lawrence, KS: University Press of Kansas pp. 169–179.

Suls, J., Martin, R. and Leventhal, H. (1997) 'Social comparison, lay referral, and the decision to seek medical care,' in B. Buunk and F.X. Gibbons (eds) *Health, Coping and Well Being: Perspectives from Social Comparison Theory*, Hillsdale, NJ: Lawrence Erlbaum Associates, pp. 195–226.

Suls, J., Martin, R. and Wheeler, L. (2000) 'Three kinds of opinion comparison: the triadic model,' *Personality and Social Psychology Review* **4**: 219–237.

Taylor, S.E. (1983) 'Adjustment to threatening events: a theory of cognitive adaptation,' *American Psychologist* **38**: 1161–1173.

Thoits, P.A. (1983) 'Multiple identities and psychological well-being: a reformulation of the social isolation hypothesis,' *American Sociological Review* **48**: 174–187.

Thoits, P.A. (1986) 'Social support and coping assistance,' *Consulting and Clinical Psychology* **154**: 416–424.

Whiting, J.W.M. and Child, I.L. (1953) *Child Training and Personality*, New Haven: Yale University Press.

Witte, K. and Allen, M. (2000) 'A meta-analysis of fear appeals: implications for effective public health campaigns,' *Health Education and Behavior* **27**: 591–615.

Zola, I.K. (1966) 'Culture and symptoms B: an analysis of patients' presenting complaints,' *American Sociological Review* **31**: 615–630.

4   Personality and self-regulation in health and disease

Toward an integrative perspective

Richard J. Contrada and Elliot J. Coups [1]

The purpose of this chapter is to discuss general approaches to understanding the role of personality in health-related self-regulation. Personality, self-regulation, and health are each associated with a large, diverse body of research. Therefore, to help focus our task, we have put the spotlight on personality. We begin with a very brief outline of the key elements of self-regulation. We then describe dispositional and social-cognitive perspectives on personality and discuss each in relation to health-related self-regulation. Although both approaches offer contributions to understanding self-regulation and health, our suggestion is that social-cognitive theory is more promising in this regard. In addition to discussing these general frameworks and associated personality constructs, we also examine the major methodological approaches involved, and discuss some of their limitations and potentials. We conclude by describing ways of extending existing models to further understand personality and health-related self-regulation.

Self-regulation: major conceptual elements

'Self-regulation' has a number of different meanings. Below, we highlight concepts and themes related to self-regulation that provide potential points of contact between personality and physical health/disease. More in-depth treatments of self-regulation may be found in Bandura (1999), Baumeister (1998), and Schwartz (1977), as well as in the chapters by Scheier and Carver, and Leventhal *et al.* in this volume (Chapters 2 and 3, respectively).

Cybernetics

Certain self-regulation concepts have counterparts in cybernetics, the science of communication and control concerned with the operation of biological and artificial systems (Wiener, 1948). A key example is the feedback loop, in which input to a system is compared to an internal reference value, which may generate corrective action depending upon the degree of discrepancy. Miller *et al.* (1960) characterized the feedback loop as the basic building block for complex behavioral processes, and numerous psychological concepts can be seen as corresponding to elements of the feedback process. For example, goals, referring to desired or undesired states or directions for change, constitute a type of internal reference (Carver and Scheier, 1999).

Psychological stress

The study of self-regulation, behavior, and health often comes into contact with psychological stress theory. Stress occurs when events and conditions tax or exceed a person's adaptive resources, activating physiologic processes that may promote physical disease, and also affecting behaviors that influence health, including substance use, eating, and sleep. *Stress-focused* research that bears upon self-regulation theory examines the impact of major life events (e.g., bereavement), minor events (e.g., daily 'hassles'), social-environmental conditions (e.g., crowding, occupational stress), and laboratory stressors (e.g., performance challenges). A psychological stress perspective typically is explicit in this work, whereas self-regulation, while potentially quite relevant, may not be referred to at all, or may be used in a narrow sense to refer to the management of affect.

In *behavior-focused* research on health-related self-regulation, theoretical analysis often begins with a hazardous exposure (e.g., proximity to environmental toxins, ingestion of dangerous substances) or a perceived health threat (e.g., acute or chronic illness). Stress-related processes may enter into responses to these exposures and threats in a number of different ways. For example, psychological processes of threat-reduction activated by psychosocial stressors may also cause inattention to hazardous exposures and health threats. In addition, certain risky actions (e.g., alcohol or tobacco use, delay in health-care seeking) may reflect the management of emotions provoked by stressors. Nonetheless, behavior-focused work on health-related self-regulation is often conceptualized without explicit reference to stress theory.

Potential stressors initiate cognitive appraisal and coping processes. Cognitive appraisal is the perception and evaluation of threatened or actual harm or loss; primary appraisal focuses on the nature and magnitude of harm or loss, and secondary appraisal focuses on coping resources and options. Problem-focused coping is cognitive or behavioral activity aimed at modifying the situation that gave rise to threat appraisal, and emotion-focused coping involves managing its subjective impact (Lazarus and Folkman, 1984). This is conceptual territory to which both psychological stress theory and self-regulation theory can lay claim. For example, cognitive appraisal reflects the evaluation of information against internal references, and coping serves to optimize the degree of discrepancy between input (threat) and reference values (goals) activated to guide and evaluate coping.

Multi-level analysis

Self-regulation involves multi-level phenomena. Cybernetic approaches in psychology view goals as varying across multiple, hierarchically organized levels of abstraction, with relatively specific goals (e.g., pain relief) nested under a series of increasingly more general goals (e.g., minimizing discomfort, maintaining quality of life) (Carver and Scheier, 1999). In illness cognition approaches (e.g., Brownlee *et al.*, 2000), a bi-level notion distinguishes between concrete-sensory mental representations, such as somatic symptoms (e.g., coughing, sneezing, headache), and abstract ones, such as disease labels (e.g., 'a cold').

Self-regulation is also multi-level in addressing phenomena of interest to more than one scientific discipline. In particular, the term 'self-regulation' is commonly used to refer to interactions between psychological and biological activity. These include alteration of physiological activity, either using behavioral techniques such as biofeedback and relaxation, or through conscious inhibition of emotion (Schwartz, 1977). Similarly, in other cross-disciplinary phenomena, self-regulative responses to physical symptoms involve the use of linguistic and conceptual categories afforded by the larger sociocultural system (e.g., 'cramp') as labels and meanings that attach to sensations emanating from the biological system (e.g., involuntary spasmodic muscle contractions), followed by corrective actions that are available and sanctioned in the culture and both physically and economically accessible (e.g., a visit to the doctor) (Leventhal *et al.*, 1998).

Major approaches to personality and their points of contact with health-related self-regulation

Personality has been subject to a variety of conceptualizations. One is a *dispositional* view focusing on '*individual differences*, or the dimensions along which people differ from each other' (Winter and Barenbaum, 1999: 6). Another is a ' "processing approach" [that] construes personality as a system of mediating units (e.g., encodings, expectancies, goals, motives) and psychological processes or cognitive-affective dynamics, conscious or unconscious, that interact with the situation' (Mischel and Shoda, 1999: 198).

Individual differences in dispositions

Trait perspectives constitute the dominant approach to conceptualizing individual differences (Winter and Barenbaum, 1999). Moreover, although not without its vocal and persuasive critics, a consensus has developed around a particular framework, the Five Factor Model (FFM), as a comprehensive account of major personality traits. In this model, personality is described in terms of five broad dispositions, one set of labels for which are extraversion, agreeableness, conscientiousness, neuroticism, and openness to experience (Costa and McCrae, 1992).

A hallmark of trait approaches is a focus on *statistical structure*. Traits correspond to *temporal* and *cross-situational* consistencies in behavior, where behavior is defined broadly in terms of thought, feeling, and action. In addition, many trait approaches posit a *hierarchical* aspect to statistical structure. For example, FFM traits describe personality at a fairly general level; each is thought to comprise a correlated set of more circumscribed facets, as where extraversion is defined in terms of gregariousness, assertiveness, activity, excitement-seeking, positive emotions, and warmth (Costa and McCrae, 1992). These facets, in turn, can be resolved into still narrower behavioral consistencies (e.g., situation-specific habits) and, conversely, the FFM traits themselves form clusters that define even broader dimensions of personality (e.g., personality types).

Research models

A large volume of research has examined individual difference factors in relation to physical health. Much of it is stress-focused, in that a disposition is thought to promote or damage health through its association with cognitive, emotional, behavioral, and, especially, physiologic responses to stressors. Salient examples are the Type A behavior pattern and its components, especially trait hostility (Contrada *et al.*, 1999). In other, behavior-focused research, personality dispositions have been examined in relation to various health-related actions and inactions, including diet, exercise, substance use, unsafe sex, health-care seeking, medical non-adherence, and adjustment to health crises (for reviews, see Contrada *et al.*, 1999; Wiebe and Christensen, 1996). Where this research has been framed within a theoretical model, it has often focused on person–situation interactions and the notions of statistical moderation and mediation.

Dispositions are commonly viewed as moderators of psychological stress. This often leads to explicit examination of the interactive effects of dispositions and stressors. However, variation in exposure to a stressor is sometimes unmeasured. For example, personality may be examined in a patient group for which disease and treatment constitute a multifaceted stressor, without comparisons to a non-patient group. This research model typically focuses on appraisal, coping, or emotional responses that may mediate effects of personality on health outcomes. Some rather novel and elegant research has focused on specific *processes of personality–stressor interaction*, testing substantive models of links between personality and cognitive appraisal (e.g., Wiebe, 1991), or coping (e.g., Bolger and Zuckerman, 1995). More often, both personality and stressor are studied as somewhat static entities, and characterization of their interplay is limited to little more than a partitioning of *statistical interaction* variance.

A more dynamic, *transactional* perspective posits reciprocal pathways of influence linking personality dispositions, environmental stressors, and coping resources (Smith, 1992). Transactional models also view traits as capable of influencing cognitive appraisal and coping. However, they additionally incorporate the notion that personality influences exposure to stressors and access to coping resources such as supportive social networks, through processes of social-environmental selection, evocation, and manipulation, and the prolongation or attenuation of exposure to demanding situations (Contrada and Guyll, 2001).

Illustrative findings

Type A behavior and trait hostility have been linked to pathophysiological responses to psychosocial stressors and to a variety of health-damaging behaviors (for reviews see Contrada *et al.*, 1999; Contrada and Guyll, 2001; Smith, 1992). However, because the Type A concept emerged from the fields of clinical cardiology and epidemiology, its status within personality theory is unclear. Other research on health-related personality dispositions includes that examining broad motives, such as stressed power motivation (e.g., Jemmott *et al.*, 1990), which have been associated with health-damaging physiologic and behavioral processes. Recent work on motivation and health has focused on more narrowly construed motives. We will discuss these and other more circumscribed personality constructs in a later section because we believe they are more fruitfully considered within a social cognitive framework.

Recent findings have linked FFM traits to appraisal, coping, and health-related behaviors. Neuroticism (or negative affectivity) is associated with a tendency to evaluate demanding situations as threatening (e.g., Gallagher, 1990), and to enter into situations that are likely to be stressful (Bolger and Zuckerman, 1995). Neuroticism appears inversely associated with adaptive forms of coping (active, problem-focused), and positively associated with maladaptive ones (e.g., self-blame, denial, wishful-thinking, disengagement) (Bolger and Zuckerman, 1995; Carver and Scheier, 1999; McCrae and Costa, 1986; Rim, 1986). Neuroticism is also inversely associated with health-enhancing behaviors such as exercise, taking vitamins, and safe driving (Booth-Kewley and Vickers, 1994). In addition, there is evidence that neurotic individuals may engage in potentially health-damaging behaviors (such as drinking alcohol) as a means of coping with negative affective states (Cooper *et al.*, 2000).

Correlates of extraversion contrast with those of neuroticism. Extraverts evaluate stressful events as challenging, rather than threatening (Gallagher, 1990). They appear inclined toward problem-focused coping and positive thinking (Rim, 1987), restraint and rational action (McCrae and Costa, 1986), and social support seeking (Amirkhan *et al.*, 1995). Extraversion has been positively linked to certain health-promoting behaviors (Booth-Kewley and Vickers, 1994), though it also has been linked to substance use, perhaps reflecting efforts to increase positive affect (Cooper *et al.*, 2000).

Conscientiousness, agreeableness, and openness to experience have been less often studied in relation to health. However, available evidence indicates that each appears associated with coping and health-related behaviors that resemble correlates of extraversion. One exception is that openness to experience has also been linked to substance use behaviors such as smoking (Booth-Kewley and Vickers, 1994; Costa, Somerfield, and McCrae, 1996; Vickers, Kolar, and Hervig, 1989; Watson and Hubbard, 1996).

Comments: statistical accounts versus substantive explanation

Transactional models of personality and health extend well beyond the simple associations that dominate the empirical literature. They require rethinking of disposition and stress constructs and of the processes whereby they influence one another. They also strain the capabilities of conventional statistical analysis. When personality and stressor constructs are placed in separate boxes in a diagram representing the ways in which they are linked with illness, it is both natural and useful as a first approximation to think of them as being related to one another in ways that correspond to statistical moderation or mediation. However, there is reason to believe that both statistical models apply, and in more than one way. Figure 4.1(a) and (b) displays four mediation models and three moderator models of the personality-stressor-illness relationship.

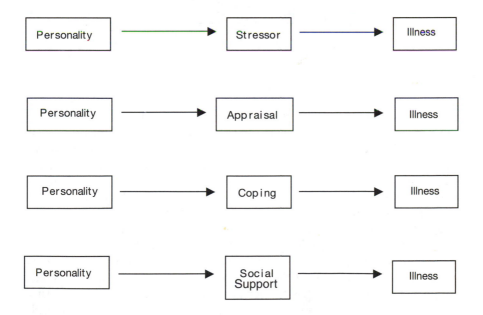

Figure 4.1(a)   Stress processes as mediators of personality effects on illness

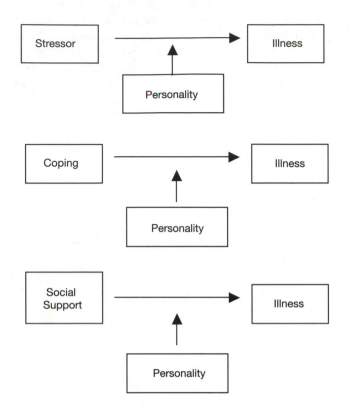

Figure 4.1(b)   Personality as moderator of stress-related effects on illness

The four diagrams in Figure 4.1(a) represent conceptual models in which personality dispositions may influence illness through effects *mediated* by four distinct stress-related processes: the disposition may influence the frequency or duration of exposures to environmental stressors; the appraisal of threat, harm, or loss following stressor exposure; the mode or effectiveness of coping activity; or the availability or helpfulness of coping resources such as social support. The three diagrams in Figure 4.1(b) represent conceptual models in which personality may influence illness by *moderating* the effects of three distinct stress-related processes: the disposition may moderate the effects of exposure to environmental stressors; the use or effectiveness of certain forms of coping activity; or the impact of available coping resources such as social support. These seven models are neither exhaustive nor mutually exclusive and two or more may operate simultaneously with respect to multiple personality dispositions in the same individuals.

Space limitations do not permit a review of evidence supporting each model; suffice it to say that most of the links implied by the models have received empirical support for one personality disposition or another, and that all are theoretically plausible, even likely (for reviews, see Contrada *et al.*, 1999; Contrada and Guyll, 2001; Hewitt and Flett, 1996; Taylor and Aspinwall, 1996). When one considers that the seven models are neither exhaustive nor mutually exclusive, and that several may operate simultaneously with respect to multiple personality dispositions in the same individuals, the task of fully capturing personality–stressor interplay within a single investigation seems truly daunting. To do so will, at a minimum, require the use of statistical methods for combining and integrating multiple instances of both mediation and moderation.

A limitation that would not be circumvented by more sophisticated application of the moderator/mediator notion is extensive reliance on statistical approaches to explanation. Separation of trait and stressor variance in multiple regression gives what may be a false impression of having isolated two independent causal factors, one person-related and one contextual. This impression is called into question by transactional models of person–situation interplay (Bandura, 1999; Smith, 1992). Similarly, separation of both trait and stressor variance from that of dependent measures of appraisal, coping, emotional state, or somatic illness gives a potentially false impression that a causal system has been isolated. To support these views, it must be shown that associations linking such measures do not reflect redundancy, or third variable causes, and it should be possible to specify and operationalize generative processes that give rise to these relationships. The problems of redundancy and third variables are well recognized with regard to the possible role of neuroticism/negative affectivity in bringing about spurious associations between measures loaded with emotional content (Watson and Pennebaker, 1989; Watson *et al.*, 1999), although statistical identification of neuroticism's role too often brings to premature foreclosure the business of specifying the underlying generating mechanism.

Less well appreciated is the possibility that measures reflecting expectancy (disposition) and behavioral (coping) content may also reflect the same underlying factor (Contrada *et al.*, 1999). Also poorly recognized are the limitations of exclusively statistical methods for validating measures. Demonstrations of internal consistency, or factorial simple structure, in measures of disposition, appraisal, or coping, beg the question of what cognitive-affective or neurobiological structure accounts for the consistencies. Statistical patterning, the hallmark of dispositional approaches, provides a starting point for causal analysis, but does not, in itself, constitute explanation. To go further, it is necessary to distinguish personality structure and statistical structure (Mischel and Shoda, 1999): cognitive-affective and/or neurobiological structures within the person must be conceptualized and operationalized separately from the consistent patterns of cognitive, affective, and behavioral activity that they produce.

Personality as process: social-cognitive approaches and middle-level units

Process perspectives on personality emphasize context, cognition, and motivation (Bandura, 1999; Mischel and Shoda, 1999). Sometimes characterized as 'social-cognitive,' or 'cognitive-social,' they make use of 'middle-level' personality units to facilitate understanding of person–situation interactions (Cantor and Zirkel, 1990). These units are intermediate with regard to degree of abstractness and generality: not as all-encompassing as more traditional personality traits and motives, but also not so narrow as to be tightly situation-bound. Middle-level units are generally cognitive in nature and often refer to beliefs about oneself and the world. They also have emotional content and motivational properties, and are at least somewhat contextualized in referring to a specific life stage or type of setting or activity. In addition, most are idiographic in that their availability within a person's cognitive-affective system, and aspects of their content, are to some extent individualized and experience-based.

Two major variants – goal constructs and self-constructs – serve as illustrations of the wide range of middle-level units that have been studied. By contrast with motive constructs such as power and affiliation, which are relatively broad and somewhat abstract, social-cognitive theorists have emphasized a variety of goal constructs that refer to a person's more immediate motives and pursuits. These include personal projects (Little, 1983), life tasks (Cantor and Kihlstrom, 1985) and personal strivings (Emmons, 1989). Each has distinctive elements, but all involve a focus on ongoing, goal-directed activities that are often accessible to consciousness and through which the individual engages in everyday living (Cantor and Zirkel, 1990).

Self and identity constructs have a rich heritage in psychology that can be traced to the discipline's inception (e.g., James, 1890). Of particular interest are self/identity constructs referring to cognitive structures that contain a person's mental representations of him/herself. These describe and organize self-knowledge (the totality of a person's self-referent beliefs), self-motives (motivational forces that guide the processing of self-referent knowledge), and self-evaluation (global self-esteem and comparative 'selves' such as the 'ideal self' involved in self-appraisal) (Baumeister, 1998).

The social-cognitive perspective on personality comes into contact with models of self-regulation and health in a number of different ways. Indeed, the work of two major social-cognitive theorists, Albert Bandura and Walter Mischel, frequently makes explicit reference to self-regulation. Here, 'self-regulation' does not refer to a circumscribed set of phenomena solely related to psychosocial stressors, hazardous exposures, or perceived health threats. It refers broadly to a set of human tendencies and capabilities, including (but not limited to) many that are highly relevant to health-related self-regulation. It also refers specifically to processes whereby sustained patterns of goal-directed activity are undertaken even when circumstances offer little support and/or pose barriers. The latter usage derives in part from research on forms of self-control (e.g., self-talk about rules and standards, self-distraction, focusing on 'cool' rather than consumatory representations of objects) through which delay of immediate gratification or tolerance of distress and discomfort may facilitate long-term goal attainment (Mischel and Shoda, 1999).

In their social-cognitive model, Mischel and Shoda (1999) view personality as a processing system in which a set of cognitive-affective units mediate situational influences on thought, feeling, and action. These include encodings, expectancies/beliefs, affects, goals/values, competencies, and self-regulatory plans. This model is highly compatible with theories of health-related self-regulation. Many specific cognitive-affective units discussed by Mischel and Shoda correspond to various phases and components of health-related self-regulation models such as those described by Carver and Scheier (1999) and Brownlee *et al.* (2000). The contextualized view of personality is well suited for conceptualizing adaptation to psychosocial stressors, hazardous exposures, and health threats. The cognitive perspective is congruent with the hypothesized role of threat appraisal, illness representations, and goals. Explicit incorporation of self-regulatory plans defines self-regulation itself as a personality process; that is, as a single set of tendencies and capabilities that operate in both health-related and non-health-related situations and contexts.

Social-cognitive theory has led to the identification of a form of statistical structure that differs from the temporal, cross-situational, and hierarchical patterns traditionally associated with personality dispositions. Rather than characteristically responding in the same manner across diverse settings and contexts, Mischel and Shoda (1999) argue that individuals display *consistent patterns of behavioral variability* across situations in the form of '*if-then*' profiles. For example, in data gathered at a summer camp, a child might consistently show high, intermediate, or low levels of verbal aggressiveness depending upon whether he or she was with a peer or an adult, and depending upon the behavior of that other person; that is, whether the peer merely approached or also teased the child, or whether the adult warned, praised, or punished the child. These patterns were stable over time and across instances of the same psychological situation (e.g., teasing peer, punishing adult). Moreover, the *if-then* profiles distinguished between children who showed the same overall level of verbal aggressiveness. Thus, in a traditional trait approach in which behavior might have been averaged across situations, the *if-then* patterns would have been treated as error variance.

In the sections that follow, we describe a set of circumscribed individual difference constructs and discuss them in relation to health-related self-regulation. Several are drawn explicitly from Mischel and Shoda's (1999) analysis. Others derive from different theoretical traditions, but are highly compatible with social-cognitive theory. We group these factors into categories relating to encoding and construal, expectancies, goals, competencies and intelligences, and response tendencies.

Encoding and construal

Aspects of construal and encoding that have been examined in social-cognitive research on personality include: selectivity of attention; categorization; assignment of personal meaning and self-relevance to situations and events; framing possible outcomes as positive states to be approached or negative ones to be avoided; and interpreting events and conditions as goal-congruent, goal-incongruent, or goal-neutral (Mischel and Shoda, 1999).

Attention to threat

A number of encoding and construal constructs describe individual differences in orientation toward threat. These dispositions can be seen as coming into play primarily at the stages of cognitive appraisal and the formation of mental representations of stressors. However, appraisal and coping are difficult to separate: perceptions of threat appraisal are subject to updating and reframing based in part on information generated by coping activity, and information gathering is itself a form of coping (Lazarus and Folkman, 1984). As a consequence, these dispositions have at times been characterized as coping styles.

One example is a threat-avoidant, 'repressive' coping style. Much work examining correlates of repressive coping has focused on emotional response patterning. Repressive copers have shown a pattern of verbal-autonomic dissociation in response to laboratory stressors in which their cardiovascular or electrodermal responses are high relative to their self-reports of negative affect (e.g., Newton and Contrada, 1992). Highly anxious subjects have also shown a contrasting pattern, with greater reactivity in the verbal response channel than in physiologic measures.

Krohne (1996) describes another construct that contrasts approach and avoidance stances toward psychological threat. Here, 'vigilance' refers to the intensity with which the individual attends to and processes threat-related information, and is conceptualized as reflecting an intolerance of uncertainty. 'Avoidance' refers to the degree to which the individual turns away from such information, and is conceptualized as reflecting intolerance of emotional arousal. Research examining vigilance and avoidance as conceptualized in this model has provided support in the form of associations with information-seeking and emotional responses to stressors (Krohne, 1996).

Yet another individual-difference factor involving a cognitive-attentional style that is activated by psychological threats is referred to as monitoring–blunting. Monitoring, a tendency to seek and to attend to threat-relevant information, forms a bipolar contrast with blunting, characterized by avoidance of such information. Monitoring amplifies threat, resulting in stronger emotional and physiological responses, whereas blunting attenuates threat and its emotional and physiological impact. Empirical research has generated results consistent with the model (e.g., Schwartz *et al.*, 1995).

Self-relevance

A second general way to conceptualize personality influences on construal or encoding involves processes through which situations are categorized or assigned meaning and significance. A variety of constructs have been examined in relation to such processes. Some involve the construal of situations in relation to self, such that the perception of an external event threatens, confirms, or otherwise interacts with a self-referent knowledge structure.

Although not explicitly conceptualized in terms of self-referent constructs, the pessimistic explanatory style might be placed into this category. A pessimistic explanatory style involves the attribution of negative events to causes that are internal ('It was something about me'), stable ('It will always be with me'), and global ('It will undermine everything I try to do') (Peterson, 2000). Thus, it transforms an external occurrence in a way that reinforces a view of the self as ineffective or otherwise doomed to a future rife with negative events. A pessimistic explanatory style has been linked both to health-damaging behaviors and to pathophysiologic processes that may account for its association with negative health outcomes (Peterson, 2000).

Self-guides, or evaluative selves, are cognitive-affective structures that operate as standards for the evaluation of the (phenomenal) actual self, and can therefore be seen as internal referents of the sort emphasized in cybernetic self-regulation models. Higgins (1987) posited that two self-guides generate different negative affective states when involved in the appraisal of self-discrepancies. The 'ought' self comprises attributes we feel we should possess, whereas the 'ideal' self is characterized by attributes that we would ideally like to possess. According to this model, situations that lead to a perceived discrepancy between actual and ought selves generate negative affect accompanied by activation, such as guilt and anxiety, whereas actual-ideal self-discrepancy generates de-activating affective states such as sadness and disappointment. Thus, the emotional impact of performing health-damaging behavior, experiencing a physical symptom, or receiving an illness diagnosis may differ depending on whether it is construed as creating an ought-self or an actual-self discrepancy.

Expectancies

Expectancy constructs play a major role in social-cognitive theory. Anticipated consequences of behavior, or outcome expectancies, were an important determinant of learning and performance in the earlier, social learning models from which social-cognitive theory evolved.

Control-related expectancies

Control may be defined abstractly in terms of contingencies between responses and outcomes. In social learning theory, and in the literature concerned with psychological stress, control, and human health, the focus has most often been on subjective response-outcome contingencies, or *perceived* control. Individual differences in perceptual, emotional, and behavioral responses to uncontrollable stressors and, in particular, research on learned helplessness (Seligman, 1975), stimulated interest in several personality constructs involving control-related expectancies.

These dispositions can be seen as being particularly relevant during secondary appraisal, as the individual considers available coping resources and options. However, as with other components of the stress process, primary and secondary appraisal are not entirely separable. Information about what is at stake in a stressful encounter, and about what can be done to cope, may be processed in parallel, or in rapid alternation, with each influencing the other and the ensuing coping process (Lazarus and Folkman, 1984). As a consequence, control-related personality dispositions may play a role in primary appraisal, secondary appraisal, and coping activity.

Rotter (1966) defined locus of control as a person's generalized expectancy regarding the causes of important outcomes, where internal causes involve actions or attributes of the person, and external causes involve factors outside the person such as the actions of others, or random factors such as chance or luck. The instrument developed by Rotter measures internal versus external locus of control as a single, bipolar dimension across a variety of life domains. However, there is now evidence of several separable dimensions, including internal locus of control, and two external dimensions, one involving powerful others and the other emphasizing chance or luck (Levenson, 1974). Internal locus of control may be associated with a general tendency to engage in problem-focused coping (e.g., Compas *et al.*, 1991). Research on the relationship between locus of control and health-related behaviors has come to be dominated by measures developed specifically with reference to the physical health domain. This work has yielded findings indicating generally positive associations between internal health locus of control and numerous health-promoting behaviors (Wallston, 2001).

Self-efficacy refers to a person's confidence that he or she can perform a particular behavior leading to a desired outcome in a particular situation (Bandura, 1999). Self-efficacy appears to influence a wide variety of phenomena, including selection of goals and activities, effort, persistence, emotional responses, and coping effectiveness (Bandura, 1999). Accordingly, self-efficacy has come to be represented in most models designed to predict and explain health-related behavior (e.g., Brownlee *et al.*, 2000) and has been incorporated into theory concerning the processes of appraising and responding to stressors (Lazarus and Folkman, 1984). Although conceived by Bandura as highly specific with regard to behavior and situation, others have examined dispositional versions of this construct that refer to the more generalized expectation that one's actions can (or cannot) bring about favorable outcomes across a variety of situations. For example, Jerusalem and Schwarzer (1992) describe a generalized perceived self-efficacy scale designed to measure a broad and stable sense of personal competence to deal efficiently with stressors. At a more intermediate level of generality are self-efficacy constructs defined with regard to a particular, health-related content domain, such as maintaining a healthy diet (Schwarzer and Renner, 2000).

Global expectancies

Several personality dispositions describe individual differences in global expectancies regarding future outcomes that are generally concerned with the valence of expectancies; that is, with the tendency to expect favorable versus unfavorable outcomes. In many cases, these constructs are defined and measured without reference to the person's role in controlling outcomes. The most extensively studied is dispositional optimism, which refers to a bipolar dimension that distinguishes individuals who generally expect positive outcomes in life from those who generally expect negative outcomes (Carver and Scheier, 1999). Dispositional optimism has been associated primarily with behavioral pathways to positive physical health outcomes, although there is also some evidence that optimists are less likely than pessimists to show strong physiological responses to stressors (for a review see Carver and Scheier, 1999). It is hypothesized that optimism fosters active engagement in goal pursuit. Supporting this view is empirical work indicating that dispositional optimism is positively associated with the use of coping responses that involve planning and taking direct action, and inversely associated with denial and avoidance.

Goals

In the social-cognitive view, much human activity is self-regulative, in that it involves the selection of goals and exercise of control over thought, motivation, affect, and action in the pursuit of goals, processes that may be characterized in terms of three phases: forethought, performance or volitional control, and self-reflection (Bandura, 1999). The parallels between this analysis and the cybernetic and illness cognition approaches to health-related self-regulation are unmistakable. They are also unsurprising given the common meta-theoretical assumptions, methodological approaches, and levels of analysis shared by these perspectives.

Goal cognition in hypochondriasis

Somatoform disorders such as hypochondriasis and somatization pose health behavior problems because they involve somatic symptoms of unknown origin that can result in overuse of health care. Hypochondriasis involves excessive worry about physical health, whereas in somatization there are actual symptoms without organic explanation. Although these syndromes are often assessed as trait-like dispositions, Karoly and Lecci (1993) offered an alternative conceptualization in terms of goal cognition. It was hypothesized that hypochondriacs would be distinguished by the number and importance of health-related goals currently being pursued. It also was expected that hypochondriacal subjects would report a pattern of stressful involvement with health-related goals. These predictions were borne out in comparisons of female college undergraduates with high and low scores on a measure of hypochondriasis. In addition, whereas the non-health-related pursuits of hypochondriacal women were not characterized with the same level of anxiety as those that were health-related, they were experienced as lacking in reward. Over-investment in health-related concerns may have undermined investment in other life pursuits, resulting in diminished progress and satisfaction.

Approach and avoidance goal-striving

Individual differences in goal-related activity have been conceptualized in terms of an approach–avoidance distinction. Approach goals refer to states or directions for change that are positive or desired, whereas avoidance goals refer to negative or undesired states or directions for change. Elliot and Sheldon (1998) assessed approach and avoidant goal-striving idiographically by asking college undergraduates to list goals they would be pursuing during the next month and then having independent judges classify them as either approach (e.g., 'To be more organized') or avoidant ('Avoid being lonely') in focus. Pursuit of avoidant goals was associated with increases in physical symptoms, controlling statistically for neuroticism, and this relationship appeared to be mediated by lower levels of perceived competence and self-determination among subjects with higher avoidance goal-pursuit scores.

Assimilative and accommodative coping

In cybernetic views of self-regulation, perception of a significant discrepancy between behavioral states and internal standards gives rise to corrective action. Brandtstäedter and Renner (1990) have conceptualized two forms of discrepancy-reducing responses as alternative coping modes. Assimilative responses involve efforts to alter conditions so as to increase conformance with goals, whereas accommodative responses involve adjusting goals to conform to conditions. In an investigation of adaptation to age-related life transitions, high scores on both 'tenacious goal pursuit' (assimilation) and 'flexible goal adjustment' (accommodation) were associated with greater life satisfaction and lower depression. Cross-sectional analysis suggested an age-related shift from assimilative to accommodative coping modes.

Self-presentation goals and risky behavior

Most models of health-related behavior focus on perceptions, beliefs, and other cognitive factors related directly to health threats or to actions that might be taken to reduce threat. Leary *et al.* (1994) reviewed wide-ranging evidence concerning the possible role of a non-health-related motive referred to as self-presentation. Self-presentation involves processes whereby individuals manage the impressions they make on others. Leary *et al.* argued that, in the interest of making a positive impression, thereby avoiding negative outcomes such as embarrassment and disturbed interpersonal relationships, a person might expose him or herself to numerous health hazards. Examples they discussed include failure to take precautions during sexual intercourse (because purchasing or using condoms may result in embarrassment), over-exposure to ultraviolet radiation (to acquire an attractive tan), unnecessary dieting, use of dangerous means of appetite suppression, and purging (to satisfy unrealistic standards for body image), and use of alcohol, tobacco, and drugs (to project an attractive social image).

Competencies and intelligences

Definitions of intelligence vary. Some focus on problem-solving ability, others on the ability to acquire new knowledge to deal with novel adaptive requirements. Most incorporate capacities that seem likely to facilitate self-regulation, whether they emphasize hierarchically inter-related abilities (Carroll, 1993), autonomous information-processing modules (Gardner, 1983), or a context-specific ability to adapt to and shape environments (Sternberg, 1997). Consider, for example, that, in his triarchic model, Sternberg (1997: 103) defines intelligence, in part, in terms of

> the core mental processes that may be key in any culture or other environmental context [that include] (a) recognizing the existence of the problem, (b) defining the nature of the problem, (c) constructing a strategy to solve the problem, (d) mentally representing information about the problem, (e) allocating mental resources in solving the problem, (f) monitoring one's solution to the problem, and (g) evaluating one's solution to the problem.

The similarity to models of health-related self-regulation is clear.

Social-cognitive approaches to personality embrace social intelligence, forms of self-control, and various forms of competence and skill as highly relevant to health-related self-regulation. Other intelligences and competencies, while not originating within social-cognitive personality research, are highly compatible with such a framework. These include emotional intelligence and higher-level intellectual abilities. In addition, there may be forms of somatic intelligence with important implications for processes of self-regulation involving the detection and interpretation of bodily sensations.

Social intelligence

One outgrowth of the social-cognitive perspective is a view of personality *as* social intelligence that emphasizes knowledge structures and cognitive skills used in everyday living to construe and discriminate among situations, formulate goals, and seek goal attainment (Kihlstrom and Cantor, 2000). Work on a variety of health-related behaviors has been guided by concepts of social competence or skill. Research on behavioral problems in children emphasizes interpersonal problem-solving skills, assertiveness, and the ability to form friendships with other children (Masten and Coatsworth, 1998). Resistance skill – the ability to refuse offers of cigarettes, alcohol, and drugs from others – has also been examined (e.g., Donaldson *et al.*, 1995). Interpersonal skills have also been studied in relation to effective communication and negotiation in safe sexual practices in the prevention of HIV/AIDS (e.g., Carey *et al.*, 2000). The communication skills of medical providers and their patients, an important element of the patient–provider relationship, have been linked to health and quality of life outcomes (Roter, 2000). Interventions have been designed to foster coping skills with interpersonal elements, such as the ability to share illness-related experiences, that allow patients to adapt to a variety of chronic medical conditions (Schneiderman *et al.*, 2001). The enhancement of interactions with social network members is one approach that has been taken in efforts to understand and promote a patient's ability to carry out medical regimens (Dunbar-Jacob and Schlenk, 2001).

With regard to stress-focused research, interpersonal skills have been implicated in the frequency with which individuals are exposed to stressors. For example, aggressive children appear to generate interpersonal conflict through negatively biased interpretations of other children's behavior (Crick and Dodge, 1994), and similar processes may operate in adults with high levels of trait hostility (Smith, 1992). Social skills are also involved in the formation of personal relationships (e.g., Masten and Coatsworth, 1998), which, in turn, may prevent or buffer the effects of stressors. Other research has demonstrated an inverse association between social competence and exposure to psychosocial stressors (e.g., Segrin, 2001). Following exposure to stressors, interpersonal skills may serve to facilitate coping and adaptation. For example, social resourcefulness has been found to predict social support and emotional well-being in caregivers of family members with dementia (Rapp *et al.*, 1998). Thus, the ability to interact effectively with others may enter into health-related stress processes at several junctures, with a high level of social intelligence contributing to the avoidance of interpersonal stress, formation of supportive relationships, and the ability to call upon others for help with stressors when they occur.

Emotional intelligence

[Emotional intelligence is the] ability to recognize the meanings of emotions and their relationships, and to reason and problem-solve on the basis of them ... [it] is involved in the capacity to perceive emotions, assimilate emotion-related feelings, understand the information of those emotions, and manage them.

(Mayer, Caruso, and Salovey, 1999: 267)

The potential relevance of emotional intelligence to health-related processes of self-regulation derives from two major considerations. First, given the importance of affect in interpersonal interactions, emotional intelligence may account for the health-promoting effects of social intelligence. Second, the importance of affect in appraisal and coping processes suggests that the capacity to deal intelligently with one's emotions may be integral to the relationship between stress and health. Literature on emotional intelligence has addressed issues of measurement, theoretical links between emotional abilities and (non-ability) emotion-related personality characteristics, and interventions. There is evidence that the perceived inability to regulate one's feelings may interact with stress to predict the need for health care visits, and that clarity in discriminating one's feelings may be associated with a tendency to ruminate less following a stressful event (Salovey *et al.*, 1999). In addition, there is support for the suggestion that emotional intelligence is a key ingredient in the formation and use of stress-buffering social connections (Salovey *et al.*, 1999).

Somatic and visceral intelligence

Physiologic processes involved in emotion, stress, and disease are associated with sensations whose accurate detection and appropriate interpretation may be crucial to practicing effective self-regulation. However, research on illness cognition has not generally been framed in terms of intelligence or ability constructs, and visceral perception has not been a major focus of theory and research on intelligence. Perceptual processes that have been examined under the rubric of intelligence have primarily involved the exteroceptive, visual, and auditory systems (e.g., Carroll, 1993), and consideration of bodily intelligence has focused on voluntary action and movement (e.g., Gardner, 1983). However, there is evidence of reliable individual differences in interoceptive ability, most involving the perception of cardiovascular processes (Wiens *et al.*, 2000). Moreover, individual differences in heartbeat detection have been associated with the intensity of emotional experience (Wiens *et al.*, 2000). There is also evidence of reliable individual differences in the ability to control autonomic processes through biofeedback training (Schwartz, 1977).

Response tendencies

Constructs discussed thus far have implications for predicting and understanding responses that represent outward manifestations of self-regulatory activity. However, although encoding strategies, expectancies, goal-related processes, and competencies may initiate and guide these responses, they can be distinguished from constructs that describe specific response tendencies. The latter may represent characteristic solutions to adaptive problems. They may also provide a readout of the state of the self-regulatory system.

Emotional response tendencies

Many individual difference constructs describe tendencies to experience emotional responses to stressors. In most cases, these have a substantial overlap with facets of the broader, neuroticism dimension of the FFM. These include trait anger, trait anxiety, and depressive symptoms (Mook *et al.*, 1990). In addition, there are stable individual differences in physiologic reactivity to stressors, which are often conceptualized in relation to emotion, but actually represent a response channel that is somewhat independent of affective systems (Brownley *et al.*, 2000). At present, little is known about the bases of reactivity. They may be located at one or more points beginning with higher-level cognitive processing centers that mediate perception and awareness of stressors, through to mid-level systems involved in automatic appraisal processes, and to yet lower-level circuits that control autonomic outflow and neuroendocrine activity. Sources of individual differences in physiologic reactivity have also been sought peripherally at the level of adrenergic receptor attributes such as density and sensitivity.

Coping styles

A rather sizeable literature surrounds the notion that individuals show characteristic coping styles; that is, temporally stable tendencies to enact certain coping responses across a broad range of stressors (Hewitt and Flett, 1996; Krohne, 1996). Coping constructs have been organized in terms of various conceptual schemes associated with particular measurement tools (Schwarzer and Schwarzer, 1996). These describe up to a dozen or more forms of coping with abstract labels (e.g., distancing, positive reappraisal, restraint) that are potentially descriptive of a wide range of specific behaviors. They cluster together empirically to form broader dimensions, such as problem-focused coping, emotion-focused coping, and approach–avoidance. Recently, comparisons of traditional retrospective measures with coping style assessments obtained in a more 'real-time' manner ('ecological momentary assessments') have raised questions about the meaning of the older generation of instruments (e.g., Schwartz *et al.*, 1999).

Comments: systematizing and operationalizing structure and process

The social-cognitive approach offers a useful framework for understanding the role of personality in health-related self-regulation. However, the signposts that it provides point in a desired direction; they do not signal arrival at a destination. Its advantages over a dispositional approach generally represent matters of degree, not differences in kind, and speak more of potential than of documented progress. Moreover, these advantages, however great, are purchased at costs in terms of parsimony and coherence. Although not without its limitations, there is something appealing about the structural simplicity of the FFM, and something solid about the convergence of supporting evidence. The proliferation of constructs pertaining to goals, selves, and other middle-level personality structures must be systematized and located within the larger sphere of personality. It remains to be seen where such efforts will lead and how they may be articulated with theory regarding psychosocial stressors, health hazards, and the management of illness and disease.

Progress here will require an assessment paradigm that is faithful to the constructs in question. Ouellette and DiPlacido (2001) noted, to their chagrin, that measures of constructs they judged to be more promising than simple traits (by virtue of context-sensitivity and process focus) make use of the very same statement-endorsement format that is employed to assess dispositions such as FFM traits. Cervone *et al.* (2001), calling attention to the general lack of broad statements regarding the implications of social-cognitive theory for personality assessment, specified a set of measurement principles derived explicitly from social-cognitive theory. Among these are recommendations to distinguish explicitly between internal personality structures and observable behavior patterns, to maintain sensitivity to the unique manifestations of personality in individuals, and to assess persons in context. Other strategies that may facilitate departure from traditional trait assessment methodology include the use of experimental priming paradigms (e.g., Higgins, 1987), implicit measurement techniques (Greenwald *et al.*, 2002), and objective assessment of intelligence (Mayer *et al.*, 1999).

For process approaches to live up to their name, greater systematization and improved measurement of social-cognitive units must be combined with new methods for modeling process. Too often the process aspect of a construct begins and ends with connotations supplied by a well-crafted label, and the work itself involves little more than correlating a conventional, self-report personality measure with health outcomes. Here, technical advances in the form of palm-held, digital recording units that permit data acquisition on what begins to approximate a real-time basis may prove useful. Kovatchev *et al.* (1998) used such methodology to acquire data on symptoms, cognitive-motor performance, subjective estimates of blood glucose, and self-regulation of glucose levels in patients with insulin-dependent diabetes. This paradigm could readily incorporate personality constructs such as approach–avoidance threat orientation or generalized self-efficacy. Developments in statistical modeling also may stimulate more process-focused research. Kovatchev *et al.* used a stochastic transitional probability model to represent self-regulation as a series of symptom-based decisions. Affleck *et al.* (1998) used a similar data-gathering strategy to examine interrelationships between personal goals and quality of life in women with fibromyalgia. In this case, a multi-level random-effects regression model permitted identification of prospective, within-subject associations linking progress toward health- and non-health-related goals to changes in symptoms and emotions.

Summary and conclusions

We conclude with a set of specific suggestions for further theoretical and empirical examination of personality in relation to self-regulatory processes whereby the individual adapts to psychosocial stressors, hazardous exposures, and illness threats. It is our view that personality theory and models of health-related self-regulation largely seek to represent the same human tendencies and capabilities. We believe that greater recognition of this state of affairs would facilitate progress in, and integration of, both fields of inquiry.

1   Cognitive, affective, behavioral, and biological aspects of self-regulation are empirically associated with personality. Available data do not permit firm statements about the magnitude or patterning of these associations, or about the generating causal mechanisms. But the clear implication is that processes governing responses to psychosocial stressors, hazardous exposures, and illness threats may reflect enduring attributes of the person. It is inadvisable to assume that these responses are stimulus-bound or reflect processes with no psychological implications outside a particular self-regulatory episode.

2   Relatively broad personality dispositions, such as Five Factor traits, will likely share only limited variance with single instances of health-related self-regulatory activity such as the appraisal of a particular threat or the use of a specific coping response. These traits may serve more usefully to predict patterns of interrelated activities aggregated across time or contexts. Predictive utility will be facilitated if temporal or cross-situational sampling of the relevant self-regulatory activity is conceptually coherent and takes into account other factors, including situational influences on self-regulation.

3   Predictive work must be followed by causal analysis to specify mechanisms that generate observed associations, including work that identifies cognitive-affective and neurobiological structures that underlie personality dispositions and their interactions with environmental demands, constraints, and resources.

4   Broad dispositions may not be ideally suited to the tasks of documenting associations between personality and health-related self-regulation and of elucidating causal process. In their discussion of social-cognitive approaches to personality assessment, Cervone *et al.*

(2001) describe a 'bottom-up' strategy in which contextualized personality units serve as a starting point for the discovery of more global patterns of personality coherence. Situated, process-focused constructs, conceptualized without making assumptions about their relationship to broader dispositions, can be examined across time and context to identify global forms of temporal and cross-situational consistency. These averaged tendencies may, or may not, correspond to broad personality constructs associated with the more conventional, 'top-down' methods for linking disposition and process.

5   In addition to 'top-down' and 'bottom-up' methods for linking broad disposition dimensions to situated, self-regulatory process, strategies that focus on middle-level personality units may also prove useful. These have merits stemming from close connection to variation in context (both situational and lifespan-related), emphasis on process and change, personal relevance (particularly when measured idiographically), motivational content, focus on functional aspects of personality, and connections to psychological activity that invests everyday life with meaning and purpose.

6   Goal-related constructs have yet to be fully exploited in the study of personality, self-regulation, and health. Regularities in the ways individuals construct, frame, and pursue goals may account for patterns of consistency across self-regulatory activities related to the pursuit of health- and non-health-related goals. Moreover, differences in health- and non-health-related forms of self-regulatory activity may constitute meaningful patterns of cross-situational variability, as in Mischel and Shoda's (1999) notion of *if-then* profiles. Table 4.1 presents a summary of ways in which goal-related processes may be involved in the interplay between personality and health-related self-regulation.

7   Models of intelligence share much with self-regulation models. They may therefore offer a valuable perspective on how, and how well, people respond to the sorts of adaptive challenges that lead to or reflect problems of physical health. For example, it is of interest to ask whether various forms of health-related self-regulation reflect a common set of abilities or involve different combinations of intelligences for dealing with social, emotional, and somatic information, and for solving abstract, higher-level problems involving such information.

8   It may be profitable to examine the cognitive, goal-directed processes of self-regulation in relation to neurobiological models of personality that emphasize motivational systems underlying goal-related behavior (e.g., Depue and Collins, 1999). This work may be particularly useful for understanding personality influences on risky behaviors such as substance use (Wills *et al.*, 1998) and unsafe sexual practices (Kalichman *et al.*, 1998).

9   The study of health-related psychological and behavioral processes should consider links to other biological factors as well. Examples include evidence in patients with functional dyspepsia of an association between

Table 4.1 Goal constructs linking personality and health-related self-regulation

Goal construct	Implication for personality and self-regulation
Goals and threat appraisal	Stress arises when important goals are challenged
Goals and coping	Threat appraisal generates goals that organize and guide coping activity, including some that represent desired and undesired states reflecting personality motives
Goals, coping appraisal, and coping style	Stable coping patterns that characterize an individual may reflect veridical or non-veridical beliefs regarding the effectiveness of previous coping responses in achieving stress-related goals in particular situations
Approach versus avoidant goal-striving	Orientations toward goal cognition such as these may extend across both health- and non-health-related domains
Accommodative versus assimilative coping	Discrepancy-reducing preferences such as these may extend across both health and non-health-related domains
Self-presentation	Pursuit of non-health-related goals such as this one may be health damaging
Goals and the statistical structure of behavior	Pursuit of qualitatively different goals (e.g., health- and non-health-related) may underlie within-person patterns of behavioral variability displayed across different situations (e.g., health-related and non-health-related)

neuroticism and cortical events produced by stimulation of the esophagus (Kanazawa *et al.*, 2001), identification of the neural circuits activated during conscious inhibition of emotion (Beauregard *et al.*, 2001), and research on genetic polymorphisms implicating dopaminergic brain reward centers in cigarette smoking and suggesting that genetic factors involved in dopamine transmission may underlie smoking patterns through which depressed smokers regulate negative affect (Lerman *et al.*, 1999).

10 Notwithstanding the substantial heritability and cross-cultural replicability of Five Factor traits (Costa and McCrae, 1992), personality is substantially 'defined, constituted, and enlivened by culture' (Cross and Markus, 1999: 392). Disease patterns, health behaviors, and stress vary geographically and as a function of socio-economic status and ethnicity,

and minority group members confront discrimination and other psycho-social stressors not usually relevant to members of the dominant majority (Contrada *et al.*, 2000). Cultures vary widely in beliefs and practices related to health, disease, and health care, in moral, religious, and spiritual dimensions, and in personal agency and interpersonal interdependence. Accordingly, there is ample reason to expect that macro-social forces qualify, color, and shape processes whereby person-ality interacts with health-related self-regulation.

Final comment

Pervin (1999) described the need for an organismic model of personality as distinguished from individual difference and social-cognitive process models discussed in this chapter. Its goal would be to show how the 'parts' of personality come together and interact within the 'whole,' single, functioning person. Problems of self-regulation as conceived by health psychologists provide an arena that is highly suitable for developing this perspective. The multiple interacting systems in which psychosocial stressors, hazardous exposures, and illness episodes are embedded provide a testing ground within which to explore self-regulation at the level of the whole person, constituted biologically, psychologically, and socioculturally. The adaptive tasks of identifying, preventing, and managing health problems throughout the life-course serve as an opportunity for modeling the person in a manner that is organismic in terms of requiring the derivation of principles to describe the organization (or disorganization) of multiple spheres of activity that make up a whole, living person. It is difficult to imagine a domain likely to be more revealing of the personality system than the human activity that surrounds the challenges of avoiding illness and disease and maintaining life.

Note

1   Preparation of this chapter was supported in part by a grant from the National Institute on Aging (AG16750). Correspondence should be addressed to Richard J. Contrada, Department of Psychology, Rutgers University, 53 Avenue E, Piscataway, NJ 08854-8040. E-mail: contrada@rci.rutgers.edu

References

Affleck, G., Tennen, H., Urrows, S., Higgins, P., Abeles, M., Hall, C., Karoly, P. and Newton, C. (1998) 'Fibromyalgia and women's pursuit of personal goals: a daily process analysis,' *Health Psychology* **17**: 40–47.
Amirkhan, J.H., Risinger, R.T. and Swickert, R J. (1995) 'Extraversion: a "hidden" personality factor in coping?' *Journal of Personality* **63**:189–212.
Bandura, A. (1999) 'Social cognitive theory of personality,' in L.A. Pervin and O.P. John (eds) *Handbook of Personality: Theory and Research*, 2nd edn, New York: Guilford, pp. 154–196.

Baumeister, R.F. (1998) 'The self,' in D.T. Gilbert, S.T. Fiske and G. Lindzey (eds) *The Handbook of Social Psychology*, vol. 2, 4th edn, Boston, MA: McGraw-Hill, pp. 680–740.

Beauregard, M., Lévesque, J. and Bourgouin, P. (2001) 'Neural correlates of conscious self-regulation of emotion,' *Journal of Neuroscience* **21**: 6993–7000.

Bolger, N. and Zuckerman, A. (1995) 'A framework for studying personality in the stress process,' *Journal of Personality and Social Psychology* **69**: 890–902.

Booth-Kewley, S. and Vickers, R.R. (1994) 'Associations between major domains of personality and health behavior,' *Journal of Personality* **62**: 281–298.

Brandtstäedter, J. and Renner, G. (1990) 'Tenacious goal pursuit and flexible goal adjustment: explication and age-related analysis of assimilative and accommodative strategies of coping,' *Psychology and Aging* **5**: 58–67.

Brownlee, S., Leventhal, H. and Leventhal, E.A. (2000) 'Regulation, self-regulation and construction of the self in the maintenance of physical health,' in M. Boekaerts, P.R. Pintrich and M. Zeidner (eds) *Handbook of Self-Regulation*, San Diego, CA: Academic Press, pp. 369–416.

Brownley, K.A, Hurwitz, B.E and Schneiderman, N. (2000) 'Cardiovascular psychophysiology,' in J.T. Cacioppo, L.G. Tassinary and G. Berntson (eds) *Handbook of Psychophysiology*, 2nd edn, New York: Cambridge University Press, pp. 224–264.

Cantor, N. and Kihlstrom, J. F. (1985) 'Social intelligence: the cognitive basis of personality,' in P. Shaver (ed.) *Review of Personality and Social Psychology*, vol. 6, Beverly Hills, CA: Sage, pp. 15–33.

Cantor, N. and Zirkel, S. (1990) 'Personality, cognition and purposive behavior,' in L.A. Pervin (ed.) *Handbook of Personality Theory and Research*, New York: Guilford, pp. 135–164.

Carey, M.P., Braaten, L.S., Maisto, S.A., Gleason, J.R., Forsyth, A.D., Durant, L.E. and Jaworski, B.C. (2000) 'Using information, motivational enhancement and skills training to reduce the risk of HIV infection for low-income urban women: a second randomized clinical trial,' *Health Psychology* **19**: 3–11.

Carroll, J.B. (1993) *Human Cognitive Abilities: A Survey of Factor-Analytic Studies*, New York: Cambridge University Press.

Carver, C.S. and Scheier, M.F. (1999) 'Stress, coping and self-regulatory processes,' in L.A. Pervin and O.P. John (eds) *Handbook of Personality: Theory and Research*, 2nd edn, New York: Guilford, pp. 553–575.

Cervone, D., Shadel, W.G. and Jencius, S. (2001) 'Social-cognitive theory of personality assessment,' *Personality and Social Psychology Review* **5**: 33–51.

Compas, B.E., Banez, G.A., Malcarne, V. and Worsham, N. (1991) 'Perceived control and coping with stress: a developmental perspective,' *Journal of Social Issues* **47**: 23–34.

Contrada, R.J. and Guyll, M. (2001) 'On who gets sick and why: the role of personality, stress and disease,' in A. Baum, T.A. Revenson and J.E. Singer (eds) *Handbook of Health Psychology*, Hillsdale, NJ: Lawrence Erlbaum Associates, pp. 59–81.

Contrada, R.J., Cather, C. and O'Leary, A. (1999) 'Personality and health: dispositions and processes in disease susceptibility and adaptation to illness,' in L.A. Pervin and O.P. John (eds) *Handbook of Personality: Theory and Research*, 2nd edn, New York: Guilford, pp. 576–604.

Contrada, R.J., Ashmore, R.D., Gary, M.L., Coups, E., Egeth, J.D., Sewell, A., Ewell, K., Goyal, T. and Chasse, V. (2000) 'Ethnicity-related sources of stress and their effects on well-being,' *Current Directions in Psychological Science* **9**: 136–139.

Cooper, M.L., Agocha, V.B. and Sheldon, M.S. (2000) 'A motivational perspective on risky behaviors: the role of personality and affect regulatory processes,' *Journal of Personality* **68**: 1059–1088.

Costa, P.T. and McCrae, R.R. (1992) 'Four ways five factors are basic,' *Personality and Individual Differences* **13**: 653–665.

Costa, P.T., Somerfield, M.R. and McCrae, R.R. (1996) 'Personality and coping: a reconceptualization,' in M. Zeidner and N.S. Endler (eds) *Handbook of Coping: Theory, Research, Applications*, New York: Wiley, pp. 44–61.

Crick, N.R. and Dodge, K.A. (1994) 'A review and reformulation of social information-processing mechanisms in children's social adjustment,' *Psychological Bulletin* **115**: 74–101.

Cross, S.E. and Markus, H.R. (1999) 'The cultural constitution of personality,' in L.A. Pervin and O.P. John (eds) *Handbook of Personality: Theory and Research*, 2nd edn, New York: Guilford, pp. 378–396.

Depue, R.A. and Collins, P.F. (1999) 'Neurobiology of the structure of personality: dopamine facilitation of incentive motivation and extraversion,' *Behavioral and Brain Sciences* **22**: 491–569.

Donaldson, S.I., Graham, J.W., Piccinin, A.M. and Hansen, W.B. (1995) 'Resistance-skills training and onset of alcohol use: evidence for beneficial and potentially harmful effects in public schools and in private Catholic schools,' *Health Psychology* **14**: 291–300.

Dunbar-Jacob, J. and Schlenk, E. (2001) 'Patient adherence to treatment regimen,' in A. Baum, T.A. Revenson and J.E. Singer (eds) *Handbook of Health Psychology*, Hillsdale, NJ: Lawrence Erlbaum Associates, pp. 571–580.

Elliot, A.J. and Sheldon, K.M. (1998) 'Avoidance, personal goals and the personality-illness relationship,' *Journal of Personality and Social Psychology* **75**: 1282–1299.

Emmons, R.A. (1989) 'The personal striving approach to personality,' in L. A. Pervin (ed.) *Goal Concepts in Personality and Social Psychology*, Hillsdale, NJ: Lawrence Erlbaum Associates, pp. 87–126.

Gallagher, D.J. (1990) 'Extraversion, neuroticism and appraisal of stressful academic events,' *Personality and Individual Differences* **11**: 1053–1057.

Gardner, H. (1983) *Frames of Mind: The Theory of Multiple Intelligences*, New York: Basic Books.

Greenwald, A.G., Banaji, M.R., Rudman, L.A., Farnham, S.D., Nosek, B.A. and Mellott, D.S. (2002) 'A unified theory of implicit attitudes, stereotypes, self-esteem and self-concept,' *Psychological Review* **109**: 3–25.

Hewitt, P.L. and Flett, G.L. (1996) 'Personality traits and the coping process,' in M. Zeidner and N.S. Endler (eds) *Handbook of Coping: Theory, Research, Applications*, New York: Wiley, pp. 410–433.

Higgins, E.T. (1987) 'Self-discrepancy: a theory relating self and affect,' *Psychological Review* **94**: 319–340.

James, W. (1890) *Principles of Psychology*, New York: Holt.

Jemmott, J.B., Hellman, C., McClelland, D.C., Locke, S.E., Kraus, L., Williams, R.M. and Valeri, C.R. (1990) 'Motivational syndromes associated with natural killer cell activity,' *Journal of Behavioral Medicine* **13**: 53–73.

Jerusalem, M. and Schwarzer, R. (1992) 'Self-efficacy as a resource factor in stress appraisal processes,' in R. Schwarzer (ed.) *Self-Efficacy: Thought Control of Action*, Washington, DC: Hemisphere, pp. 195–213.

Kalichman, S.C., Tannenbaum, L. and Nachimson, D. (1998) 'Personality and cognitive factors influencing substance use and sexual risk for HIV infection among gay and bisexual men,' *Psychology of Addictive Behaviors* **12**: 262–271.

Kanazawa, M., Fukudo, S., Nomura, T. and Hongo, M. (2001) 'Electrophysiological correlates of personality influences in visceral perception,' *Journal of the American Medical Association* **286**: 1974–1975.

Karoly, P. and Lecci, L. (1993) 'Hypochondriasis and somatization in college women: a personal projects analysis,' *Health Psychology* **12**: 103–109.

Kihlstrom, J.F. and Cantor, N. (2000) 'Social intelligence,' in R.J. Sternberg (ed.) *Handbook of Intelligence*, New York: Cambridge University Press, pp. 359–379.

Kovatchev, B., Cox, D., Goder-Frederick, L., Schlundt, D. and Clarke, W. (1998) 'Stochastic model of self-regulation decision making exemplified by decisions concerning hypoglycemia,' *Health Psychology* **17**: 277–284

Krohne, H.W. (1996) 'Individual differences in coping,' in M. Zeidner and N.S. Endler (eds) *Handbook of Coping: Theory, Research, Applications*, New York: Wiley, pp. 381–409.

Lazarus, R.S. and Folkman, S. (1984) *Stress, appraisal and coping*, New York: Springer.

Leary, M.R., Tchividijian, L.R. and Kraxberger, B.E. (1994) 'Self-presentation can be hazardous to your health: impression management and health risk,' *Health Psychology* **13**: 461–470.

Lerman, C., Caporaso, N.E., Audrain, J., Main, D., Bowman, E.D., Lockshin, B., Boyd, N. R. and Shields, P.G. (1999) 'Evidence suggesting the role of specific genetic factors in cigarette smoking,' *Health Psychology* **18**: 14–20.

Levenson, H. (1974) 'Activism and powerful others: distinctions within the concept of internal-external control,' *Journal of Personality Assessment* **38**: 377–383.

Leventhal, H., Leventhal, E.A. and Contrada, R.J. (1998) 'Self-regulation, health and behavior: a perceptual-cognitive approach,' *Psychology and Health* **13**: 717–733.

Little, B. (1983) 'Personal projects: a rationale and methods for investigation,' *Environment and Behavior* **15**: 273–309.

Masten, A.S. and Coatsworth, J.D. (1998) 'The development of competence in favorable and unfavorable environments: lessons from research on successful children,' *American Psychologist* **53**: 205–220.

Mayer, J.D., Caruso, D. and Salovey, P. (1999) 'Emotional intelligence meets traditional standards for an intelligence,' *Intelligence* **27**: 267–298.

McCrae, R.R. and Costa, P.T. (1986) 'Personality, coping and coping effectiveness in an adult sample,' *Journal of Personality* **54**: 385–405.

Miller, G., Galanter, E. and Pribram, K. (1960) *Plans and the Structure of Behavior*, New York: Henry Holt & Co.

Mischel, W. and Shoda, Y. (1999) 'Integrating dispositions and processing dynamics within a unified theory of personality: the cognitive-affective personality system,' in L.A. Pervin and O.P. John (eds) *Handbook of Personality: Theory and Research*, 2nd edn, New York: Guilford, pp. 197–218.

Mook, J., Van der Ploeg, H.M. and Kleijn, W.C. (1990) 'Anxiety, anger and depression: relationships at the trait level,' *Anxiety Research* **3**: 17–31

Newton, T.L. and Contrada, R.J. (1992) Verbal-autonomic response dissociation in repressive coping: the influence of social context,' *Journal of Personality and Social Psychology* **62**: 159–167.

Ouellette, S.C. and DiPlacido, J. (2001) 'Personality's role in the protection and enhancement of health: where the research has been, where it is stuck, how might it move,' in A. Baum, T.A. Revenson and J.E. Singer (eds) *Handbook of Health Psychology*, Hillsdale, NJ: Lawrence Erlbaum Associates.

Pervin, L.A. (1999) 'Epilogue: constancy and change in personality theory and research,' in L.A. Pervin and O.P. John (eds) *Handbook of Personality: Theory and Research*, 2nd edn, New York: Guilford, pp. 689–704.

Peterson, C. (2000) 'The future of optimism,' *American Psychologist* **55**: 44–55.

Rapp, S.R., Shumaker, S., Schmidt, S., Naughton, M. and Anderson, R. (1998) 'Social resourcefulness: its relationship to social support and wellbeing among caregivers of dementia victims,' *Aging and Mental Health* **2**: 40–48.

Rim, Y. (1986) 'Ways of coping, personality, age, sex and family structural variables,' *Personality and Individual Differences* **7**: 113–116.

—— (1987) 'A comparative study of two taxonomies of coping styles, personality and sex,' *Personality and Individual Differences* **8**: 521–526.

Roter, D. (2000) 'The enduring and evolving nature of the patient–physician relationship,' *Patient Education and Counseling* **39**: 5–15.

Rotter, J.B. (1966) 'Generalized expectancies for internal versus external control of reinforcement,' *Psychological Monographs* **80**: 1, whole no. 609.

Salovey, P., Bedell, B.T., Detweiler, J.B. and Mayer, J.D. (1999) 'Coping intelligently: emotional intelligence and the coping process,' in C.R. Snyder (ed.) *Coping: The Psychology of What Works*, New York: Oxford University Press, pp. 141–164.

Schneiderman, N., Antoni, M.H., Saab, P.G. and Ironson, G. (2001) 'Health psychology: psychosocial and biobehavioral aspects of chronic disease management,' *Annual Review of Psychology* **52**: 555–580.

Schwartz, G.E. (1977) 'Psychosomatic disorders: psychosomatic disorders and biofeedback: a psychobiological model of disregulation,' in J.D. Maser and M.E.P. Seligman (eds) *Psychopathology: Experimental Models*, New York: W.H. Freeman, pp. 270–307.

Schwartz, J.E., Neale, J.M., Marco, C., Shiffman, S. and Stone, A.A. (1999) 'Does trait coping exist? A momentary assessment approach to the evaluation of traits,' *Journal of Personality and Social Psychology* **77**: 360–369.

Schwartz, M.D., Lerman, C., Miller, S.M., Daly, M. and Masny, A. (1995) 'Coping disposition, perceived risk and psychological distress among women at increased risk for ovarian cancer,' *Health Psychology* **14**: 232–235.

Schwarzer, R. and Renner, B. (2000) 'Social-cognitive predictors of health behavior: action self-efficacy and coping self-efficacy,' *Health Psychology* **19**: 487–495.

Schwarzer, R. and Schwarzer, C. (1996) 'A critical survey of coping instruments,' in M. Zeidner and N.S. Endler (eds) *Handbook of Coping: Theory, Research, Applications*, New York: Wiley, pp. 107–132.

Segrin, C. (2001) 'Social skills and negative life events: testing the deficit stress generation hypothesis,' *Current Psychology: Developmental, Learning, Personality, Social*, **20**: 19–35.

Seligman, M.E.P. (1975) *Helplessness: On Depression, Development and Death*, San Francisco: W.H. Freeman.

Smith, T.W. (1992) 'Hostility and health: current status of a psychosomatic hypothesis,' *Health Psychology* **11**: 139–150.

Sternberg, R.J. (1997) 'The concept of intelligence and its role in lifelong learning and success,' *American Psychologist* **52**: 1030–1037.

Taylor, S.E. and Aspinwall, L.G. (1996) 'Mediating and moderating processes in psychosocial stress: appraisal, coping, resistance and vulnerability,' in H.B. Kaplan (ed.) *Psychosocial Stress: Perspectives on Structure, Theory, Life-Course and Methods*, San Diego, CA: Academic Press, pp. 71–110.

Vickers, R.R., Kolar, D.W. and Hervig, L.K (1989) 'Personality correlates of coping with military basic training,' *U.S. Naval Health Research Center Report*, report no. 89-3, San Diego, CA: U.S. Naval Health Research Center.

Wallston, K.A. (2001) 'Conceptualization and operationalization of perceived control,' in A. Baum, T.A. Revenson and J.E. Singer (eds) *Handbook of Health Psychology*, Hillsdale, NJ: Lawrence Erlbaum Associates, pp. 49–58.

Watson, D. and Hubbard, B. (1996) 'Adaptational style and dispositional structure: coping in the context of the five-factor model,' *Journal of Personality* **64**: 737–774.

Watson, D. and Pennebaker, J.W. (1989) 'Health complaints, stress and distress: exploring the central role of negative affectivity,' *Psychological Review* **96**: 234–254.

Watson, D., David, J.P. and Suls, J. (1999) 'Personality, affectivity and coping,' in C.R. Snyder (ed.) *Coping: The Psychology of What Works*, New York: Oxford University Press, pp. 119–140.

Wiebe, D.J. (1991) 'Hardiness and stress moderation: a test of proposed mechanisms,' *Journal of Personality and Social Psychology* **60**: 89–99.

Wiebe, D.J. and Christensen, A.J. (1996) 'Patient adherence in chronic illness: personality and coping in context,' *Journal of Personality* **64**: 815–835.

Wiener, N. (1948) *Cybernetics; or, Control and Communication in the Animal and the Machine*, Cambridge, MA: Technology Press.

Wiens, S., Mezzacappa, E.S. and Katkin, E.S. (2000) 'Heartbeat detection and the experience of emotions,' *Cognition and Emotion* **14**: 417–427.

Wills, T.A., Windle, M. and Cleary, S.D. (1998) 'Temperament and novelty seeking in adolescent substance use: convergence of dimensions of temperament with constructs from Cloninger's theory,' *Journal of Personality and Social Psychology* **74**: 387–406.

Winter, D.G. and Barenbaum, N.B. (1999) 'History of modern personality theory and research,' in L.A. Pervin and O.P. John (eds) *Handbook of Personality: Theory and Research*, 2nd edn, New York: Guilford, pp. 3–27.

Part II

Representations of illnesses and health actions

5 Representations of chronic illnesses

*Adrian A. Kaptein, Margreet Scharloo,
Desirée I. Helder, Wim Chr. Kleijn, Inez
M. van Korlaar and Maaike Woertman*[1]

> Illness is the night-side of life, a more onerous citizenship. Everyone who is
> born holds dual citizenship, in the kingdom of the well and in the kingdom
> of the sick.
>
> (Sontag, 1979: 3)

The great majority of human beings hold citizenship in the kingdom of the
well for the most part of their lives. Major episodes of significant morbidity
come into play, on average, in the last few years of our existence on earth
(Hoffman *et al.*, 1996). However, for an increasing number of people, chronic
illness becomes part of their citizenship. Given the epidemiological transition
that is taking place in industrialised countries (Olshansky and Ault, 1986), no
longer are acute illnesses the most serious threats to our lives; chronic illnesses
have become the primary challenges that we will have to accommodate in our
existence.

Being chronically ill implies involvement with health care professionals in a
health care system. Usually, however, this involvement is of a quite limited
nature: most patients with chronic somatic illnesses will have approximately
four appointments per year in an out-patient clinic where they will spend
approximately ten minutes per appointment; an hour a year seems a fair estimate of the duration of the direct contact between patient and various
representatives of the health care system. This fairly simple arithmetic clearly
demonstrates how it is almost impossible to underestimate the importance of
how patients themselves have no choice but to incorporate their chronic illness
into their daily lives. Patients with chronic illness must find ways to make
sense of complaints, symptoms and signs; they must adjust their daily lives in
virtually every respect in order to maintain some sense of equilibrium and
'quality of life'. Health care professionals are important in trying to keep the
medical condition at bay, yet support from important others, information on
how to live with the chronic condition from patient organisations or media
and self-management skills seem to be at least as important (Lorig, 2002).

Various scientific disciplines, especially those in the social and behavioural sciences, provide the student of chronic illnesses with theories and

empirical data that elucidate how patients with chronic somatic disorders respond to their affliction. This chapter focuses on how people with chronic somatic disorders make sense of their illnesses. It will use the common-sense model (CSM), developed by Leventhal and colleagues over the past two decades, as a guiding theoretical system (Leventhal *et al.*, 2001; Leventhal *et al.*, 1980). A short excursion to other disciplines and theoretical models aims to outline the position of the CSM in relation to the work of others. We will start with a description of 'chronic illness', noting that defining chronic illness seems to be, surprisingly enough, an impossible task. Some epidemiological data on prevalence, incidence, morbidity and mortality regarding chronic (somatic) disorders are briefly discussed. Theoretical approaches on chronic illness in medical sociology, medical anthropology and health psychology will be briefly introduced. Within the health psychology domain, theories on chronic illness – those developed by Lazarus and Folkman (1984), Leventhal *et al.* (2001) and Moos and Tsu (1977) – will be our guiding perspectives in introducing the concept of illness representations. A selective review of empirical data on illness representations in five major chronic illnesses – asthma, chronic obstructive pulmonary disease, neurological disorders, cancer and cardiovascular disorders – will be the basis for some remarks on representations of chronic illness. We end this chapter by giving some suggestions for future research on representations of chronic illness and by briefly considering the clinical implications of this research for improving health care delivery.

Chronic illness

The word 'chronic' comes from the Greek 'chronos' which stands for 'time'; 'chronikos' in Greek stands for 'during a long period of time'. The element of time, therefore, is a core concept in most descriptions of chronic illness. A generally accepted definition of 'chronic illness' is not available. Even in important books on this subject, the central concept is not defined (e.g., Burish and Bradley, 1983; Nicassio and Smith, 1995). It should be noted that 'disease', 'illness' and 'sickness' are three words from different disciplines – medicine, psychology and sociology, respectively – reflecting the medical basis of any physiological dysfunction, the impact of the dysfunction on a person and the societal response to those with medical problems, respectively (Bury, 2001).

Verbrugge and Patrick provide a definition of 'chronic conditions' that encompasses the core elements of most other descriptions of the concept:

> long-term diseases, injuries with long sequelae, and enduring structural, sensory, and communication abnormalities. They are physical or mental (cognitive and emotional) in nature, and their onset time ranges from before birth to late in life. Their defining aspect is duration. Once they are past certain symptomatic or diagnostic thresholds, chronic conditions are

essentially permanent features for the rest of life. Medical and personal regimens can sometimes control but can rarely cure them.

(Verbrugge and Patrick, 1995: 173)

In epidemiological studies of chronic illness, three characteristics from this definition are usually operationalised: (1) duration – the condition should last for a minimum of a given time period (usually three months), or should occur a number of times (usually three times or more); (2) severity of functional limitations – being unable to perform work, household chores or daily activities for, usually, four months or longer; and (3) use of health care services – medical care is required for a continued period of time (Van den Bos, 1995).

'Most people reading this chapter will probably die of a chronic disease' – this is how Burish and Bradley (1983: 3) start the introduction to their book on coping with chronic disease. Some twenty years later, this statement is more true than ever. Data from the Global Burden of Disease study clearly demonstrate the transition of acute illness to chronic conditions in causing morbidity and mortality. Globally, lower respiratory infections, diarrhoeal diseases, and conditions arising during the perinatal period were the top three disease categories in the 1990 list of disease burden, as measured in disability-adjusted life years (Murray and Lopez, 1996). The authors predict that by 2020, the chronic illness conditions of ischaemic heart disease (including cerebrovascular disease) and chronic obstructive pulmonary disease (COPD) will make up the top of that list.

Two myths deserve attention in the context of chronic (somatic) disorders. First, it is too simplistic to assume that medical care has contributed greatly to the increased longevity in industrialised societies. In a recent paper, Bunker (2001) debunks this myth by demonstrating how 'age-adjusted death rates were reported to be greater in countries with greater numbers of doctors, and presumably with more medical care. … death rates for diseases amenable to treatment were reported to be greatest in areas with the most medical care resources' (p. 1260). Behavioural scientists who claim that behavioural interventions for high-risk health behaviour produce meaningful gains in life expectancy create myths as well: 'with about a quarter of the population smoking, the population as a whole would gain about one and a half years if every smoker quit' (Bunker, 2001: 1262). Mortality due to chronic illness remains a problem that will not be resolved easily, despite optimistic expectations regarding the efficacy of medical care and behavioural interventions.

Chronic illness: a behavioural perspective

Discussing the definitions and prevalence of chronic illness does not touch upon the suffering of those afflicted. Anyone who has visited 'the night-side of life' and then returned 'to the kingdom of the well' or who currently suffers a chronic illness has first-hand experience of the pervasive effects of such a condition on virtually all realms of life. Social and behavioural scientists have described and developed theories to capture this suffering and to delineate potential responses to chronic illnesses by those afflicted; in addition to these scholars, students of chronic illness can turn to other sources of knowledge on chronic illness. Poems and novels on chronic illness offer great insights into the kingdom of the sick. *The Plague* by Camus (1948) describes individual and collective responses to a highly contagious infectious disease; Mann in *The Magic Mountain* (1952) portrays the complicated interactions between patients and staff in a high-altitude clinic for sufferers of tuberculosis; and Solzhenitzyn (1971) gives a moving account of patients and staff living in a cancer ward. Any student of health psychology will benefit from reading these novels. Increasingly, courses in 'Medicine and Literature' are being offered to medical students (Skelton *et al.*, 2000). The journal *Literature and Medicine* is a fascinating source for students of illness representations in patients with chronic illnesses (see also Trautmann and Pollard, 1982).

In the area of medical anthropology, Kleinman (1988) developed his theory of 'explanatory models' in an attempt to categorise the responses of persons with a (chronic) illness to their condition. His work has a qualitative approach, which is why we discuss it here first: his empirical work functions as a link between, on the one hand, purely qualitative accounts in poems and novels written by or focusing on ill persons, and, on the other, the more formal, quantitative work on assessing illness representations and coping carried out by medical sociologists (e.g., Bury, 2001; Mechanic, 1966; Radley, 1994), psychiatrists (e.g., Lipowski, 1970) and psychologists (e.g., Lazarus and Folkman, 1984; Leventhal *et al.*, 2001; Moos and Tsu, 1977).

Explanatory models are 'the notions about an episode of sickness and its treatment that are employed by all those engaged in the clinical process' (Kleinman, 1988: 121). In his qualitative research, in various countries and cultures, Kleinman demonstrated that explanatory models are ordered along a distinct number of dimensions. Patients with chronic illnesses, when asked about their views, described their conditions in terms of the nature of the medical problem, why it had affected them, why now, what course it would follow, how it affected their body and what treatments they desired. It is remarkable and fascinating to note how the dimensions of these illness perceptions resemble those identified by others in quantitative research in patients in other (Western) cultures: identity (its label and associated symptoms), cause, timeline (expected duration), consequences (likely outcomes) and potential for cure/control (cf. Leventhal, 1995; Weinman *et al.*, 1996).

Other research has addressed the concept of illness behaviour (Mechanic, 1966), defined as 'the varying perceptions, thoughts, feelings, and acts affecting the personal and social meaning of symptoms, illness, disabilities and their consequences' (Mechanic, 1977: 79). Here, perceptions of symptoms are conceptualised as determinants of the decision by individuals as to whether to use health services or act in another way in response to (perceived) disturbances in bodily functioning. Bury and Radley continue in this line of research, using more qualitative accounts ('illness narratives') of illness behaviour as determinants of medical outcomes in patients with chronic somatic illnesses (Bury, 2001; Radley, 1994). In liaison-psychiatry, Lipowski (1970) also emphasised the importance of the subjective meaning of illness-related information in the process of adjustment to a chronic, somatic, disorder.

Moos and Tsu (1977) put their analyses of adapting to a chronic illness into the framework of crisis theory, conceptualising a serious physical illness as a life crisis. Adaptive tasks that follow from trying to restore some equilibrium (physical, psychological, social) are divided into 'illness-related' and 'general' categories; in the context of the current chapter, the work by Lazarus and Folkman (1984) on coping deserves discussion. Central to the concept of coping is the *appraisal* of stimuli that are associated with the stressors brought on by chronic illness. As discussed in various publications, the stress-coping model by Lazarus and Folkman has been and still is extremely influential in empirical studies in the area of clinical health psychology (e.g., Coyne and Racioppo, 2000). At the same time, many criticisms have been raised regarding the relative absence of evidence to suggest that coping explains a substantial amount of variance in outcomes and the relatively unspecified nature of the stressors and their meanings associated with the process of coping with a chronic illness (Coyne and Racioppo, 2000; De Ridder, 1997). A fairly simple and straightforward illustration of the lack of attention to the nature and meaning of stressors is the number of pages dedicated to these components of the stress-coping model in a chapter of an introductory health psychology textbook (Forshaw, 2002): four pages on appraisal and coping, yet less than a page on the stressors and their perceived meaning. This underlines one of the conclusions of Somerfield and McCrae (2000: 624) in their evaluation of stress and coping research: 'in place of general coping strategies, researchers must focus on responses specific to each stressful context'. Or, formulated somewhat differently and more critically, by Coyne and Racioppo (2000: 657): 'even when asked to report on a relatively well-defined class of stressors, respondents may draw upon very different stressful episodes with very different goals, options for coping, and prior probabilities of particular outcomes'. Critical analyses of the assessment of coping are in line with the issues raised above (e.g., Kleijn *et al.*, 2000; De Ridder and Schreurs, 2001; Schwarzer and Schwarzer, 1996).

The CSM developed by Leventhal *et al.* (2001) is more precise in outlining the stimuli associated with health threats and coping tasks. The CSM is described in detail in other chapters in this volume. Of particular relevance to the present chapter is the CSM's delineation of identity, cause, consequences, timeline and control/cure as the primary dimensions of illness representations; moreover, the CSM proposes that illness representations are primary guides to coping behaviour. Our concern here is to focus on illness representations of patients with chronic somatic disorders, their assessment and their relation with various aspects of illness outcomes; in an earlier work, we analysed the history of the assessment of illness representations (Kaptein *et al.*, 2001). The upshot of our exposé was that: (1) despite the relatively short history of empirical research on illness representations, a considerable number of assessment approaches have been applied; and (2) the publication of the Illness Perception Questionnaire (IPQ; Weinman *et al.*, 1996) greatly stimulated further empirical work in this area. The recent publication of the IPQ-R (revised) will only strengthen this development (Moss-Morris *et al.*, 2002).

In order to explore the issue of representations of chronic illness and their relation to outcomes in some empirical detail, we decided to review the empirical literature on this topic for five medical conditions: asthma, chronic obstructive pulmonary disease (COPD), neurological disorders, cancer and cardiovascular diseases.

Representations of chronic illness: a selective review

The authors of this chapter are involved with studies on representations of the five chronic illnesses reviewed here. For the purpose of writing this chapter, each author conducted a literature search using the Medline, PsycInfo and Current Contents databases. The medical subject headings of the five illnesses or illness categories were combined with the following key words: 'illness representation', 'illness perception', 'illness belief', 'illness cognition', 'illness attributions' and 'illness attitudes'; in addition, our personal files on illness representations were checked for papers that matched the selection criteria. The papers selected are summarized in Tables 5.1 to 5.5. They are not exhaustive reviews: studies are included when illness representations were explicitly assessed as such and when relations between illness representations and a dependent variable in some sense were included. More extensive discussions on this topic can be found in Helder (2002), Van Korlaar *et al.* (in review), Scharloo (2002) and Scharloo and Kaptein (1997).

Asthma

Asthma typically is a cyclical disorder: reversibility of breathlessness is the hallmark of asthma (Kaptein and Creer, 2002) and the primary characteristic with which a patient with asthma must deal. The literature search on asthma and illness representations produced some twenty papers, six of which were selected and summarized in Table 5.1.

All six studies applied a descriptive design, exploring illness representations via various types of interviews or questionnaires. All studies report associations between illness representations and the patient's attempt to control the medical problem (coping procedure) or to appraise outcomes.

Table 5.1 Review of studies on illness representations and outcome in patients with asthma

First author (year)	Objective	Method and subjects	Instruments; dimensions	Results
Adams (1997)	To explore how patients with asthma conceptualise and use their prescribed medication.	Cross-sectional study of 30 adults.	In-depth interview; self-presentation and disclosure, notions of asthma and medication.	Representation of asthma as an acute condition was associated with greater use of reliever medication, and non-use of adequate medication. Representations of asthma as a chronic, controllable condition were associated with use of adequate medication.
Chambers (1999)	To explore relations between patients' beliefs about asthma and use of medication.	Cross-sectional study of 349 adults.	Survey; use of and attitudes to inhaled corticosteroids, health beliefs (Health Belief Model dimensions).	Identity (high) and consequences (high) predicted use of inhaled corticosteroids.
Hand (1996)	To examine the relationship between beliefs about asthma medication and inhaler use.	Cross-sectional study of 40 adults.	Interview on attitudes to asthma and asthma medication.	Consequences (high) predicted use of inhaled corticosteroids, irrespective of objective asthma severity.
Horne (2002)	To evaluate the degree to which variations in reported adherence to preventer medication for asthma could be predicted by representations of asthma and asthma medication.	Cross-sectional study of 100 community-based adults.	IPQ (Illness Perception Questionnaire); identity, causal beliefs, timeline, consequences, cure/control. BMQ (Beliefs about Medicines Questionnaire); treatment necessity and treatment concerns.	Illness identity predicted use of health care services; treatment beliefs predicted use of preventer medication.
Paterson (1999)	To investigate the relative contribution of personal illness experience to the sophistication of children's illness conceptualisations of colds and asthma.	Cross-sectional study of 182 children (35 with asthma).	Structured interview, with dimensions from IPQ.	Children with asthma had somewhat more sophisticated conceptualisations of asthma than did children without asthma.
Priel (1994)	To explore the relationships of negative affectivity with patients' perceptions of and responses to asthma attacks.	Cross-sectional study of 47 adults with asthma in an outpatient clinic.	Negative affect, perceived asthma severity, use of medication and use of health care services.	High negative affectivity was associated with asthma being perceived as more severe, and with higher use of asthma medication.

Only the study by Horne and Weinman (2002) explicitly tested the CSM. Representations of identity (high) and consequences (high) generally appear to be associated with greater use of medication and health care services. Although illness representations of asthma have been the subject of a fairly large number of studies, they have not yet been specifically targeted in intervention studies on the self-management of asthma.

Chronic obstructive pulmonary disease (COPD)

As the diagnostic label of COPD implies, this respiratory disorder entails all characteristics of a chronic condition. Studies on representations of COPD were identified in the manner outlined above. Only studies that listed the assessed illness perception dimensions as separate concepts and examined relationships between these concepts and outcomes were included in the review. A total of seven studies matched the criteria (see Table 5.2). The search revealed that over a period of twenty years, only seven studies have been published on the subject, which suggests illness perceptions in patients with COPD are an underdeveloped area of research. Also, only one study used a longitudinal design and in most studies, only one or two dimensions were measured. Leventhal's CSM was used as a theoretical framework in three studies.

Self-report outcome measures were used in four studies (Kellner *et al.*, 1987; Scharloo *et al.*, 1998; Scharloo *et al.*, 2000; Weaver and Narsavage, 1992), while four studies also employed behavioural measures of functioning: return visits to the emergency department (Stehr *et al.*, 1991); nursing unit managers' ratings of adjustment (Lacroix *et al.*, 1991); 12-minute walking distance (Morgan *et al.*, 1983); and the number of visits to the outpatient clinic and strength of medication (Scharloo *et al.*, 2000). In four studies, beliefs accounted for more variance in the outcome measures than did the physiologic variables (Lacroix *et al.*, 1991; Morgan *et al.*, 1983; Scharloo *et al.*, 1998; Stehr *et al.*, 1991) and in all studies, beliefs were related to functioning. Across studies, negative outcome appeared to be associated with negative beliefs about treatment control and consequences, negative emotional representations, inaccurate identity beliefs/more perceived symptoms and inaccurate causal beliefs/having causal beliefs/less belief in emotional causes of illness. The results from the reviewed studies suggest that beliefs deserve to be given a more prominent place in research and treatment in patients with COPD (cf. Kaptein and Dekker, 2000).

Neurological diseases

Search terms as described above were combined with 'neurological disease', 'neurology' and 'brain injury'. Seven papers focusing on illness representations in neurological disease were identified (Fabbri *et al.*, 2001; Helder *et al.*, in

Table 5.2 Review of studies on illness representations and outcome in patients with chronic obstructive pulmonary disease (COPD)

First author (year)	Objective	Method and subjects	Instruments; dimensions	Results
Kellner (1987)	To examine attitudes and fears about disease, and their relationships with anxiety, depression, anger-hostility, and somatic symptoms.	Cross-sectional study evaluating differences between 50 patients with chronic airflow obstruction (CAO) and 50 age- and gender-matched family practice patients with other chronic diseases.	Illness Attitude Scales (IAS); emotional representations (worry about illness, concern about pain).	No differences between patient groups on 'worry' or 'concern' sub-scales. In CAO patients, worry and concern correlated with depression, and worry with anger-hostility. The sub-scales were unrelated to somatic symptoms in CAO patients.
Lacroix (1991)	To explore the utility of the Schema Assessment Instrument (SAI) with respect to patients 'level of functioning.	Cross-sectional study evaluating relationships between the accuracy of illness beliefs and level of adaptive functioning in 31 patients with chronic respiratory conditions.	SAI: identity, causes.	Accuracy of patients' knowledge correlated positively with ratings of adaptive functioning. No relationship was observed between severity and prognosis of patients' medical condition and functioning.
Morgan (1983)	To examine mood, psychiatric disturbance, patients' illness beliefs and attitudes, and their relationship to physical performance.	Cross-sectional study identifying factors that contributed significantly to variance in the 12-minute walking test in 50 patients with chronic bronchitis.	Semantic differential; control (treatment control), consequences (bronchitis consequences).	Negative beliefs about treatment and consequences correlated negatively with walking distance.
Scharloo (1998)	To examine illness perceptions and coping, and their relationship to functioning in patients with different chronic illnesses.	Cross-sectional study identifying factors that contributed to functional disability in 80 patients with COPD.	Illness Perception Questionnaire (IPQ); identity, causes, timeline, consequences, control/cure.	In patients with COPD, having fewer perceived symptoms was associated with better role and social functioning and less disability in activities of daily life.
Scharloo (2000)	To study the contribution of coping and illness perceptions to outcome 1 year later.	Longitudinal study identifying factors that contributed significantly to variance in functional disability, number of hospital visits, and strength of medication in 64 patients with COPD.	IPQ: identity, causes, timeline, consequences, control/cure.	Having fewer perceived symptoms was associated with better social functioning and better perceived health. Less belief in emotional attributions (others and stress) was associated with more hospital visits.
Stehr (1991)	To determine if psychosocial and physiologic factors were associated with unscheduled return visits to the emergency department.	Retrospective study identifying variables distinguishing 21 patients with COPD who relapse from 12 non-relapsers.	Semantic differential; control (treatment control).	A negative belief about treatment was identified as characteristic of return visits to the emergency department.
Weaver (1992)	To identify physiological and psychological variables that affect the functional status of patients.	Cross-sectional study examining relationships among causal attributions, depressed mood, self-esteem, pulmonary function, exercise capacity, and functional status in 140 patients with COPD.	AIS, open-ended questions, judges coding recorded answers into categories; causes.	Differences between those who did/did not ask 'why me': those who had not asked were more functional.

Table 5.3 Review of studies on illness representations and outcome in patients with neurological disorders

First author (year)	Objective	Method and subjects	Instruments; dimensions	Results
Fabbri (2001)	To examine the relationship between emotional, cognitive, and behavioural factors in outpatients attending neurology and cardiology clinics.	Self-report questionnaire study with 65 consecutive new patients attending general neurology or cardiology outpatient clinics.	Hospital Anxiety and Depression Scale, Illness Perception Questionnaire (IPQ), Somatosensory Amplification Scale, Health Anxiety Questionnaire.	Depressed patients had negative perceptions about their illness; they believed that their illness would last a long time, have serious consequences, and probably could not be cured or controlled. Depressed patients indicated that their illness caused them considerable disability and they were apathetic about seeking reassurance from their doctors. There were no differences between neurology and cardiology patient groups in these associations.
Helder (in press)	To describe the illness perceptions and coping mechanisms of patients with Huntington's disease (HD), and to assess the role of illness perceptions in the well-being of these individuals.	A cross-sectional, questionnaire-guided interview study of 77 HD patients.	Unified Huntington Disease Rating Scale (UHDRS), Mini-Mental State (MMS), IPQ, COPE, Medical Outcome Study 36-item Short Form Health Survey (MOS SF-36).	HD patients' illness perceptions were characterised by a strong illness identity combined with beliefs about a long duration of HD, perceived negative consequences for their daily lives, and little hope for cure or improvement of their symptoms. Both illness perceptions and coping mechanisms significantly predicted well-being.
Helder (in review)	To investigate differences between the illness perceptions and coping mechanisms of HD patients and their partners, and to assess whether these differences influence the well-being of HD patients.	A cross-sectional, questionnaire-guided interview study with 51 HD patients and their partners.	UHDRS, MMS, IPQ, COPE, MOS SF-36.	In contrast with their partners, HD patients reported experiencing significantly fewer symptoms of HD and more control over the disease process. These differences did however not predict HD patients' well-being.

	Aim	Method	Measures	Findings
Kemp (1999)	To determine the relative contributions of neuroepilepsy, coping, and illness representation variables to psychological adjustment.	A cross-sectional, interview study of 94 patients with epilepsy.	Measure devised to assess the distinct components of illness representations, Revised Ways of Coping Checklist, Mental Health Inventory, self-esteem scale, Social Avoidance and Distress Scale.	After controlling for the effects of group membership and neuroepilepsy variables, coping and illness representations each explained significant additional variance in psychological adjustment.
Roberts (2000)	To examine attitudes, beliefs, and experiences regarding Alzheimer disease (AD) among patients' first-degree relatives.	Mailed questionnaire study with 203 first-degree relatives of AD patients.	Questionnaire devised to assess: AD knowledge, AD cause beliefs, AD treatment optimism, and perceived AD threat.	Relatives were knowledgeable about AD, had an accurate sense of their disease risk, and endorsed etiologically significant factors as causes. Many participants held misconceptions about HD, and unrealistic expectations for future treatment developments.
Schiaffino (1998)	To investigate the relationship of illness representations to concurrent and later mood in patients with rheumatoid arthritis (RA) and in patients with multiple sclerosis (MS)	A longitudinal, questionnaire study of 63 patients with RA and 66 adults with MS.	20-item self-report measure of depression, Implicit Models of Illness Questionnaire (IMIQ).	For MS patients, beliefs in symptom variability were associated with a higher depressed mood.
Swift (2001)	To investigate the lack of knowledge and misconceptions concerning brain injury, as perceived by individuals having personal and/or professional experience of brain injury.	A cross-sectional, qualitative, semi-structured interview study with 2 persons who suffered a traumatic brain injury (TBI), 1 person who suffered a non-TBI, 2 spousal caregivers, 3 parental caregivers, and 14 rehabilitation professionals.	A semi-structured interview based on Leventhal et al.'s CSM.	Individuals had inaccurate beliefs regarding: timeline/duration of recovery, diversity of consequences, symptom identity. The knowledge gaps and misconceptions provide a focus for information provision and educational interventions.

press; Helder *et al.*, in review; Kemp *et al.*, 1999; Roberts and Connell, 2000; Schiaffino *et al.*, 1998; Swift and Wilson, 2001). Leventhal's CSM was the focus of all the studies and the IPQ was used in three studies (Fabbri *et al.*, 2001; Helder *et al.*, in press; Helder *et al.*, in review).

Four studies dealt with the illness perceptions of patients suffering from neurological disease (Fabbri *et al.*, 2001; Helder *et al.*, in press; Kemp *et al.*, 1999; Schiaffino *et al.*, 1998), one study focused on the illness perceptions of couples dealing with Huntington's disease (Helder *et al.*, in review), one study focused on the illness perceptions of first-degree relatives of patients suffering from Alzheimer disease (Roberts and Connell, 2000) and another study focused on misconceptions about brain injury among the general public and among individuals with experience of the condition (Swift and Wilson, 2001).

In the area of neurological disorders, illness representations were assessed in a fairly theory-driven manner. Relationships between representations and various aspects of health outcomes have not yet been examined in great detail. Helder *et al.* (in press) report significant associations between illness identity (high) and poorer functional status in Huntington's disease patients (Helder *et al.*, in press). In patients with multiple schlerosis, Schiaffino *et al.* (1998) report high symptom variability – a reflection of identity – to be associated with subsequent depression. No empirical work has been done up to now on interventions targeting illness representations for patients with neurological disorders.

Cancer

The term 'cancer' was combined with the terms described above. Approximately 100 references were found that comprised instances of illness perceptions as defined in the previous section. Only ten references were found within the medically oriented Medline database, while the remaining ninety were identified through the psychological database PsycINFO. Not all references were of practical use for the purposes of this review because not all matched the mentioned criteria. Thus, those *not* used were references to theoretical studies, review studies, cancer screening studies, studies of illness perceptions by only non-patients, prevention studies, or book chapters. Only five references proved useful. They are summarized in Table 5.4.

All studies investigated adult patients. One study used heterogeneous groups of patients with different forms of cancer and the rest assessed homogeneous groups (patients with breast cancer, gynecological cancer and cervical abnormalities).

Although the selected studies examined the role of psychological variables in relation to the experience of being a cancer patient, and all used one or more elements of our definition of illness perception, hardly any of the selected studies explicitly used Leventhal's CSM. Only the Cameron *et al.*

Table 5.4 *Review of studies on illness perceptions and outcome in patients with cancer*

First author (year)	Objective	Method and subjects	Instruments; dimensions	Results
Bradley (2001)	To examine the relationships between illness representations and health behaviour.	Interviews with 12 women with early stage gynaecological cancer.	CSM dimensions of illness representation.	Illness identity (high) maintained fears of recurrence and predicted greater use of seeking medical care.
Cameron (1998)	To explore the associations of trait anxiety with sensitivity and biases in symptom reports and attributions, and with emotional responses and protective behaviour.	Double-blind, placebo-controlled trial of tamoxifen therapy. Longitudinal questionnaire study; 140 patients (breast cancer in remission).	General Anxiety sub-scale (Multiple Affect Adjective Checklist), self-rated symptoms, side effects expectancies and beliefs, self-rated cancer worries, frequency of breast self-examination.	Trait anxiety was associated with activation of illness-related representations that trigger attentiveness to sensations, worry, and protective coping in response to somatic cues.
Elliott (1996)	To assess the hypothesis that beliefs and knowledge about cancer pain management would be related to lower pain intensity scores.	Randomised community trial; 314 patients (different cancer) and family members.	Structured interviews and self-rated scales: Brief Pain Inventory, Eastern Cooperative of Oncology Groups (ECOG) performance status, knowledge and attitude/belief items.	Patients' and family members' reports of patient pain and performance status were highly correlated. Cognitive factors are related to family members' reports of cancer pain in the patients, but not to the level of pain reported by the patients themselves.
Marteau (2002)	To describe women's beliefs about the role of smoking in the causation of cervical abnormalities, and their explanatory models for any such perceived risk.	36 women with cervical abnormalities .	Interview eliciting perceived causes and perceived control/cure	Causal beliefs were related to sexual activity, not to smoking.
Petrie (1999)	To examine positive changes reported in their lives by myocardial infarction (MI) and cancer patients.	Longitudinal questionnaire study; 143 patients (MI), 52 patients.	Sickness Impact Profile (SIP), open-ended question, self-rated items on health and life.	Seven major positive themes were identified. Positive changes (60 %) were unrelated to illness severity. Most reported common theme (by cancer patients) was improved close relations with others. Explanatory models are suggested in explaining individual differences.

Table 5.5 Review of studies on illness representations and outcome in patients with cardiovascular diseases

First author (year)	Objective	Method and subjects	Instruments	Results
Cooper (1999)	To determine whether illness beliefs could predict cardiac rehabilitation attendance.	Prospective study of 152 patients with myocardial infarction (MI) or coronary artery bypass graft surgery (CABG).	Illness Perception Questionnaire (IPQ); control/cure, consequences, timeline, causal attribution.	Attenders scored significantly higher than non-attenders on perception of control and causal attribution of MI to lifestyle.
Dammen (1999)	To assess the factorial structure of the Illness Attitude Scales (IAS).	Questionnaire study of 199 patients with chest pain.	IAS	Factor analysis revealed three sub-scales: health anxiety (HA), illness behaviour (IB), and health habits (HH). Respective internal consistency: $\propto$ = .92, .80, .49. The HH sub-scale did not correlate with HA and IB and did not discriminate between patients with and without panic disorder.
Gump (2001)	To determine if illness representations differ as a function of age and how representations predict postoperative health behaviours in conjunction with age.	Prospective study of 309 patients undergoing CABG surgery.	Interview on illness representations; causes, timeline, control.	Older patients were more likely to see old age as a cause for their disease and less likely to attribute their illness to genetics, health behaviour, and emotions. They also perceived less control over the disease.
Haugbolle (2002)	To examine medication- and illness-related factual knowledge and perceptions of angina pectoris patients.	Qualitative research interviews with 123 angina pectoris patients.	Semi-structured interview on illness perceptions.	Three categories were established to describe the patients' perception of illness: 'positive', 'acceptance', and 'negative'. The results do not indicate that a negative illness perception is related to limited knowledge about the illness.

Study	Aim	Sample	Measure	Results
Petrie (1996)	To examine whether patients' initial perceptions of their MI predict attendance at a cardiac rehabilitation course, return to work, disability, and sexual dysfunction.	Study of 143 patients with MI.	Questionnaire with items from Illness Perception Questionnaire (IPQ).	Attendance at rehabilitation course was correlated with stronger cure/control beliefs; return to work within 6 weeks was correlated with the belief that the illness would last a short time and have fewer consequences. Belief in serious consequences was related to later disability in work, and recreational and social activities. Strong illness identity was related to greater sexual dysfunction.
Van Tiel (1998)	To explore sex differences in illness beliefs and behaviour in patients with suspected coronary artery disease (CAD).	Interviews with 28 patients with chest pain and suspected CAD.	Semi-structured interview with items about illness beliefs (susceptibility, risk factors, symptom attribution).	Both men and women think of CAD as 'men's disease', have equal knowledge of risk factors. Men consider their own CAD risk to be lower than estimated probability for men and as low as estimated risk for women.
Veldtman (2000)	To evaluate illness knowledge and understanding in children and adolescents with congenital and acquired heart disease.	Interviews with 63 children and adolescents (7–18 years old) with heart diseases.	Semi-structured interview based on Leventhal's illness representation model.	Illness understanding was poor: 30 % had a good understanding; 77 % did not know the medical name of their condition; 33 % had wrong belief or poor understanding of their illness. Understanding was unrelated to age, sex or nature of the disease. Understanding of illness duration was significantly related to age.

(1998) study cites Leventhal's work in this field and no study used a standardized illness representations questionnaire.

Two studies used a cross-sectional design (Marteau *et al.*, 2002; Bradley *et al.*, 2001); associations between illness beliefs at one stage of the illness and outcome variables (such as illness behaviour, quality of life) at a later stage were observed in the three longitudinal studies. Illness identity was associated with health behaviour (Bradley *et al.*, 2001; Cameron *et al.*, 1998). All five studies are theory-based, thereby facilitating the development of a research agenda for future work, including intervention studies.

Cardiovascular disorders

The literature search combined the terms described above with 'cardiovascular diseases' (explode). A total of seven articles matched the criteria; they are summarized in Table 5.5.

One study (Dammen *et al.*, 1999) focused on assessing the factorial structure of a questionnaire – the Illness Attitude Scales (IAS) – in patients with chest pain. The other six studies used questionnaires and standardised interviews to measure illness perceptions in patients with various cardiovascular diseases.

Of these six, one focused on illness representations in children with various heart diseases (Veldtman *et al.*, 2000), while the other five investigated adult patients with myocardial infarction (Cooper *et al.*, 1999; Petrie *et al.*, 1996), chest pain (Dammen *et al.*, 1999; Van Tiel *et al.*, 1998), coronary artery bypass graft surgery (Cooper *et al.*, 1999; Gump *et al.*, 2001) and angina pectoris (Haugbølle *et al.*, 2002).

Most studies measured illness representations based on Leventhal's CSM. Two studies used items from the IPQ. In the study by Cooper *et al.* (1999), timeline, control/cure, consequences and causal attribution to lifestyle and stress were measured. Petrie *et al.* (1996) also used the IPQ items in their study but did not include the causal attribution sub-scale. Both studies investigated the role of illness perceptions in attendance at a cardiac rehabilitation course in London, UK, and Auckland, New Zealand, respectively, and both found a strong correlation between attendance and high cure/control beliefs. Two studies attempted to assess age differences in illness perceptions. Gump *et al.* (2001) measured cause, timeline and control with self-constructed questions in the only study that measured age differences in adults. Veldtman *et al.* (2000) conducted semi-structured interviews based on Leventhal's CSM representational attributes in children. Only one study explored gender differences in beliefs about cardiovascular disease (Van Tiel *et al.*, 1998).

General discussion

Representations of chronic illness appear to be the focus of considerable research interest in the field of health psychology, with the CSM serving as a highly stimulating theoretical framework. The availability of the IPQ has initiated an impressive number of empirical studies on representations of (chronic) illnesses in recent years. Given the central focus of this volume, we have attempted to illustrate in this chapter how the CSM is being used to describe illness attributes and representations in patients with various chronic illnesses and to examine associations between illness representations and various aspects of medical, psychological, and social outcome. Based on the selective literature reviews on illness representations in patients with five different chronic illnesses, and on relationships between those representations and outcome, some cautionary remarks seem in order.

Only a limited number of empirical papers have explicitly studied the predictive power of different dimensions of illness representations for well-defined outcome variables. Those studies are all very recent; sophisticated assessment methods for measuring representations have been published only recently. Given the positive responses of the health psychology community to the CSM, it seems safe to predict a rapidly increasing number of empirical publications on the topic of this chapter. It follows that publications on the effects of intervention in illness representations will be a fascinating area to watch.

Some cautious conclusions can be drawn on the basis of the findings summarised in the tables in this chapter. With asthma, identity and consequences predict outcome to some extent (Horne and Weinman, 2002). These dimensions are associated with more distal outcomes in COPD patients (Scharloo *et al.*, 2000a), such as well-being and functional status. In the selected studies on neurological disorders, identity and timeline stand out as being associated with depression and well-being (Helder *et al.*, in press; Schiaffino *et al.*, 1998). With cancer, identity turns up as an important correlate of aspects of outcome (Bradley *et al.*, 2001; Cameron *et al.*, 1998). Finally, control, causes, consequences and timeline predict outcomes in patients with cardiovascular diseases (Cooper *et al.*, 1999; Petrie *et al.*, 1996). Interestingly, only a few studies explicitly address the theoretical issue of the relative importance of illness representations and coping as predictors of outcome (e.g., Scharloo *et al.*, 1998; Scharloo *et al.* 2000b). In those few studies, however, the authors suggest that illness representations explain greater amounts of variance in outcome than coping. Systematic reviews of these topics seem highly relevant.

Further research into the intercorrelations of the representation dimensions, and their associations with various outcome measures is not only theoretically relevant and interesting, it is also instrumental in defining targets for interventions by attempting to change (dimensions of) illness representations. As far as outcomes are concerned, we feel more attention should be given to observable, behavioural outcomes (Kaplan, 1990) – for example, returning to work, length of hospitalisation, survival – rather than to predicting self-reported psychological variables – for example, anxiety, depression – on the basis of self-reported illness representations.

In the chapter by Petrie *et al.* (this volume, Chapter 13), the issue of interventions in illness representations is discussed in detail, so for this topic the reader is referred there. Regarding clinical implications, it seems important to increase the sensitivity of physicians and other health care professionals to the relevance of illness representations of patients with chronic illnesses. Pachter (1994) makes a strong case for this in his paper on folk illness beliefs and behaviours and their implications for health care delivery. Hunt *et al.* (2001) point out that by ignoring 'folk epidemiology' (which is a concept quite similar to 'illness representations'), health care professionals can impede medical care and attempts to educate patients (cf. Kaptein, 2000). It will take excellent scientific and social skills to seduce physicians (and psychologists!) to incorporate the patient's story about his/her illness into the clinical encounter.

Listening to patients talk about their chronic illness gives us an insight into how they make sense of their stay in 'the kingdom of the sick'. They appear to be trying to adjust to their plight by cognitively (and emotionally) making sense of their experiences. As their representations of their illness predict aspects of outcome, and as illness representations apparently are amenable to clinical health psychology interventions with positive effects on outcome, continuing and intensifying this type of research will help patients with chronic somatic disorders during their stay 'in the nightside of life'.

Note

1   Correspondence concerning this chapter should be addressed to Adrian A. Kaptein, Unit of Psychology, Leiden University Medical Centre (LUMC), PO Box 1251 2340 BG OEGSTGEEST, The Netherlands. E-mail: a.a.kaptein@umail.leidenuniv.nl

References

Adams, S., Pill, R. and Jones, A. (1997) 'Medication, chronic illness and identity: the perspective of people with asthma', *Social Science and Medicine* **45**: 189–201.

Bradley, E.J., Calvert, E., Pitts, M.K. and Redman, C.W.E. (2001) 'Illness identity and the self-regulatory model in recovery from early stage gynaecological cancer', *Journal of Health Psychology* **6**: 511–521.

Bunker, J.P. (2001) 'The role of medical care in contributing to health improvements within societies', *International Journal of Epidemiology* **30**: 1260–1263.

Burish, T.G. and Bradley, L.A. (eds) (1983) *Coping with Chronic Illness: Research and Applications*, New York: Academic Press.

Bury, M. (2001) 'Illness narratives: fact or fiction?, *Sociology of Health and Illness* **23**: 263–285.

Cameron, L.D., Leventhal, H. and Love, R. R. (1998) 'Trait anxiety, symptom perceptions, and illness-related responses among women with breast cancer in remission during a tamoxifen clinical trial', *Health Psychology* **17**: 459–469.

Camus, A. (1948) *The Plague*, New York: Alfred A. Knopf.

Chambers, C.V., Markson, L., Diamond, J.J. and Berger, M. (1999) 'Health beliefs and compliance with inhaled corticosteroids by asthmatic patients in primary care practices,' *Respiratory Medicine* **93**: 88–94.

Cooper, A., Lloyd, G., Weinman, J. and Jackson, G. (1999) 'Why patients do not attend cardiac rehabilitation: role of intentions and illness beliefs', *Heart* **82**: 234–236.

Coyne, J.C. and Racioppo, M.W. (2000) 'Never the twain shall meet? Closing the gap between coping research and clinical intervention research', *American Psychologist* **55**: 655–664.

Dammen, T., Friis, S. and Ekeberg, Ø. (1999) 'The Illness Attitude Scales in chest pain patients: a study of psychometric properties', *Journal of Psychosomatic Research* **46**: 335–342.

de Ridder, D.T.D. (1997) 'What is wrong with coping assessment? A review of conceptual and methodological issues', *Psychology and Health* **12**: 417–431.

de Ridder, D. and Schreurs, K. (2001) 'Developing interventions for chronically ill patients: is coping a helpful concept?' *Clinical Psychology Review* **21**: 205–240.

Elliott, B.A., Elliott, T.E., Murray, D.M., Braun, B.L. and Johnson, K.M. (1996) 'Patients and family members: the role of knowledge and attitudes in cancer pain', *Journal of Pain and Symptom Management* **12**: 209–220.

Fabbri, S., Kapur, N., Wells, A. and Creed, F. (2001) 'Emotional, cognitive, and behavioral characteristics of medical outpatients', *Psychosomatics* **42**: 74–77.

Forshaw, M. (2002) *Essential Health Psychology*, London: Arnold.

Gump, B.B., Matthews, K.A., Scheier, M.F., Schulz, R., Bridges, M.W. and Magovern, G.J. (2001) 'Illness representations according to age and effects on health behaviors following coronary artery bypass graft surgery', *Journal of the American Geriatric Society* **49**: 284–289.

Hand, C.H. and Bradley, C. (1996) 'Health beliefs of adults with asthma: toward an understanding of the difference between symptomatic and preventive use of inhaler treatment', *Journal of Asthma* **33**: 331–338.

Haugbølle, L.S., Sørensen, E.W. and Henriksen, H.H. (2002) 'Medication- and illness- related factual knowledge, perceptions and behaviour in angina pectoris patients', *Patient Education and Counseling* **47**: 281–289.

Helder, D.I. (2002) 'Huntington's disease: a study on illness perceptions, coping mechanisms, and well-being of patients and their partners', unpublished Ph.D. thesis, Leiden, The Netherlands.

Helder, D.I., Kaptein, A.A., van Kempen, G.M.J., Weinman, J., van Houwelingen, J.C. and Roos, R.A.C. (in press) 'Living with Huntington's disease: illness perceptions, coping mechanisms and patients' well-being', *British Journal of Health Psychology*.

Helder, D.I., Kaptein, A.A., van Kempen, G.M.J., Weinman, J., van Houwelingen, J.C. and Roos, R.A.C. (in review) 'The impact of spouses' illness perceptions on the well-being of a sample of 51 patients with Huntington's disease'.

Hoffman, C., Rice, D. and Sung, H.Y. (1996) 'Persons with chronic conditions. Their prevalence and costs', *Journal of the American Medical Association* **276**: 1473–1479.

Horne, R. and Weinman, J. (2002) 'Self-regulation and self-management in asthma: exploring the role of illness perceptions and treatment beliefs in explaining non-adherence to preventer medication,' *Psychology and Health* 17, 17–32.

Hunt, K., Emslie, C. and Watt, G. (2001) 'Lay constructions of a family history of heart disease: potential for misunderstandings in the clinical encounter?' *Lancet* **357**: 1168–1171.

Kaplan, R.M. (1990) 'Behavior as the central outcome in health care', *American Psychologist* **45**: 1211–1220.

Kaptein, A.A. (2000) 'On psychology in medicine,' in A.A. Kaptein, A. Appels and K. Orth-Gomér (eds) *Psychology in Medicine*, Houten: Bohn Stafleu van Loghum, pp. 1–17.

Kaptein, A.A. and Creer, T.L. (eds) (2002) *Respiratory Disorders and Behavioural Medicine*, London: Martin Dunitz.

Kaptein, A.A. and Dekker, F.W. (2000) 'Psychosocial support', *European Respiratory Monograph* **5**: 58–69.

Kaptein, A.A., Scharloo, M. and Weinman, J. (2001) 'Assessment of illness perceptions,' in A. Vingerhoets (ed.) *Assessment in Behavioral Medicine*, Hove, UK: Brunner-Routledge, pp. 179–194.

Kellner, R., Samet, J.M. and Pathak, D. (1987) 'Hypochondriacal concerns and somatic symptoms in patients with chronic airflow obstruction', *Journal of Psychosomatic Research* **31**: 575–582.

Kemp, S., Morley, S. and Anderson, E. (1999) 'Coping with epilepsy: do illness representations play a role?' *British Journal of Clinical Psychology* **38**: 43–58.

Kleijn, W.C., van Heck, G.L. and van Waning, A. (2000) 'Experiences with a Dutch adaptation of the COPE-questionnaire' (in Dutch), *Gedrag and Gezondheid* **28**: 213–226.

Kleinman, A. (1988) *The Illness Narratives*, New York: Basic Books.

Lacroix, J.M., Martin, B., Avendano, M. and Goldstein, R. (1991) 'Symptom schemata in chronic respiratory patients', *Health Psychology* **10**: 268–273.

Lazarus, R.S. and Folkman, S. (1984) *Stress, Appraisal, and Coping*, New York: Springer.

Leventhal, H. (1995) 'Latino folk illnesses: why they are just like ours!' *Psychology and Health* **10**: 349–352.

Leventhal, H., Leventhal, E.A. and Cameron, L. (2001) 'Representations, procedures, and affect in illness self-regulation: a perceptual-cognitive model,' in A. Baum, T.A. Revenson and J.E. Singer (eds) *Handbook of Health Psychology*, Mahwah, NJ: Lawrence Erlbaum Associates, pp. 19–47.

Leventhal, H., Meyer, D. and Nerenz, D.R. (1980) 'The common sense representation of illness danger,' in S. Rachman (ed.), *Contributions to Medical Psychology*, vol. 2, New York: Pergamon Press, pp 7–30.

Lipowski, Z.J. (1970) 'Physical illness, the individual and the coping processes,' *International Journal of Psychiatry in Medicine* **1**: 91–102.

Lorig, K. (2002) 'Partnership between expert patients and physicians', *Lancet* **359**: 814–815.

Mann, T. (1952) *The Magic Mountain*, New York: Modern Library.

Marteau, T.M., Rana, S. and Kubba, A. (2002) 'Smoking and cervical cancer: a qualitative study of the explanatory models of smokers with cervical abnormalities', *Psychology, Health and Medicine* **7**: 107–109.

Mechanic, D. (1966) 'Response factors in illness: the study of illness behavior', *Social Psychiatry* **1**: 11–20.

—— (1977) 'Illness behavior, social adaptation, and the management of illness', *The Journal of Nervous and Mental Diseases* **165**: 79–87.

Moos, R.H. and Tsu, V.D. (eds) (1977) *Coping with Physical Illness*, New York: Plenum.

Morgan, A.D., Peck, D.F., Buchanan, D.R. and McHardy, G.J.R. (1983) 'Effect of attitudes and beliefs on exercise tolerance in chronic bronchitis', *British Medical Journal* **286**: 171–173.

Moss-Morris, R., Weinman, J., Petrie, K.J., Horne, R., Cameron, L.D. and Buick, D. (2002) 'The Revised Illness Perception Questionnaire (IPQ-R)', *Psychology and Health* **17**: 1–16.

Murray, C.J.L. and Lopez, A.D. (eds) (1996) *The Global Burden of Disease*, Boston, MA: Harvard University Press.

Nicassio, P.M. and Smith, T.W. (eds) (1995) *Managing Chronic Illness. A Biopsychosocial Perspective*, Washington, DC: American Psychological Association.

Olshansky, S.J. and Ault, A.B. (1986) 'The fourth stage of the epidemiologic transition: the age of delayed degenerative disease', *The Milbank Quarterly* **64**: 355–391.

Pachter, L.M. (1994) 'Culture and clinical care', *Journal of the American Medical Association* **271**: 690–694.

Paterson, J., Moss-Morris, R. and Butler, S.J. (1999) 'The effect of illness experience and demographic factors on children's illness representations', *Psychology and Health* **14**: 117–129.

Petrie, K.J., Buick, D.L., Weinman, J. and Booth, R.J. (1999) 'Positive effects of illness reported by myocardial infarction and breast cancer patients', *Journal of Psychosomatic Research* **47**: 537–543.

Petrie, K.J., Weinman, J., Sharpe, N. and Buckley, J. (1996) 'Role of patients' view of their illness in predicting return to work and functioning after myocardial infarction: longitudinal study', *British Medical Journal* **312**: 1191–1194.

Priel, B., Heimer, D., Rabinowitz, B. and Hendler, N. (1994) 'Perceptions of asthma severity: the role of negative affectivity', *Journal of Asthma* **31**: 479–484.

Radley, A. (1994) *Making Sense of Illness*, London: Sage.

Roberts, J.C. and Connell, C.M. (2000) 'Illness representations among first-degree relatives of people with Alzheimer disease,' *Alzheimer Disease and Associated Disorders* **14**: 129–136.

Scharloo, M. (2002) 'Illness perceptions, coping and functional status in chronic illness', unpublished Ph.D. thesis, Leiden, The Netherlands.

Scharloo, M. and Kaptein, A.A. (1997) 'Measurement of illness perceptions in patients with chronic somatic disorders: a review,' in K.J. Petrie and J.A. Weinman (eds) *Perceptions of Health and Illness*, Amsterdam: Harwood Academic, pp. 103–154.

Scharloo, M., Kaptein, A.A., Weinman, J.A., Willems, L.N.A. and Rooijmans, H.G.M. (2000a) 'Physical and psychological correlates of functioning in patients with chronic obstructive pulmonary disease,' *Journal of Asthma* **37**: 17–29.

Scharloo, M., Kaptein, A.A., Weinman, J., Bergman, W., Vermeer, B.J. and Rooijmans, H.G.M. (2000b) 'Patients' illness perceptions and coping as predictors of functional status in psoriasis: a 1-year follow-up', *British Journal of Dermatology* **142**: 899–907.

Scharloo, M., Kaptein, A.A., Weinman, J.A., Hazes, J.M., Willems, L.N.A., Bergman, W. and Rooijmans, H.G.M. (1998) 'Illness perceptions, coping and functioning in patients with rheumatoid arthritis, chronic obstructive pulmonary disease and psoriasis', *Journal of Psychosomatic Research* **44**: 573–585.

Schiaffino, K.M., Shawaryn, M.A. and Blum, D. (1998) 'Examining the impact of illness representations on psychological adjustment to chronic illnesses,' *Health Psychology* **17**: 262–268.

Schwarzer, R. and Schwarzer, C. (1996) 'A critical survey of coping instruments,' in M. Zeidner and N.S. Endler (eds) *Handbook of Coping*, New York: Wiley, pp. 107–132.

Skelton, J.R., Thomas, C.P. and Macleod, J.A.A. (2000) 'Teaching literature and medicine to medical students. Part I: the beginning,' *Lancet* **356**: 1920–1922.

Solzhenitsyn, A. (1971) *Cancer Ward;* Harmondsworth, UK: Penguin.

Somerfield, M.R. and McCrae, R.R. (2000) 'Stress and coping research. Methodological challenges, theoretical advances, and clinical applications,' *American Psychologist* **55**: 620–625.

Sontag, S. (1979) *Illness as Metaphor*, New York: Vintage Books.

Stehr, D.E., Klein, B.J. and Murata, G.H. (1991) 'Emergency department return visits in chronic obstructive pulmonary disease: the importance of psychosocial factors', *Annals of Emergency Medicine* **20**: 1113–1116.

Swift, T. L. and Wilson, S. L. (2001) 'Misconceptions about brain injury among the general public and non-expert health professionals: an exploratory study', *Brain Injury* **15**: 149–165.

Trautmann, J. and Pollard, C. (1982) *Literature and Medicine*, Pittsburgh: Pittsburgh University Press.

van den Bos, G.A.M. (1995) 'The burden of chronic diseases in terms of disability, use of health care and healthy life expectancies', *European Journal of Public Health* **5**: 29–34.

van Korlaar, I.M., Vossen, C.Y., Cameron, L.D., Rosendaal, F.R., Bovill, E.G. and Kaptein, A.A. (in review) 'Quality of life in venous thromboembolic disease: a review'.

van Tiel, D., van Vliet, K.P. and Moerman, C.J. (1998) 'Sex differences in illness beliefs and illness behaviour in patients with suspected coronary artery disease', *Patient Education and Counseling* **33**: 143–147.

Veldtman, G.R., Matley, S.L., Kendall, L., Quirk, J., Gibbs, J.L., Parsons, J.M. and Hewison, J. (2000) 'Illness understanding in children and adolescents with heart disease', *Heart* **84**: 395–397.

Verbrugge, L.M. and Patrick, D.L. (1995) 'Seven chronic conditions: their impact on US adults' activity levels and use of medical services', *American Journal of Public Health* **85**: 173–182.

Weaver, T.E. and Narsavage, G.L. (1992) 'Physiological and psychological variables related to functional status in chronic obstructive pulmonary disease', *Nursing Research* **41**: 286–291.

Weinman, J., Petrie, K. J., Moss-Morris, R. and Horne, R. (1996) 'The Illness Perception Questionnaire: a new method for assessing the cognitive representation of illness', *Psychology and Health* **11**: 431–445.

6 Representational beliefs about functional somatic syndromes

Rona Moss-Morris and Wendy Wrapson[1]

Envisage experiencing a range of unpleasant symptoms such as sharp muscle pains, persistent stomach upsets, bad headaches and intense fatigue following a relatively minor illness or injury. As time goes by your symptoms get worse and although you visit your family doctor and various specialists a number of times, they cannot find anything wrong with you. You are convinced you are ill, but nobody seems to believe you. Undoubtedly it would be an extremely worrying and frustrating situation for you, feelings that are shared by a substantial number of patients. Recent surveys suggest that as many as 50 per cent of patients newly referred to outpatient specialist clinics present with medically unexplained symptoms such as these (Gureje *et al.*, 1997; Nimnuan *et al.*, 2001a). 'Medically unexplained symptoms' is a term used to describe physical symptoms which cannot be explained by observable biomedical pathology. When these symptoms are severe enough to significantly interfere with the patient's daily functioning, he or she may be diagnosed with a functional somatic syndrome (FSS).

A number of different FSS have been described. The names of some of the most common syndromes and their key features are presented in Table 6.1. Some of the syndromes, such as chronic fatigue syndrome (CFS) (Fukuda *et al.*, 1994), fibromyalgia (Wolfe *et al.*, 1990) and irritable bowel syndrome (IBS) (Thompson *et al.*, 1999), have well-researched, published diagnostic criteria. These diagnoses are based on a specified symptom profile together with the exclusion of certain medical or psychiatric conditions that may be contributing to the symptoms. The diagnosis of other conditions such as hyperventilation syndrome are more controversial, with some insisting it should be diagnosed using physiological tests of hyperventilation, while others believe a specified symptom profile is more valid (Spinhoven *et al.*, 1993; Vansteenkiste *et al.*, 1991). At the extreme end of the spectrum are illnesses such as multiple chemical sensitivity, which are not recognized as legitimate syndromes by the international medical organizations despite the fact that the diagnosis is popular with patients and with some health care professionals, particularly those who practise alternative medicine (Terr, 1998).

Table 6.1   Common functional somatic syndromes and their key characteristic symptoms

Syndrome	Characteristic symptoms
Chronic fatigue syndrome	Persistent or relapsing fatigue which is not substantially reduced by rest
Fibromyalgia	Persistent musculoskeletal aches, pains and stiffness in specified multiple sites
Irritable bowel syndrome	Abdominal pain and/or bloating that is relieved by defecation and is associated with a change in frequency/consistency of stools
Temporomandibular joint dysfunction	Pain in the face, jaw, or mouth and limitation of jaw movement
Tension headache	Headache or neck pain which is tight or pressing and gets worse as the day progresses
Non-cardiac chest pain	Chest pain which occurs at rest and is not associated with exertion
Hyperventilation	Breathing more than normal in conjunction with symptoms such as dizziness, a pounding heart, numbness or tingling
Premenstrual syndrome	Mood swings, food cravings, breast tenderness and abdominal bloating which occur just before menstruation and disappear soon afterwards
Chronic pelvic pain	Pain in the lower abdomen which is not specifically related to the menstrual cycle
Multiple chemical sensitivity	Adverse symptom reactions to chemical substances at lower levels of exposure than commonly tolerated

The past two decades have seen a sharp increase in the number of published studies on FSS. Most of these studies focus on a particular condition. However, there is increasing recognition of the substantial overlap in the presentations of these illnesses. A recent review of the case definitions of these disorders found that eight definitions contained bloating, abdominal distention, or headache as core symptoms, while six contained fatigue (Wessely *et al.*, 1999). Patients with one FSS frequently meet diagnostic criteria for others (Aaron and Buchwald, 2001). While some argue that the overlap is substantial enough to suggest that the existence of distinct FSS should be re-considered (Nimnuan *et al.*, 2001b), others provide tentative evidence that illnesses such as fibromyalgia, IBS and CFS can be discriminated from one another using latent variable models (Robbins *et al.*, 1997).

The argument concerning 'one or many' FSS is reflected in researchers' beliefs about the aetiology of these conditions (for a review, see Manu,

1998). Proponents of psychological models generally support the idea that FSS reflect common psychopathological processes, while proponents of biological models argue that FSS are distinct entities that are underpinned by specific genetic and biological abnormalities.

An in-depth discussion of the merits of each of these models is beyond the scope of this chapter. It is sufficient to note that although there is some support for each approach, neither provides a complete explanation. The aetiology of FSS may be better understood in terms of more complex biopsychosocial models which incorporate predisposing, precipitating and perpetuating factors. Surawy and colleagues (Suraway *et al.*, 1995) initially developed this model around a series of case studies on CFS patients. They propose that predisposed people may be highly achievement orientated, basing their self-esteem and the respect of others on their abilities to live up to certain high standards. When these people are faced with precipitating factors which affect their ability to perform, such as a combination of excessive stress and an acute biological illness, their initial reaction is to press on and keep coping. This behaviour leads to the experience of ongoing symptoms that may be more closely related to pushing too hard than to the initial illness. However, in making sense of the situation, patients attribute the ongoing symptoms to physiological factors. The common response to a physical illness is rest. However, reduced activity conflicts with achievement orientation and may result in bursts of activity in an attempt to meet expectations. These periodic bursts of activity inevitably exacerbate symptoms and result in failure, which further reinforces the belief that they have a serious illness. As time goes by, efforts to meet previous standards of achievement are abandoned and patients become increasingly preoccupied with their symptoms and illness. This results in chronic disability and the belief that one has an ongoing incurable illness that may eventually be diagnosed as an FSS.

This interactional model has the potential to accommodate both the differences and the overlap between the conditions. The factors that precipitate the disorders may be different. It may be a viral or bacterial infection, an adverse reaction to a particular substance, a musculoskeletal overuse pattern, or a specific injury. Patients may also have different predisposing genetic or biological vulnerabilities for certain disorders (Gillespie *et al.*, 2000), while other predisposing factors such as social desirability and/or high levels of stress may be more common across disorders. However, the necessary common features of these disorders appear to be the perpetuating factors. These factors essentially form part of an illness self-regulatory system as described by Leventhal and colleagues (Leventhal *et al.*, 1997). According to their common-sense model the self-regulatory system is activated by a patient's tendency to attribute symptoms to disease rather than to other factors. This attributional style results in the development of an illness schema, which directs coping behaviours that perpetuate the extent of the symptoms and disability experienced by the patient.

In the following sections we review the literature that has investigated the role of the self-regulatory model in FSS. Much of this research has been conducted on patients with CFS, so this is a focus of the chapter. However, as far as possible we have incorporated findings from other FSS into our discussion. We begin by examining cognitive illness representations in FSS. This is followed by discussions of the relationships between cognitive illness representations, coping and disability, and emotional representations of illness, coping and outcome. In the final sections we provide a brief discussion of the link between self-concept and illness representations in FSS and the role that sociocultural factors play in the development of the illness representations.

Cognitive illness representations in functional somatic syndromes

As described in Chapter 3, patients cluster their ideas about an illness around five components: identity, cause, control/cure, timeline and consequences. Each of these components appears to have specific features in FSS.

Illness identity

Illness identity refers to the label of the illness and the symptoms the patient views as being part of the illness label (Leventhal *et al.*, 1997). It forms the starting point for the development of the illness representation, which typically begins with the experience of symptoms that then triggers a search for an illness label. This search is often fraught with problems for patients with FSS. They frequently describe lengthy delays, disputes or confusion over their diagnosis and a great sense of relief when a diagnosis of a FSS is finally made (Ax *et al.* 1997; Broom and Woodward, 1996). The relief is associated with having something concrete to tackle as well as a legitimisation of suffering. For instance, one patient described how a diagnosis of CFS made her feel better as it let her know what she was up against (Broom and Woodward, 1996). Another felt that the diagnosis proved to others that she was definitely ill (Ax *et al.*, 1997).

The striking feature of most FSS is the large number of symptoms that sufferers associate with the illness. Studies which have compared chronic pelvic pain, fibromyalgia, IBS and CFS patients with matched patient groups with identified medical pathology have found that the functional groups consistently report a significantly higher number of general symptoms (Gomborone *et al.* 1995; McGowan *et al.*, 1998; Weinman *et al.*, 1996; Robbins and Kirmayer, 1990). Why does this happen, when clearly the patients have less medical pathology than the other groups? One explanation in line with Leventhal *et al.*'s (1997) concept of symmetry is that when given a diagnostic label, the individual will seek symptoms consistent with the diagnosis. FSS are associated with a large number of diffuse, ambiguous symptoms so that any normal symptom or bodily sensation such as a sore throat, headache or fatigue may be inadvertently attributed to the illness. A similar misattribution process may occur when patients experience various negative mood states. For instance, non-cardiac chest pain patients may misattribute signs of anxiety such as a pounding heart and sweating to signs of cardiac illness (Avia, 1999). Similar symptoms could be misattributed by hyperventilation patients as signs of a respiratory disorder. In other situations the misattribution may be more concrete whereby negative moods themselves are seen to be symptoms of the illness. For instance, patients with premenstrual syndrome have been shown to experience negative moods throughout the month, but during the premenstrual period they label these mood states as symptoms of their problem (Veeninga and Kraaimaat, 1995).

Examples such as these suggest that it is not only the labelling of symptoms that is important for building up the illness identity in FSS, but also the patients' general interpretation of the meaning of symptoms. A number of studies have shown that FSS patients have a preference for attributing common symptoms to physical factors, rather than to psychological or normative factors (Butler *et al.*, 2001; Dendy *et al.*, 2001; Robbins and Kirmayer, 1991). This tendency appears to be a risk factor for developing an FSS in the first place. Cope *et al.* (1994) found that the most important risk factor for developing CFS after a viral infection was the tendency to make physical attributions for symptoms. A population-based study found that pain-free individuals who reported a wide range of physical symptoms were more at risk of developing fibromyalgia symptoms six months later (McBeth *et al.*, 2001).

Patients with FSS also have a tendency to exaggerate or distort the meaning of symptoms. Studies which have compared CFS patients' performance on concentration and memory tasks with their subjective reports of cognitive symptoms have invariably found that the reports of cognitive difficulty are far greater than the objective test data would suggest (Moss-Morris *et al.*, 1996b). Both chronic pain and CFS patients demonstrate a greater tendency to overgeneralise or catastrophise the consequences of experiencing somatic symptoms when compared to healthy controls (Moss-Morris and Petrie, 1997).

Hypervigilance to symptoms may help to explain the strong illness identity in FSS. Fibromyalgia patients have a significantly lower threshold and tolerance to pain and noise stimuli when compared to patients with rheumatoid arthritis and healthy controls (McDermid *et al.*, 1996), while IBS patients show a hypersensitivity to visceral sensations (Naliboff *et al.*, 1998). Some theorists argue that this hypervigilance is a biological sensory phenomenon. Others suggest that the belief or fear that one has a serious physical illness may lead the perceiver to focus undue attention on somatic information, which in turn may result in a misinterpretation of the symptoms (Naliboff *et al.*, 1998). Certainly, there is some experimental evidence that chronic pain, IBS and CFS patients have an information processing bias for somatic information (Gibbs-Gallagher *et al.*, 2001; Moss-Morris and Petrie, in press; Pincus and Morley, 2001).

Taken together, the literature suggests that FSS patients' strong illness identity may be a function of a tendency to label symptoms in a somatic fashion and to exaggerate the meaning of symptoms. Because FSS labels are often more ambiguous than illnesses with medically recognised symptoms, a large range of physical and emotional symptoms can be misattributed to the patient's disease label. These cognitive processes may be related to a hyper-vigilance to bodily sensations which in itself strengthens the illness identity, by helping patients to notice or identify symptoms in the first place.

Causal beliefs

The label a patient has for his or her illness is crucially important, as it acts as the catalyst around which the other illness representation domains develop. For instance, once people have a label or a diagnosis, they tend to spontaneously develop ideas about the cause of their illness. The difficulty for patients with FSS is that not only are the causes of the illnesses unknown, they are also hotly debated by health professionals. Patients often feel that doctors dismiss the extent of their symptoms because their medical tests invariably come back negative (Peters *et al.*, 1998). There is a strong sense that they are not believed or, worse still, that the doctors see the symp-toms as 'all in the mind'. For the patients, however, the symptoms are real, therefore they must have a cause.

A number of studies have shown that most patients with FSS have a strong conviction that they have a serious physical disease (Gomborone *et al.*, 1995; McGowan *et al.*, 1998; Trigwell *et al.*, 1995). However, the causal models are often quite complex and multifactorial. Typically they include an immune or nervous system that has been damaged in some way, thus allowing the entry of an unidentified or mysterious pathogen (Peters *et al.*, 1998). The damage may occur because of factors such as a virus, stress, injury, or a reaction to allergens or pollutants. Although these models incor-porate psychosocial factors, these tend to be viewed as external rather than internal to the individual and less important than the physical factors. For instance, CFS patients frequently attribute part of their illness to overwork, family and job stress, but they are significantly less likely to make internal attributions for their illness such as 'my own behaviour' or 'my emotional state' when compared with medically ill and depressed patients (Moss-Morris, 1997; Weinman *et al.*, 1996). Only 30 per cent of the illness is attributed to psychosocial factors while the remaining 70 per cent is explai-ned by biological factors (Moss-Morris and Petrie, 2001).

The specific attribution made depends to some extent on the nature of the syndrome, although causal beliefs such as stress and overwork appear to be common to almost all of the FSS. The most popular causal beliefs in chronic headache sufferers include heredity factors, emotional distress, menopause or menstrual problems, diet and an overactive lifestyle (Kraaimaat and Van Schevikhoven, 1988). Patients with temporomandibular disorders attribute their conditions to injury, dental work, inherent structural problems, teeth grinding/clenching and stress (Garro *et al.*, 1994), while CFS patients attribute their condition to a virus, immune dysfunction, pollution or environmental chemicals, diet, overwork and stress (Moss-Morris, 1997). Thus, in making sense of their symptoms, patients may reflect back to possible precipitants of the condition. However, as discussed at the beginning of the chapter, the ongoing symptoms may be more closely associated with perpetuating rather than precipitating factors.

Although most FSS patients will provide definitive statements when asked about what caused their condition, there is a sense that they are seeking a more complete explanation in the hope that this will provide an ultimate cure (Peters *et al.*, 1998). Their dissatisfaction with the causal explanations given to them by doctors leads them to turn to the lay literature, self-help groups or the Internet for support and answers. This literature tends to provide a rather rigid biological view of the illness and is often intolerant of other formulations. Davison and Pennebaker (1997), in their analysis of linguistic patterns of patients' groups on the Internet, found that, when compared with patients with medically explained symptoms, CFS sufferers had the most rigidly defined boundaries about illness prototypes. They were intolerant of any suggestion that psychological factors might be involved in their illness or that psychological treatments such as cognitive behavioural therapy might be helpful.

Timeline and consequences dimensions

Because patients have an illness identity that incorporates a wide range of disparate symptoms, the experience of any symptom or bodily change serves as a constant reminder that their illness is still present. It is not surprising, therefore, that most patients with FSS hold chronic timeline beliefs (Peters *et al.*, 1998; Weinman *et al.*, 1996). Cyclical timeline models are also common. This is particularly evident in premenstrual syndrome, where the condition is by medical definition determined by monthly fluctuations in symptoms (Veeninga and Kraaimaat, 1995). Other patients talk about more random day-to-day fluctuations in symptoms. For example, a patient with chronic pelvic pain told us that she could be feeling fine on one day and then for no apparent reason on the following day she would be unable to move because of the pain.

The cyclical model of the illness appears to be associated with beliefs about the consequences of overactivity. In one study we asked CFS patients what they thought would be the consequence of pushing themselves beyond their present physical state (Petrie *et al.*, 1995). Almost all of the patients reported that their symptoms would be exacerbated and one-third of the patients had highly exaggerated expectations, such as having a total collapse, being bed-ridden for weeks, or even dying.

In general, illnesses that are viewed as chronic are seen by patients as having serious consequences (Moss-Morris *et al.*, 2002). This also appears to be the case in FSS, but in many instances these patients perceive the consequences of their illness to be even more profound than do patients with medically explained symptoms. A study of chronic headache patients showed that patients generally believed that their headaches had a major impact on their lives and that this was not likely to change (Narduzzi *et al.*, 1998). A study comparing fibromyalgia patients with rheumatoid arthritis patients found that although the arthritis group reported significantly higher levels of physical disability, the fibromyalgia group reported that their illness had a greater impact on their ability to perform their daily activities (Robbins and Kirmayer, 1990). Similarly, when compared with patients with rheumatoid arthritis and diabetes, CFS patients perceived the consequences of their illness to be more serious (Weinman *et al.*, 1996).

For many patients, the perception that the illness has profound consequences mirrors reality. A recent review of prognostic studies in CFS found that fewer than 10 per cent of patients appear to return to their pre-morbid levels of functioning with the majority remaining significantly impaired (Joyce *et al.*, 1996). Similarly, follow-up studies of fibromyalgia and non-cardiac chest pain patients show that the majority still experience significant symptomatology with as few as 2 per cent having no symptoms (Potts and Bass, 1993; Wallace, 1997). However, some patients do see aspects of their illness as having had more positive consequences; for example, where the illness has given them the opportunity to disengage from an unpleasant or unsatisfactory lifestyle and a chance to do things in a different way (Ware, 1992).

Control/cure

The control/cure dimension includes beliefs about how one recovers from, or controls, the illness. Although a number of studies have looked at what FSS patients do to control or cope with their illness, few have explored their beliefs in this area. There is some evidence that CFS patients' beliefs in the controllability of their illness and symptoms are equivalent to that of patients with other chronic medical illnesses (Weinman *et al.*, 1996). However, the important factor may not be so much whether or not they believe they can control their illness, but rather what they believe controls their illness. The work by Ray *et al.* (1995) suggests that CFS patients believe that rest and reduced activity is helpful in controlling symptoms, while maintaining activity is unhelpful. Patients often believe that if they don't stop and rest, they will go downhill. This belief tends to develop after a period during which they tried to keep going despite the symptoms, but failed (Ware, 1998).

As with the causal beliefs, patient information may help to maintain the control beliefs. The website www.cfs-news.org advises sufferers that 'the most beneficial program is for the patient to avoid stress and to get lots of rest ... Failure to avoid stress often leads to short-term and long-term set-backs which may be serious.'

The use of alternative medicines is another major theme in sufferers' views of how to control FSS. A plethora of Internet sites exist which offer solutions such as magnetic relaxation pads, the chi machine and an array of natural remedies. A website, www.Odisease.com, claims that MPS-Gold balances the immune system and heals fibromyalgia. Another, www.fibromyalgiacure.com, claims that mercury poisoning causes fibromyalgia and offers a new natural cure.

The data from these sites suggest that beliefs about cure or control closely mirror causal beliefs. The treatments offered fit with sufferers' perceptions that the illness is caused by some sort of physiological imbalance, and so many feel drawn to these medicines that claim to boost their immune system and return them to full health. As traditional medicine is often seen as having no recognised treatment for FSS, it is not surprising that many patients turn to help from alternative practitioners who make promises of miracle cures or dramatic improvements.

The impact of cognitive representations on coping and disability

As mentioned earlier, the self-regulatory model proposes that illness represen-tations guide the ways in which patients cope with their illness, which in turn influence adaptive outcomes. In the case of FSS, illness representations appear to play an even more significant role, insofar as cross-sectional, longitudinal and prospective studies have shown that they influence both the onset of the condition itself as well as the perpetuation of the level of disability and symp-toms experienced by patients (Chalder and Williams, 1998; Cope *et al.*, 1994; Heijmans, 1998; McBeth *et al.*, 2001; Moss-Morris *et al.*, 1996a; Moss-Morris and Petrie, 2001; Robbins and Kirmayer, 1990; Schwartz and Gramling, 1997). The relationship between illness beliefs and ongoing disability is largely accounted for by illness identity, serious consequences and a bias for inter-preting symptoms as physical in nature. The specific causal beliefs appear to be less important in relation to disability, but attributing the illness to external factors appears to protect against feelings of depression and failure (Moss-Morris, 1997; Powell *et al.*, 1990).

FSS patients' behavioural responses to their illness have also been shown to be significant in determining adaptive outcome. We have already seen that most patients believe that limiting activity and stress is an effective way of control-ling the illness. These beliefs are reflected in the protective behaviours common in FSS sufferers (Kraaimaat and Van Schevikhoven, 1988; Mello-Goldner and Jackson, 1999; Moss-Morris and Petrie, 2001; Ray *et al.*, 1997; Van Dulmen *et al.*, 1996). A study of CFS patients showed that 70 per cent had stopped all forms of physically active pastimes, while the remaining 30 percent had substantially reduced such activities because of a possible exacerbation of symptoms (Schweitzer *et al.*, 1995). Limiting behaviours extend to many areas of people's lives, including social interactions. A study of patients with temporomandibular disorders showed that they avoided activities not only to avoid the perceived negative consequences of doing too much, but because of the unpredictability of symptoms (Garro *et al.*, 1994). Avoidance of social commitments and plans was often judged as preferable to letting people down.

Although FSS sufferers may perceive that they are limiting or controlling their symptoms by reducing activity levels, avoidance behaviour does not seem to be an effective way of controlling symptoms. For example, in a study of chronic headache sufferers the level of avoidance behaviour increased with chronicity, even though the level of pain remained constant, suggesting that avoidance behaviour was not instrumental in reducing pain (Philips and Jahanshahi, 1986). CFS studies have shown that limiting activities results in higher levels of functional impairment (Moss-Morris and Petrie, 2001; Ray *et al.*, 1995, 1997; Sharpe *et al.*, 1992). Furthermore, changes in avoidance behaviours and beliefs are strong predictors of improvement following cognitive behavioural therapy for IBS and CFS (Deale *et al.*, 1998; Van Dulmen *et al.*, 1996). Another important feature of reducing or avoiding activity is that these behavioural strategies will help to maintain and strengthen the patient's illness representation. The less patients do the more disabled they feel, which serves to reinforce the belief that the illness has serious consequences. Thus, illness beliefs and coping behaviours become mutually reinforcing.

It is important to note that limiting activity because you believe it is an effective way of controlling illness is not the same as avoiding activity because you have given up dealing with the problem. Our work on CFS suggests that two separate pathways from illness perceptions, to coping and through to disability may exist (Moss-Morris, 1997; Moss-Morris *et al.*, 1996b). CFS patients who hold excessively negative beliefs about the identity, consequences and timeline of their illness tend to give up or withdraw from dealing with the illness. Rather than actively choosing to limit their activity, their negative illness beliefs and stable, external attributions may lead to feelings of helplessness and loss of control, resulting in a passive withdrawal from activity and a heightened negative affect. Conversely, CFS patients with less pessimistic illness beliefs, who nevertheless experience a number of symptoms which they strongly attribute to signs of a physical disease, believe that rest is the effective way of dealing with their symptoms, and as a result choose to limit their exposure to stress and activity. They feel more in control of their illness, are psychologically better adjusted to their condition, but are still unduly disabled.

Emotional representations, coping and disability

Up until now we have focused on patients' cognitive models of their illness and how these may ultimately impact on their adjustment to their condition.

However, patients also have parallel emotional responses or representations of their illness that may have an independent effect on self-regulatory behaviour (Leventhal *et al.*, 1997)

There is some evidence that illness anxiety plays a significant role in determining FSS patients' responses to seeking treatment and the way in which they manage their symptoms. In light of the uncertainty surrounding the aetiology of a FSS sufferer's symptoms, it is not unexpected that anxiety should be a common emotional response. As noted previously, the delay in being given a diagnosis can be extremely distressing to patients. The inability of the medical profession to explain symptoms does not necessarily alleviate this distress. Instead, patients tend to seek a multitude of medical opinions, in an effort to find an explanation for their symptoms (Peters *et al.*, 1998). Treatment seeking is often associated with anxiety about the possible seriousness of the symptoms; for example, the possibility of having cancer (Kettell *et al.*, 1992).

The role of fear in influencing avoidance behaviour has received substantial attention from researchers, particularly in the area of chronic pain. The nature of the fear may well be specific to the particular FSS. In chronic pain, the fear that activity will exacerbate the pain and that the experience of pain signals harm or damage in some way, results in patients avoiding certain activities or guarding and bracing certain parts of the body (Sharp, 2001). Avoidance of activities clearly lead to a disability, while guarding or bracing has a direct effect on the musculature that may in itself aggravate the pain. In the case of IBS, fear of embarrassment rather than fear of the consequences of activity may be more important in determining behaviour. For example, a common symptom of IBS is flatus that can be so embarrassing as to deter sufferers from engaging in social situations. Patients may also be anxious that, in unfamiliar surroundings, if they experience urgency to reach a toilet they will not be able to do so in time (Salkovskis, 1992).

There is sound evidence that fear avoidance beliefs are associated with ongoing disability and unemployment in chronic pain patients (Vlaeyen *et al.*, 1995; Vlaeyen and Linton, 2000). We have also seen that concrete beliefs about the need to rest and avoid stress are related to avoidance behaviours and subsequent disability. As far as we are aware there is no literature investigating the interrelationship between fear avoidance and cognitive avoidance. However, data from cognitive behavioural treatment studies suggest that it is important to address both the fear and the cognition. Treatments that use a carefully graded approach to increasing activity or exercise levels in these patients have shown good results and minimal dropouts (Deale *et al.*, 1997; Fulcher and White, 1997). These studies started at a low level of intensity in keeping with the patients' current levels of activity. Patients were reassured that this level of activity was safe, and the graded process can be seen as a process of desensitisation to the fear of activity. Interventions aimed at restoring function which have tried to get patients to exercise without using a controlled graded approach generally show less dramatic improvement and high drop-out levels (Meyer and Lemley, 2000; Wearden *et al.*, 1998).

The social construction of illness representations in functional somatic syndromes

The data reviewed so far suggest that patients with FSS have a characteristic illness representation, which in many instances differentiates them from patients with other medical illnesses. The question that now arises is where do these representations come from? Self-regulation theory suggests that illness episodes are imbedded within a larger personal and sociocultural context. In the final two sections of this chapter we take a brief look at how self-concept and sociocultural factors may influence the development of the characteristic illness representation in FSS.

Self-schema and illness representations in functional somatic syndromes

At the beginning of this chapter we discussed how an achievement orientation and high personal expectations may predispose people to developing FSS (Surawy *et al.*, 1995). These personality features may be a product of underlying assumptions that form part of a person's self-schema or self-concept (Beck, 1991). Such assumptions might include an underlying belief that in order to be acceptable to others and oneself one needs to achieve at high levels. There is some evidence to support this idea. Retrospective reports from CFS patients and their spouses suggest that prior to their illness the patients were hard-driving individuals (Van Houdenhove *et al.*, 2001). CFS patients also tend to interpret mistakes as equivalent to failure and to believe that failure means losing the respect of others (White and Schweitzer, 2000), while chronic facial pain patients have an unrealistically high expectation of themselves and a strong sense of obligation to others (Schwartz and Gramling, 1997). For these people, integrating their self-concept into a situation where their ability to perform or to help others is threatened, such as an acute illness during a time of stress, is clearly going to pose difficulties. If they attribute their inability to cope to something about themselves then this may lead to a perception of failure, self-criticism and a lowering of self-esteem. One way to protect this from happening is to attribute the symptoms to an external cause. This has the positive effect of protecting the person from feeling they are in any way responsible for failing to live up to expectations.

We have already seen that patients with FSS have a definite tendency to attribute their symptoms to external biological causes and that these attributions are positively related to self-esteem. The protective process of these attributions was also demonstrated in a study that showed how women with

PMS use their symptoms as a strategy to justify failure in academic performance (Mello-Goldner and Jackson, 1999). More work is clearly needed in this area, but it suggests that illness representations in FSS form an integral part of a patient's self-concept. Perceiving oneself as a physically ill person can help to integrate a self which is not coping with the self-concept of one as a competent achievement orientated person.

Sociocultural factors which shape illness representations in functional somatic syndromes

Patients who need to protect themselves by attributing their illness to disease factors can be seen as a reflection of Western society's attitude towards, and misconceptions of, psychological illness. The attitude that a physical disease is more 'valid and deserving' than a psychological one pervades the current media coverage of illnesses such as CFS (MacLean and Wessely, 1994). The opinion that people with depression are just unmotivated, lazy individuals is not uncommon and the lay literature is full of such inaccurate stereotypes. Health professionals are also not immune to such opinions. Engel (2000) argues that the practise of medicine is still dominated by mythical 'either/or' thinking – if symptoms are not viewed as entirely physical then they must be psychological, which also implies that they are less acceptable. The fact that almost all psychological illnesses have biological features is ignored. Furthermore, once a somatic illness is seen to be psychological, doctors frequently make the assumption that the symptoms are imaginary. It is not surprising therefore that FSS patients avoid a psychological label at all costs.

Other social factors such as support groups and the family may help to maintain certain illness beliefs. Examples in earlier parts of this chapter have shown how information on the Internet and from 'chat groups' helps to shape illness beliefs. Similarly, FSS patient support groups represent a strong political movement sanctioning the organic nature of the condition. Active lobbying against psychiatric research is not uncommon and may include anonymous denunciations and allegations sent to funding bodies and medical journals (Wessely, 1997).

The family also plays an important role, as illness perceptions are not restricted to just the person suffering from the illness. The patient's spouse and family have perceptions that influence the way they respond to the patient. For instance, partners who are very solicitous may encourage the patient to accommodate to their illness by taking on the roles the patient feels they can no longer perform (Schmaling and DiClementi, 1995). Thus, supportive partners may unintentionally collude with patients in maintaining their disability.

In summary, sociocultural factors that shape illness representations can occur at multiple levels. Beliefs inherent within our current culture, broader political movements such as patient support groups, and the more immediate family social environment can all play a role. These factors presumably interact with the patients' need to find a way of understanding their illness that will protect their vulnerable self-concept.

Summary and future directions

The data reviewed in this chapter suggest that FSS patients' cognitive illness representations contain a strong illness identity and a belief that the illness is caused primarily by a biological agent. Patients see their illness as serious and chronic, and believe that the best way to keep the illness under control is to avoid stress and activity. Avoidance is also related to affective responses such as fear of embarrassment or fear of overdoing things. These self-regulatory processes appear to be related to ongoing disability and symptom experience in these disorders.

Taken together these data provide support for our initial argument: that core common self-regulatory processes might mediate between a precipitating event and the experience of ongoing symptoms and disability in patients with FSS. However, in drawing conclusions, some important caveats need to be made. First, although individual studies in this area suggest that overlap exists, there is almost no literature comparing self-regulatory processes across FSS. Studies showing overlap between these illnesses have almost exclusively focused on the symptom presentations of these disorders. Future work needs to focus not only on the similarity of the perpetuating self-regulatory factors, but on some of the differences, particularly in relation to possible predisposing or precipitating factors.

Secondly, how these changes in beliefs and behaviour may impact on physiology have been largely omitted from this review. There are a number of studies which have shown that FSS are accompanied by a range of small but significant changes to the neuroendocrine and immune systems (for reviews see Moss-Morris and Petrie, 2000; Manu, 1998). These changes may be a result of prolonged inactivity, or an erratic routine that is a consequence of accommodating to the symptoms on a day-to-day basis. Thus a vicious cycle of events may arise, whereby behaviours lead to changes in physiology which themselves result in symptoms, once again confirming the belief that the illness is serious and ongoing. However, to date there is no empirical literature in this area and this is clearly an important area for future investigation.

Note

1   Correspondence should be addressed to Rona Moss-Morris, Health Psychology, Faculty of Medical and Health Sciences, The University of Auckland, Private Bag 92019, Auckland, New Zealand. E-mail: r.moss-morris@auckland.ac.nz

References

Aaron, L.A. and Buchwald, D. (2001) 'A review of the evidence for overlap among unexplained clinical conditions', *Annals of Internal Medicine* **134**: 868–881.

Avia, M.D. (1999) 'The development of illness beliefs', *Journal of Psychosomatic Research* **47**: 199–204.

Ax, S., Gregg, V.H. and Jones, D. (1997) 'Chronic fatigue syndrome: sufferers' evaluation of medical support', *Journal of the Royal Society of Medicine* **90**: 250–254.

Beck, A.T. (1991) 'Cognitive therapy: a 30-year retrospective', *American Psychologist* **46**: 368–375.

Broom, D.H. and Woodward, R.V. (1996) 'Medicalisation reconsidered: toward a collaborative approach to care', *Sociology of Health and Illness* **18**: 357–378.

Butler, J.A., Chalder, T. and Wessely, S. (2001) 'Causal attributions for somatic sensations in patients with chronic fatigue syndrome and their partners', *Psychological Medicine* **31**: 97–105.

Chalder, T. and Williams, C. (1998) 'Illness attribution, illness behaviour and personality in chronic fatigue syndrome', *Bailliere's Clinical Psychiatry* **3**: 407–417.

Cope, H., David, A., Pelosi, A. and Mann, A. (1994) 'Predictors of chronic "postviral" fatigue', *The Lancet* **344**: 864–868.

Davison, K.P. and Pennebaker, J.W. (1997) 'Virtual narratives: illness representations in online support groups', in K.J. Petrie and J. Weinman (eds) *Perceptions of Health and Illness*, Amsterdam: Harwood Academic, pp. 463–486.

Deale, A., Chalder, T. and Wessely, S. (1998) 'Illness beliefs and treatment outcome in chronic fatigue syndrome', *Journal of Psychosomatic Research* **45**: 77–83.

Deale, A., Chalder, T., Marks, I. and Wessely, S. (1997) 'Cognitive behavior therapy for chronic fatigue syndrome: a randomized controlled trial', *American Journal of Psychiatry* **154**: 408–414.

Dendy, C., Cooper, M. and Sharpe, M. (2001) 'Interpretation of symptoms in chronic fatigue syndrome', *Behaviour Research and Therapy* **39**: 1369–1380.

Engel, C.C., Jr (2000) 'Unexplained physical symptoms: medicine's "dirty little secret" and the need for prospective studies that start in childhood', *Psychiatry: Interpersonal and Biological Processes* **63**: 153–159.

Fukuda, K., Straus, S.E., Hickie, I., Sharpe, M.C., Dobbins, J.G., Komaroff, A. and International Chronic Fatigue Syndrome Study Group (1994) 'The chronic fatigue syndrome: a comprehensive approach to its definition and study', *Annals of Internal Medicine* **121**: 953–959.

Fulcher, K.Y. and White, P.D. (1997) 'Randomised controlled trial of graded exercise in patients with the chronic fatigue syndrome', *British Medical Journal* **314**: 1647–1652.

Garro, L.C., Stephenson, K.A. and Good, B.J. (1994) 'Chronic illness of the temporomandibular joints as experienced by support-group members', *Journal of General Internal Medicine* **9**: 372–378.

Gibbs-Gallagher, N., Palsson, O.S., Levy, R.L., Meyer, K., Drossman, D.A. and Whitehead, W.E. (2001) 'Selective recall of gastrointestinal-sensation words: evidence for a cognitive-behavioral contribution to irritable bowel syndrome', *American Journal of Gastroenterology* **96**: 1133–1138.

Gillespie, N.A., Zhu, G., Heath, A., Hickie, I.B. and Martin, N.G. (2000) 'The genetic aetiology of somatic distress', *Psychological Medicine* **30**: 1051–1061.

Gomborone, J., Dewsnap, P., Libby, G. and Farthing, M. (1995) 'Abnormal illness attitudes in patients with irritable bowel syndrome', *Journal of Psychosomatic Research* **39**: 227–230.

Gureje, O., Simon, G.E., Ustun, T.B. and Goldberg, D.P. (1997) 'Somatization in cross-cultural perspective: a World Health Organization study in primary care', *American Journal of Psychiatry* **154**: 989–995.

Heijmans, M. (1998) 'Coping and adaptive outcome in chronic fatigue syndrome – importance of illness cognitions', *Journal of Psychosomatic Research* **45**: 39–51.

Joyce, E., Blumenthal, S. and Wessely, S. (1996) 'Memory, attention, and executive function in chronic fatigue syndrome', *Journal of Neurology, Neurosurgery and Psychiatry* **60**: 495–503.

Kettell, J., Jones, R. and Lydeard, S. (1992) 'Reasons for consultation in irritable bowel syndrome: symptoms and patient characteristics', *British Journal of General Practice* **42**: 459–461.

Kraaimaat, F.W. and van Schevikhoven, R.E.O. (1988) 'Causal attributions and coping with pain in chronic headache sufferers', *Journal of Behavioral Medicine* **11**: 293–302.

Leventhal, H., Benyamini, Y., Brownlee, S., Diefenbach, M., Leventhal, E.A., Patrick-Miller, L. and Robitaille, C. (1997) 'Illness representations: theoretical foundations', in K.J. Petrie and J. Weinman (eds) *Perceptions of Health and Illness*, Amsterdam: Harwood Academic, pp. 19–45.

MacLean, G. and Wessely, S. (1994) 'Professional and popular views of chronic fatigue syndrome', *British Medical Journal* **308**: 776–777.

Manu, P. (1998) *Functional Somatic Syndromes: Etiology, Diagnosis and Treatment*, Cambridge: Cambridge University Press.

McBeth, J., Macfarlane, G.J., Benjamin, S. and Silman, A.J. (2001) 'Features of somatization predict the onset of chronic widespread pain: results of a large population-based study', *Arthritis and Rheumatism* **44**: 940–946.

McDermid, A.J., Rollman, G.B. and McCain, G.A. (1996) 'Generalized hypervigilance in fibromyalgia: evidence of perceptual amplification', *Pain* **66**: 133–144.

McGowan, L.P.A., Clark-Carter, D.D. and Pitts, M.K. (1998) 'Chronic pelvic pain: a meta-analytic review', *Psychology and Health* **13**: 937–951.

Mello-Goldner, D. and Jackson, J. (1999) 'Premenstrual syndrome (PMS) as a self-handicapping strategy among college women', *Journal of Social Behavior and Personality* **14**: 607–616.

Meyer, B.B. and Lemley, K.J. (2000) 'Utilizing exercise to affect the symptomology of fibromyalgia: a pilot study', *Medicine and Science in Sports and Exercise* **32**: 1691–1697.

Moss-Morris, R. (1997) 'The role of illness cognitions and coping in the aetiology and maintenance of the chronic fatigue syndrome', in K.J. Petrie and J. Weinman (eds) *Perceptions of Health and Illness*, Amsterdam: Harwood Academic, pp. 411–439.

Moss-Morris, R. and Petrie, K.J. (1997) 'Cognitive distortions of somatic experiences: revision and validation of a measure', *Journal of Psychosomatic Research* **43**: 293–306.

—— (2000) *Coping with Chronic Fatigue Syndrome*, London: Routledge.

—— (2001) 'Discriminating between chronic fatigue syndrome and depression: a cognitive analysis', *Psychological Medicine* **31**: 469–479.

—— (in press) 'Experimental evidence for interpretative but not attention biases toward somatic information in patients with chronic fatigue syndrome', *British Journal of Health Psychology*.

Moss-Morris, R., Petrie, K.J. and Weinman, J. (1996a) 'Functioning in chronic fatigue syndrome: do illness perceptions play a regulatory role?' *British Journal of Health Psychology* **1**: 15–25.

Moss-Morris, R., Petrie, K.J., Large, R.G. and Kydd, R.R. (1996b) 'Neuropsychological deficits in chronic fatigue syndrome – artifact or reality?' *Journal of Neurology, Neurosurgery and Psychiatry* **60**: 474–477.

Moss-Morris, R., Weinman, J., Petrie, K.J., Horne, R., Cameron, L.D. and Buick, D. (2002) 'The Revised Illness Perception Questionnaire (IPQ-R)', *Psychology and Health* **17**: 1–6.

Naliboff, B.D., Munakata, J., Chang, L. and Mayer, E.A. (1998) 'Toward a biobehavioral model of visceral hypersensitivity in irritable bowel syndrome', *Journal of Psychosomatic Research* **45**: 485–492.

Narduzzi, K.J., Nolan, R.P., Reesor, K., Jackson, T., Spanos, N.P., Hayward, A.A. and Scott, H.A. (1998) 'Preliminary investigation of associations of illness schemata and treatment-induced reduction in headaches', *Psychological Reports* **82**: 299–307.

Nimnuan, C., Hotopf, M. and Wessely, S. (2001a) 'Medically unexplained symptoms: an epidemiological study in seven specialities', *Journal of Psychosomatic Research* **51**: 361–367.

Nimnuan, C., Rabe-Hesketh, S., Wessely, S. and Hotopf, M. (2001b) 'How many functional somatic syndromes?' *Journal of Psychosomatic Research* **51**: 549–557.

Peters, S., Stanley, I., Rose, M. and Salmon, P. (1998) 'Patients with medically unexplained symptoms: sources of patients' authority and implications for demands on medical care', *Social Science and Medicine* **46**: 559–565.

Petrie, K., Moss-Morris, R. and Weinman, J. (1995) 'The impact of catastrophic beliefs on functioning in chronic fatigue syndrome', *Journal of Psychosomatic Research* **39**: 31–37.

Philips, H.C. and Jahanshahi, M. (1986) 'The components of pain behaviour report', *Behaviour Research and Therapy* **24**: 117–125.

Pincus, T. and Morley, S. (2001) 'Cognitive-processing bias in chronic pain: a review and integration', *Psychological Bulletin* **127**: 599–617.

Potts, S.G. and Bass, C.M. (1993) 'Psychosocial outcome and use of medical resources in patients with chest pain and normal or near-normal coronary arteries: a long term follow-up study', *Quarterly Journal of Medicine* **86**: 583–593.

Powell, R., Dolan, R. and Wessely, S. (1990) 'Attributions and self-esteem in depression and chronic fatigue syndromes', *Journal of Psychosomatic Research* **34**: 665–673.

Ray, C., Jefferies, S. and Weir, W.R.C. (1995) 'Coping with chronic fatigue syndrome: illness responses and their relationship with fatigue, functional impairment and emotional status', *Psychological Medicine* **25**: 937–945.

—— (1997) 'Coping and other predictors of outcome in chronic fatigue syndrome – a 1-year follow-up', *Journal of Psychosomatic Research* **43**: 405–415.

Robbins, J.M. and Kirmayer, L.J. (1990) 'Illness worry and disability in fibromyalgia syndrome', *International Journal of Psychiatry in Medicine* **20**: 49–63.

—— (1991) 'Attributions of common somatic symptoms', *Psychological Medicine* **21**: 1029–1045.

Robbins, J.M., Kirmayer, L.J. and Hemami, S. (1997) 'Latent variable models of functional somatic distress', *The Journal of Nervous and Mental Disease* **185**: 606–615.

Salkovskis, P.M. (1992) 'Somatic problems', in K. Hawton, P.M. Salkovskis, J. Kirk and D.M. Clark (eds) *Cognitive Behaviour Therapy for Psychiatric Problems: A Practical Guide*, Oxford: Oxford University Press, pp. 235–276.

Schmaling, K.B. and DiClementi, J.D. (1995) 'Interpersonal stressors in chronic fatigue syndrome: a pilot study', *Journal of Chronic Fatigue Syndrome* 1: 153–157.

Schwartz, S.M. and Gramling, S.E. (1997) 'Cognitive factors associated with facial pain', *Cranio – The Journal of Craniomandibular Practice* 15: 261–266.

Schweitzer, R., Kelly, B., Foran, A., Terry, D. and Whiting, J. (1995) 'Quality of life in chronic fatigue syndrome', *Social Science and Medicine* 41: 1367–1372.

Sharp, T.J. (2001) 'The "safety seeking behaviours" construct and its application to chronic pain', *Behavioural and Cognitive Psychotherapy* 29: 241–244.

Sharpe, M., Hawton, K., Seagroatt, V. and Pasvol, G. (1992) 'Follow up of patients presenting with fatigue to an infectious diseases clinic', *British Medical Journal* 305: 147–152.

Spinhoven, P., Onstein, E. J., Sterk, P.J. and Le Haen-Versteijnen, D. (1993) 'Discordance between symptom and physiological criteria for the hyperventilation syndrome', *Journal of Psychosomatic Research* 37: 281–289.

Surawy, C., Hackmann, A., Hawton, K. and Sharpe, M. (1995) 'Chronic fatigue syndrome: a cognitive approach', *Behaviour Research and Therapy* 33: 535–544.

Terr, A.I. (1998) 'Multiple chemical sensitivities', in P. Manu (ed.) *Functional Somatic Syndromes: Etiology, Diagnosis and Treatment*, Cambridge: Cambridge University Press, pp. 202–218.

Thompson, W.G., Longstreth, G.F., Drossman, D.A., Heaton, K.W., Irvine, E.J. and Müller-Lissner, S.A. (1999) 'Functional bowel disorders and functional abdominal pain', *Gut* 45: 43–47.

Trigwell, P., Hatcher, S., Johnson, M., Stanley, P. and House, A. (1995) ' "Abnormal" illness behaviour in chronic fatigue syndrome and multiple sclerosis', *British Medical Journal* 311: 15–18.

van Dulmen, A.M., Fennis, J.F.M. and Bleijenberg, G. (1996) 'Cognitive-behavioral group therapy for irritable bowel syndrome: effects and long term follow-up', *Psychosomatic Medicine* 58: 508–514.

van Houdenhove, B., Neerinckx, E., Lysens, R., Vertommen, H., van Houdenhove, L., Onghena, P., Westhovens, R. and D'Hooghe, M.B. (2001) 'Victimization in chronic fatigue syndrome and fibromyalgia in tertiary care – a controlled study on prevalence and characteristics', *Psychosomatics* 42: 21–28.

Vansteenkiste, J., Rochette, F. and Demedts, M. (1991) 'Diagnostic tests of hyperventilation syndrome', *European Respiratory Journal* 4: 393–399.

Veeninga, A. and Kraaimaat, F.W. (1995) 'Causal attributions in premenstrual syndrome', *Psychology and Health* 10: 219–228.

Vlaeyen, J.W.S. and Linton, S.J. (2000) 'Fear-avoidance and its consequences in chronic musculoskeletal pain: a state of the art', *Pain* 85: 317–332.

Vlaeyen, J.W.S., Kole-Snijders, A.M.J., Boeren, R.G.B. and van Eek, H. (1995) 'Fear of movement/(re)injury in chronic low back pain and its relation to behavioral performance', *Pain* 62: 363–372.

Wallace, D.J. (1997) 'The fibromyalgia syndrome', *Annals of Medicine* 29: 9–21.

Ware, N.C. (1992) 'Suffering and the social construction of illness: the delegitimation of illness experience in chronic fatigue syndrome', *Medical Anthropology Quarterly* 6: 347–361.

—— (1998) 'Sociosomatics and illness course in chronic fatigue syndrome', *Psychosomatic Medicine* **60**: 394–401.

Wearden, A.J., Morriss, R.K., Mullis, R., Strickland, P.L., Pearson, D.J., Appleby, L., Campbell, I.T. and Morris, J.A. (1998) 'Randomised, double-blind, placebo-controlled treatment trial of fluoxetine and graded exercise for chronic fatigue syndrome', *British Journal of Psychiatry* **172**: 485–490.

Weinman, J., Petrie, K.J., Moss-Morris, R. and Horne, R. (1996) 'The Illness Perception Questionnaire: a new method for assessing the cognitive representation of illness', *Psychology and Health* **11**: 431–445.

Wessely, S. (1997) 'Chronic fatigue syndrome: a twentieth century illness?' *Scandinavian Journal of Work, Environment and Health* **23**: 17–34.

Wessely, S., Nimnuan, C. and Sharpe, M. (1999) 'Functional somatic syndromes: one or many?' *The Lancet* **354**: 936–939.

White, C. and Schweitzer, R. (2000) 'The role of personality in the development and perpetuation of chronic fatigue syndrome', *Journal of Psychosomatic Research* **48**: 515–524.

Wolfe, F., Smythe, H.A., Yunus, M.B., Bennett, R.M., Bombardier, C., Goldenberg, D.L., Tugwell, P., Campbell, S.M., Abeles, M. and Clark, P. (1990) 'The American College of Rheumatology 1990 criteria for the classification of fibromyalgia. Report of the Multicenter Criteria Committee', *Arthritis and Rheumatism* **33**: 160–172.

7 Treatment perceptions and self-regulation

Robert Horne[1]

In affluent countries, the biggest slice of the health care pie is consumed by the management of chronic diseases such as coronary heart disease, diabetes and asthma. Here, good outcomes depend as much on self-management as on good medical care and, for most of these conditions, self-management hinges on the appropriate use of medicines. But it is thought that over a third of prescribed medicines are not taken as directed (Horne, 1997). Non-adherence is a concern for those providing, receiving or funding care because it not only entails a waste of resources but also a missed opportunity for therapeutic benefit. However, few effective interventions to facilitate adherence have been developed (Haynes *et al.*, 1996) and there is increasing interest in understanding why so many patients do not adhere to treatment and in finding ways of helping patients get the most from prescribed medication.

Using medication appropriately is essentially dependent on two factors: *ability* and *motivation*. A variety of barriers may reduce one's ability to follow treatment instructions as intended, such as a misunderstanding of the instructions, difficulties fitting the regimen into one's daily schedule, forgetting to take doses, an inability to use the treatment because of impaired manual dexterity or other problems, and so on. These factors are undoubtedly important and were the main focus of much of the early adherence research. However, one reason why interventions to promote adherence have met with little success is that they tend to target ability issues and ignore motivation. Psychologists have developed several theoretical models to explain how people initiate and maintain actions to preserve or improve health status. These models share the common assumption that the motivation to engage in and maintain health-related behaviours arises from beliefs that influence the interpretation of information and experiences and guide behaviour (see Conner and Norman (1996) for a review of social cognition models, and Horne and Weinman (1998) for an overview of theoretical approaches to adherence).

In social cognition models, the antecedents of behaviour are specified at the *process* level (e.g., attitudes inform intentions and behaviour). However, if these models are to be used to develop interventions then they are likely to be more effective if they also specify *content* (e.g., the *beliefs* that contribute to the positive or negative evaluations that constitute the *attitude* towards the behaviour). This is recognised within the common-sense model of self-regulation (CSM) where the content as well as the process of illness representations is specified (see Leventhal *et al.*, this volume, Chapter 3). However, theoretical models of health behaviour are likely to be more explanatory as their contents become more specific to the behaviour in question (Fishbein and Ajzen, 1975). Although representations of coping procedures are implicit within the CSM (Leventhal *et al.*, 1998), a more explicit consideration of treatment perceptions is warranted when the model is applied to adherence. A better understanding of how people perceive treatments will improve our ability to operationalise theories of social cognition and self-regulation and enhance their power to explain variations in adherence and to guide the development of interventions to improve use of health care resources. This chapter presents a simple framework for conceptualising the specific treatment beliefs that may be particularly salient to adherence and summarises empirical evaluations of this framework in relation to medication adherence. It will then consider the role of treatment beliefs in the self-regulation of illness and outline the implications for future research and practice.

Beliefs about medicines

Given the importance of medicines in health care and the apparently widespread problem of non-adherence, surprisingly little attention has focused on how people perceive and make decisions about medicines. There are a few notable exceptions (for a review see Horne, 1997). A dozen or so interview-based studies have focused on people's perceptions of medications (Arluke, 1980; Coulter, 1985; Gabe and Lipshitz Phillips, 1982; Morgan and Watkins, 1988). It was striking that certain representations of medicines (e.g., that medicines are addictive and accumulate within the body to produce 'long-term' effects) seemed to be common across locations and cultures (USA, UK and Europe) and illness/treatment categories (Horne, 1997).

These studies and our own preliminary interviews conducted with people with chronic medical problems (cardiovascular disease and renal impairment) led us to question whether or not the commonly expressed beliefs about prescribed medicines could be summarised as simple core themes. We therefore began our investigation of medication beliefs by exploring the principal components underlying representations of prescribed medication. These analyses showed that, although patients' ideas about medicines are often complex and diverse, many of the beliefs relating to prescribed medication could be grouped under two categories: perceptions of *necessity* or personal need for the treatment, and *concerns* about negative effects. This analysis formed the basis for the development and validation of the Beliefs about Medicines Questionnaire (BMQ; Horne *et al.*, 1999a). This provided a valid and reliable way of quantifying the perceived need for prescribed medication (the Specific Necessity scale) and common concerns about potential adverse effects (the Specific Concerns scale), and facilitated research into how these beliefs relate to uptake and adherence to medication. The BMQ also assesses more general beliefs about the extent to which medicines are perceived as intrinsically harmful substances that are overused by doctors (the General Harm and General Overuse scale); the topic of beliefs about medicines in general will be dealt with in more detail later.

Necessity and concerns: common-sense representations of prescribed medication

Necessity

Our initial studies of over 500 patients with a range of chronic medical conditions showed that people who were prescribed the same medication for the same condition differed in their perceptions of personal need for it. Necessity beliefs are operationalised by statements such as 'My health depends on this medicine', 'These medicines protect me from becoming worse', and 'Without these medicines I would be very ill'. Although scores on the Necessity scale tended to be positively skewed, there was considerable variation, with about 20 per cent reporting doubts about the necessity of their medication (scores below the scale mid-point).

It is worth noting that perceived necessity is not a form of efficacy belief. Although views about efficacy are likely to contribute to perceived need, the constructs are not synonymous. We might believe that a treatment will be effective but yet not perceive a personal need for it. In a recent study of beliefs about anti-retroviral medication, the belief that it would be effective at controlling HIV progression explained about 25 per cent of the variance in perceived need (Horne *et al.*, 2002). Conversely, we might perceive a strong need for a treatment that we perceive to be only moderately effective, because we know that it is the only treatment that is available. We can anticipate that necessity beliefs are more closely related to adherence than beliefs about treatment efficacy.

Concerns

The Specific Concerns scale of the BMQ assesses core concerns regarding concrete experiences of unpleasant symptoms as medication 'side effects' and the disruptive effects of medication on daily living, as well as more abstract worries that regular use could lead to dependence or that the medication would accumulate within the body and lead to obscure, long-term effects. These core concerns seem to be fairly generic and relevant across a range of disease states and cultures, and they are typically endorsed by over a third of participants (as indicated by scores above the scale mid-point; Horne *et al.*, 2001a; Horne *et al.*, 2001c; Horne and Weinman, 1999, 2002; Webb *et al.*, 2001). In recent studies, we have augmented the core items of the Concerns scale with additional items (elicited during pilot interviews) representing concerns that are specific to the particular class of medicine (Horne and Weinman, 2002); for example, worries that corticosteroid inhalers prescribed for asthma will result in weight gain (Hand and Bradley, 1996) or that regular use of analgesic medication now will make it less effective in the future (Gill and Williams, 2001).

Costs and benefits, pros and cons, and treatment efficacy

Necessity beliefs and concerns are evaluative summations of the personal *salience* of the potential benefits and costs identified in the health belief model (Rosenstock, 1974) and pros and cons specified in the transtheoretical model (Prochaska and DiClemente, 1984). To arrive at a necessity belief we ask the question: 'To what extent do I need this benefit?' The concerns construct includes the impact of costs (e.g., 'I worry about side effects'). Likewise, we might identify a number of pros and cons about a treatment but we then need to decide how important these pros and cons are: 'How much do I need the pros and how worried am I about the cons?'

Do necessity beliefs and concerns influence uptake and adherence to treatment?

Initial studies of asthma, kidney disease, coronary heart disease, cancer (Horne and Wienman, 1999) and HIV/AIDS (Horne *et al.*, 1999c) confirmed our simple hypothesis that reported adherence would be positively correlated with *necessity* beliefs and negatively correlated with *concerns*. The correlations were moderate in size (*r*'s ranging from 0.2–0.4), but given the complexity of adherence with its many potential antecedents and the considerable measurement error present in the studies, they suggested the relationships were worthy of further investigation. Other researchers have also found that necessity beliefs and concerns relate to adherence (e.g., Chambers *et al.*, 1999; Ezzy *et al.*, 1998). Subsequent regression analyses of combined data from four illness groups (asthma, renal, cardiac and cancer) revealed that medication beliefs were stronger predictors of reported adherence than clinical or demographic variables and accounted for 19 per cent of the explained variance in adherence (Horne and Wienman, 1999). In a separate sample of 100 community-based asthma patients, hierarchical regression analysis showed that medication necessity and concerns added a further 17 per cent to the explained variance in reported adherence after taking account of the effects of demographic and clinical variables (6 per cent explained variance) and illness perceptions (13 per cent explained variance; Horne and Weinman, 2002).

The cross-sectional design of the studies meant that we could not be sure about causality, but in prospective studies necessity beliefs and concerns elicited at baseline were predictive of medication adherence following myocardial infarction (Horne *et al.*, 1999b), and in studies of initial uptake (Horne *et al.*, 2001a) and subsequent adherence to HAART for HIV/AIDS (Horne *et al.*, in review). Preliminary analyses of data from on-going studies, in which we have used other methods for assessing adherence (such as electronic monitors and prescription redemption rates), also suggest that adherence is related to the necessity-concerns construct (Dr Janet Butler, personal communication, 2002; James, 1999; Waller and Weinman, 2001). In studies where we have controlled for the effects of negative affect, we found that it does not significantly alter the observed relationship between medication beliefs and reported adherence (Horne *et al.*, 2002). We now need to test these relationships in experimental studies. If the relationship is causal, and assuming other factors are held constant, then a change in beliefs should result in a change in adherence.

Balancing necessity against concerns: the common-sense logic of non-adherence

The research outlined above suggests that many patients are faced with a *necessity-concerns dilemma* when deciding whether or not to adhere to treatment advice. Medication can be perceived as a 'double-edge sword' whereby the potential benefit is compromised by the tendency to harm. For some, the dilemma is made more acute by the fact that efficacy and toxicity appear to go hand in hand and that more effective medicines implicitly have more severe side effects (Gabe and Lipshitz Phillips, 1982; Leventhal *et al.*, 1986).

The separate effect of necessity beliefs and concerns on medication usage is illustrated in Figure 7.1, which shows the mean scores for BMQ necessity and concerns scales for HIV-positive individuals offered highly active anti-retroviral treatment (HAART; Horne *et al.*, 2001a). Uptake and refusal of HAART was predicted by perceived need and concerns elicited shortly after the treatment offer (as part of routine clinical practice, patients were offered treatment and then had about fourteen days in which to consider whether or not to accept). It was interesting that the relative difference between mean concerns and mean necessity scores was much greater for those refusing HAART than for those accepting.

This pattern raises interesting questions about the interplay between perceived necessity and concerns in adherence decisions at the individual level. In deciding whether or not to follow treatment advice, strong perceptions of personal need might 'override' concerns about adverse effects. Conversely, moderate levels of concern might stimulate avoidance of medication if necessity beliefs are relatively low. We surmised that the way in which individuals judged their personal need for treatment *relative* to their concerns would have a greater influence on adherence and uptake than

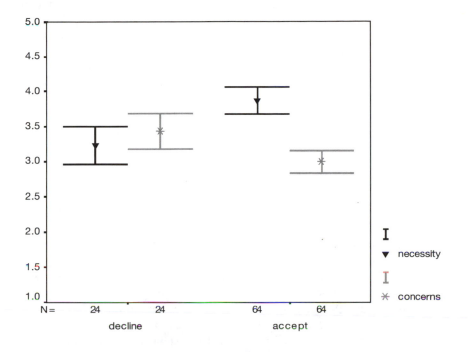

Figure 7.1 Beliefs about HAART (necessity and concerns) among consecutive HIV-positive individuals who chose either to accept (*N* = 64) or to decline (*N* = 24) the treatment

Source: Horne *et al.* (in review).

necessity beliefs and concerns considered in isolation. We have begun to explore how individuals rate their level of concern about medication *relative* to their perceived need for it by computing a simple necessity–concerns differential (NCD) for each participant (obtained by subtracting the individual's scores on the necessity and concerns scales). Although the NCD provides a crude indicator of the relative importance of needs and concerns, the measure has methodological limitations. The separate scales are scored from 1–5, but we cannot be sure that a score on one scale equates to the same score on the other; or indeed that the distances between scores are equivalent within and between the scales.

Nevertheless, NCD scores (which were normally distributed) were more strongly correlated with reported adherence than necessity beliefs and concerns considered in isolation (Horne and Weinman, 1999). Moreover, patients who attained higher scores on the concerns scale than on the necessity scale were significantly less adherent. These preliminary results justify further research designed to develop more robust numerical representations of how individuals balance the risks and benefits of medication and how this process might influence adherence. We expect the relationship to be complex and to vary between and within individuals. The 'cost-benefit analysis' may be implicit rather than explicit. In some situations, non-adherence could be the result of a deliberate strategy to minimise harm by taking less medication. Alternatively, it might simply reflect the fact that patients who do not perceive their medication to be important (low scores on the necessity scale) may be more likely to forget to take it. The impact of perceptions of treatment on adherence is also likely to be influenced by beliefs about adherence, such as the importance of strict adherence to achieve the desired outcome. A key question here is 'What can I get away with?' (Siegel *et al.*, 2000)

Treatment beliefs and self-regulation theory

This section focuses on implications for self-regulation theory of the work discussed above. Although most of the research has focused on medication, the theoretical implications are likely to extend to other treatments such as surgery, physiotherapy and rehabilitation classes. Here I suggest a symbiotic relationship between the necessity-concerns framework and the CSM in explaining variations in treatment uptake and adherence. The CSM helps us to understand the process by which treatment perceptions influence adherence. Moreover, the *contents* of illness representations relate to the perceptions of treatment necessity. Equally, treatment perceptions and the necessity-concerns framework can be used to extend the explanatory power of the CSM in relation to treatment adherence (Horne, 1997; Horne and Weinman, 2002).

Deciding that we need a treatment

We can differentiate between two stages in the process by which we arrive at our views about our need for a particular treatment. First, we must be convinced that our condition warrants treatment. Here perceptions of treatment necessity are intimately bound up with representations of the illness as the individual attempts to achieve common-sense coherence. If we agree that our condition warrants treatment, then we have to decide whether the specific treatment is the one that we need as opposed to some other treatment. In order to make this decision we must judge the relative necessity of different treatment options – for example, our prescribed medication versus alternative options such as receiving acupuncture, a homeopathic remedy or a pill made from powdered dolphin's penis (these are apparently available at several retail outlets in London; Richardson, 1995). Treatments such as medication or surgery that are perceived to carry risks or costs must be balanced against perceived need as previously discussed. These evaluations are likely to be influenced by a range of factors including our 'prototypic' beliefs about classes of treatments, the past experiences of ourselves and others, social and cultural norms, and information we receive from various sources. These factors are likely to influence perceptions of both necessity and concerns, as well as judgments of need relative to concerns, and will be considered in more detail later.

Does the condition warrant treatment? Perceptions of illness inform beliefs about treatment necessity

Symptom perceptions

Initial perceptions of treatment necessity and subsequent appraisal are influenced by symptom experiences and expectations. At one level, symptoms may stimulate medication use by acting as a reminder or by reinforcing beliefs about its necessity. Conversely, the absence of severe symptoms might cause one to interpret one's condition as more benign that it actually is and hence to doubt the need for treatment (Horne *et al.*, 2001a; Siegel and Gorey, 1997). Moreover, symptoms may stimulate concerns if they are interpreted as side effects or, alternatively, as evidence that the medication is not working (Leventhal *et al.*, 1986).

Consequences and timeline

As the person searches for a coherent explanatory model of the illness, symptom experiences inform representations of timeline and personal consequences and also perceptions of treatment necessity (Horne and Weinman, 2002). People strive to attain 'common-sense' coherence between their perceptions of illness and treatment. For example, patients who perceive their asthma to be a cyclical rather than a chronic disease are likely to doubt the necessity of their preventer inhaler and thus not use it sufficiently (Horne and Weinman, 2002). Messages about treatment necessity are likely to be more convincing if they are consistent with the individual's representation of their illness.

Causal attributions

One might expect perceptions of personal need for individual treatment options to be influenced by beliefs about the putative causes of the illness. Changing diet may be perceived to be more necessary than taking medication if the person believes that diet causes the illness. However, we have not found causal beliefs to be strongly related to medication necessity in our studies of chronic illness. This may be because we have found relatively little variation in causal beliefs between patients with the same chronic illness.

Control/cure

The relationship between treatment beliefs and beliefs about illness control are specific to the type of control belief. Necessity beliefs are positively correlated with beliefs that the illness will be controlled by treatment (a form of efficacy belief) but not with other control beliefs (e.g. chance/fate or personal control over illness; Horne and Weinman, 2002). The relationship between beliefs about illness controllability and treatment need is conditional on the perception that the particular treatment is appropriate.

Prototypic beliefs about diseases influence perceptions of treatment necessity

Bishop and Converse (1986) suggest that people's schemata of diseases can be thought of as idealised representations of the symptoms and attributes associated with different diseases. These prototypes serve as standards against which people match and evaluate information about experienced symptoms. Prototypic beliefs about diseases are also likely to influence perceptions of treatment necessity. Patients will be less convinced of their need for treatment if their experience of symptoms and perceptions of cause, timeline, consequences and controllability do not match expectations derived from prototypic beliefs about the illness. This point is illustrated by a recent study exploring the reasons why people with HIV refused treatment with HAART. Evidence-based guidelines for the optimum time at which to initiate HAART stipulate viral load (a marker for disease activity) and CD4 count (an indicator of immune status) as key indicators for when HAART is clinically indicated. However, receiving 'abstract' information about personal CD4 and viral load lab results was less persuasive than more 'concrete' symptom experiences. A common reason given by interviewees for refusing HAART was that they were experiencing few, if any, of the symptoms that they associated with late-stage HIV/AIDS (Cooper *et al*.., in press). Their experiences (of feeling fine) did not match their prototypic beliefs about when HAART would be necessary.

Treatment as a health threat: processing concerns about adverse effects

Medication concerns are evaluative summations of representations of the threat posed by medication. In common with illness representations, they have a cognitive and an emotional dimension. Cognitive representations of treatment threat are likely to share a similar structure to illness representations. Unpleasant symptoms may be (correctly or incorrectly) labelled as side effects of the medication and the expectation of medication side effects may initiate a search for confirmatory symptoms. This is demonstrated by the 'nocebo' effect whereby people report symptomatic 'side effects' after taking a pharmacologically inert placebo (Crow *et al.*, 1999).

Representations of the risks (and benefits) of medication will also comprise beliefs about the timeline for the onset and duration of effects, their likely consequences and the potential for control or cure (Leventhal *et al.*, 1998). The need to take treatments may also be interpreted as a threat to self-identity, as compromising fundamental notions of self-reliance (Conrad, 1985) or self-efficacy in being able to resist the progress of disease (Cooper *et al.*, 2002).

Parallel processing of cognitive and emotional representations of treatment

Just as with illness representations, cognitive and emotional aspects of treatment representations are processed in parallel. Beliefs that taking medication will result in unpleasant side effects may be a source of anxiety and worry. In some situations, such as the prescription of intensive cancer chemotherapy or radical surgery, people may fear the treatment more than the illness. They may therefore decide that it is better to reject treatment that might prolong life, on the grounds that it might diminish the quality of life.

An extended self-regulation model

Figure 7.2 shows the relevance of treatment perceptions to the CSM. It suggests that, when the coping procedure in question involves decisions about treatment, then the model should be extended to include treatment perception as well as illness representations. There is preliminary empirical support for the utility of the approach in explaining adherence to medication (Horne et al., 2001a). The key to the numbered paths shown in the diagram is as follows: (1) symptom experiences and information trigger treatment perceptions, depending on attribution of cause – for example, illness attribution reinforces treatment necessity, attribution to side-effects reinforces concerns; (2) parallel processing of cognitive and emotional representations of treatment – for example, 'Having to take this treatment worries me'; (3) illness perceptions and treatment beliefs have an internal logic as the individual strives for common-sense coherence; (4) treatment perceptions influence adherence – adherence and non-adherence are both types of coping procedures; (5) the outcome of adherence/non-adherence is appraised with subsequent reinforcement or change in treatment representations.

Origins of perceived need and concerns

General beliefs about classes of treatment: 'treatment prototypes'

Perceptions of specific medicines are related to more general beliefs about medicines as a whole (Horne *et al.*, 1999a). When asked to talk about medicines, people appear to access schema relating to medicines as a *class* of treatments that share certain general properties (Britten, 1994; Echabe *et al.*, 1992). Many patients and student volunteers have a fairly negative view of medicines as a whole, perceiving them as generally harmful substances that are overused by doctors (Horne *et al.*, 1999a; Horne *et al.*, 2001b). Moreover, the dangerous aspects of medication are often linked to their chemical/

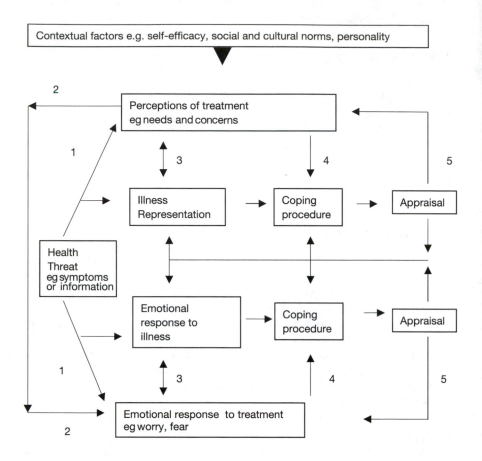

Figure 7.2 Treatment perceptions and the common-sense model of self-regulation

unnatural origins and a greater concern about the potential adverse effects of prescribed medication (Horne *et al.*, 1999a) and are also related to non-adherence (Peters *et al.*, 2001). General beliefs about a class of treatments might inform a patient's expectations of a newly prescribed treatment and represent a source of bias in the attribution of symptom causes in situations of symptom ambiguity (e.g., where the symptoms may be medication side effects, illness-related, or signs of ageing; Siegel *et al.*, 1999).

We can only speculate on the origins of this schema. One possibility is that information about a particular medicine (e.g., speculation in the press that anti-depressants are 'addictive') might feed into a 'general schema' from which the conclusion 'most medicines are addictive' is then extrapolated. Negative experiences with medicines in the past (one's own or those of significant others) are also likely to have an effect. Negative views about medicines in general appear to be related to a broader world-view that is suspicious of chemicals in food and the environment (Gupta and Horne, 2001), and that perceives complementary therapies (e.g. homeopathy/herbalism) as safer and more 'natural' (Horne *et al.*, 1999a). This world-view appears to be related to an increasing suspicion of science, medicine and technology in general within Western culture (Horne *et al.*, 2001b; Petrie and Wessely, 2002). Suspicions of medicines, chemicals and related 'modern health worries' are associated with the use of complementary therapies and with the rejection of medication (Gupta and Horne, 2001; New and Senior, 1991; Petrie *et al.*, 2001).

General schema about medicines also influence perceptions of specific necessity. Positive views about medication may lead to inappropriate demands for prescriptions. This could be particularly problematic in developing countries if expensive pharmaceuticals (such as antibiotics) are purchased for the treatment of routine or self-limiting conditions (such as uncomplicated diarrhoea) for which simpler and cheaper treatments are adequate (Haak, 1988).

Perceptions of personal sensitivity to medication

Leventhal and colleagues (personal communication, 2002) have developed a *sensitive soma* scale to measure individual differences in perceptions of personal sensitivity and susceptibility to the adverse effects of medication. People who view themselves as being particularly sensitive to the adverse effects of medication have stronger concerns about their prescribed medication and tend to perceive medicines in general as intrinsically harmful and overused by doctors (Horne, 1997). We know little about the origins of sensitive soma beliefs, but they may arise from more general perceptions of oneself and one's hardiness, and from past experiences (of oneself and of others).

Perceptions of personal resilience

Determining the necessity of a treatment may also be influenced by notions of self. There has been disappointingly little research in this area, but perceptions that one can resist the progress of disease by drawing on sources of 'inner strength', 'hardiness' or by keeping a 'positive outlook' all emerged as reasons for rejecting HAART in interviews with over 100 HIV-positive men (Cooper *et al.*, 2002). At present, we know little about the role of optimistic bias in treatment decisions.

Demographic variables

In studies to date, medication beliefs do not appear to be strongly or consistently influenced by age and gender. There are some exceptions. In a recent survey of over 1300 people with inflammatory bowel disease, those over 45 years old had stronger medication concerns and greater doubts about necessity than those under 45 years old. Older patients were also more adherent. We do not know whether this reflects an age-related tendency to risk aversion or simply an age-related reporting bias (paper in preparation). Cultural factors appear to be important. In one study, British students who identified themselves as having an Asian (rather than European) cultural background had more negative beliefs about medicines (paper in preparation). Although the investigation of dispositional variables as antecedents of beliefs and adherence is interesting, we have focused our attention on variables that are more likely to be amenable to change.

Conclusions and implications

Medication beliefs are important determinants of adherence. The necessity-concerns construct provides a simple framework for operationalising key beliefs relating to adherence within the context of theories of social cognition and self-regulation. However, our understanding is by no means complete. For example, we know little about how people process information about the risks of treatment and about how this is balanced against perceived need. Moreover, the argument for a treatment belief approach has so far focused on the patient and yet the practitioners' perceptions of treatment may also affect behaviour outcomes. Research on practitioner beliefs is clearly warranted.

Clinicians must recognise that many patients start with considerable suspicions about modern medicines and these beliefs may influence how information about medicines is interpreted and acted upon (Berry *et al.*, 1998). Knowledge about how people perceive medication could also inform the type of written information provided to patients. Patients' perceptions of their illness and treatment may not readily emerge in medical consultations, and we need brief interventions that help clinicians to elicit and respond to patients' perceptions of their illness and treatment. We are currently evaluating approaches based on the necessity-concerns and self-regulatory framework. An awareness of patients' perceptions of treatment offers the potential for a better understanding of patients' response to illness and treatment with major implications for research and practice.

Notes

1   Thanks to Carol, Eddie and Oscar for supporting the production of this chapter with liberal doses of family time. I am also grateful to Vanessa Cooper, Jane Clatworthy and Grace Gallantry for helpful comments on an earlier draft. Correspondence concerning this chapter should be addressed to Robert Horne, Centre for Health Care Research, University of Brighton, BN1 9PH, UK. E-mail: r.horne@brighton.ac.uk

References

Arluke, A. (1980) 'Judging drugs: patients' conceptions of therapeutic efficacy in the treatment of arthritis', *Human Organization* **39**: 84–88.

Berry, D.C., Michas, I.C. and De Rosis, F. (1998) 'Evaluating explanations about drug prescriptions: effects of varying the nature of information about side effects and its relative position in explanations', *Psychology and Health* **13**: 767–784.

Bishop, G.D. and Converse, S.A. (1986) 'Illness representations: a prototype approach', *Health Psychology* **5**: 95–114.

Britten, N. (1994) 'Patients' ideas about medicines: a qualitative study in a general practice population', *British Journal of General Practice* **44**: 465–468.

Chambers, C.V., Markson, L., Diamond, J.J., Lasch, L. and Berger, M. (1999) 'Health beliefs and compliance with inhaled corticosteroids by asthmatic patients in primary care practices', *Respiratory Medicine* **93**: 88–94.

Conner, M. and Norman, P. (1996) *Predicting Health Behaviour: Research and Practice with Social Cognition Models*, Buckingham: Open University Press.

Conrad, P. (1985) 'The meaning of medications: another look at compliance', *Social Science and Medicine* **20**: 29–37.

Cooper, V., Horne, R., Gellaitry, G., Lambert, N. and Fisher, M. (2002) 'Perceptions of HAART among HIV-positive men who have been recommended treatment', *HIV Medicine* **3**: 186.

Cooper, V., Buick, D., Horne, R., Lambert, N., Gellaitry, G. and Leake, H. (2002) 'Perceptions of HAART among those who have declined a treatment offer: preliminary results from an interview-based study,' *AIDS Care* **14**: 319–328.

Coulter, A. (1985) 'Decision making and the pill: the consumer's view', *British Journal of Family Planning* **11**: 98–103.

Crow, R., Gage, H., Hampson, S., Hart, J., Kimber, A. and Thomas, H. (1999) 'The role of expectancies in the placebo effect and their use in the delivery of health care: a systematic review', *Health Technology Assessment* **3**: 1–96.

Echabe, A.E., Guillen, C.S. and Ozmaiz, J.A. (1992) 'Representations of health, illness and medicines: coping strategies and health promoting behaviour', *British Journal of Clinical Psychology* **31**: 339–349.

Ezzy, D.E., Bartps, M.R., O de Visser, R. and Rosenthal, D. (1998) 'Antiretroviral uptake in Australia: medical attitudinal and cultural correlates', *International Journal of STD and AIDS* **9**: 579–586.

Fishbein, M. and Ajzen, I. (1975) *Belief, Attitude, Intention and Behavior: An Introduction to Theory and Research*, Reading, MA: Addison Wesley.

Gabe, J. and Lipshitz Phillips, S. (1982) 'Evil necessity? The meaning of benzodiazepine use for women patients from one general practice', *Sociology of Health and Illness* **4**: 201–209.

Gill, A. and Williams, A.C.D. (2001) 'Preliminary study of chronic pain patients' concerns about cannabinoids as analgesics', *The Clinical Journal of Pain* **17**: 245–248.

Gupta, K. and Horne, R. (2001) 'The influence of health beliefs on the presentation and consultation outcome in patients with chemical sensitivities,' *Journal of Psychosomatic Research* **50**: 131–137.

Haak, H. (1988) 'Pharmaceuticals in two Brazilian villages: lay practices and perceptions', *Social Science and Medicine* **27**: 1415–1427.

Hand, C.H. and Bradley, C. (1996) 'Health beliefs of adults with asthma: toward an understanding of the difference between symptomatic and preventive use of inhaler treatment', *Journal of Asthma* **33**: 331–338.

Haynes, R.B., McKibbon, K.A. and Kanani, R. (1996) 'Systematic review of randomised clinical trials of interventions to assist patients to follow prescriptions for medications', *Lancet* **348**: 383–386.

Horne, R. (1997) 'Representations of medication and treatment: advances in theory and measurement', in K.J. Petrie and J.A. Weinman (eds) *Perceptions of Health and Illness*, Amsterdam: Harwood Academic, pp. 155–188.

Horne, R. and Weinman, J. (1998) 'Predicting treatment adherence: an overview of theoretical models', in L. Myers and K. Midence (eds) *Adherence to Treatment in Medical Conditions*, London: Harwood Academic, pp. 25–50.

—— (1999) 'Patients' beliefs about prescribed medicines and their role in adherence to treatment in chronic physical illness', *Journal of Psychosomatic Research* **47**: 555–567.

—— (2002) 'Self-regulation and self-management in asthma: exploring the role of illness perceptions and treatment beliefs in explaining non-adherence to preventer medication', *Psychology and Health* **17**: 17–32.

Horne, R., Cooper, V. and Fisher, M. (in review) 'Predicting non-adherence to HAART: the role of patients' doubts about personal need and concerns about potential adverse effects'.

Horne, R., Weinman, J. and Hankins, M. (1999a) 'The beliefs about medicines questionnaire: the development and evaluation of a new method for assessing the cognitive representation of medication', *Psychology and Health* **14**: 1–24.

Horne, R., Cooper, V., Fisher, M. and Buick, D. (2001a) 'Beliefs about HIV and HAART and the decision to accept or reject HAART', *HIV Medicine* **2**: 195.

Horne, R., Cooper, V., Weinman, J. and Fisher, M. (2002) 'Predicting acceptance of highly active antiretroviral treatment (HAART): the role of the patients' perceptions of illness and treatment', in *Proceedings of XIV International AIDS Conference*, Barcelona 7–12 July, Monduzzi Editore: 251–254.

Horne, R., Frost, S., Hankins, M. and Wright, S. (2001b) ' "In the eye of the beholder": pharmacy students have more positive perceptions of medicines than students of other disciplines', *International Journal of Pharmacy Practice* **9**: 85–89.

Horne, R., James, D., Weinman, J. and Vincent, R. (1999b) 'Patients' beliefs about medicines predict adherence to treatment following first myocardial infarction (MI)', in *Proceedings of the Annual Conference, Division of Health Psychology*, University of Leeds, UK: British Psychological Society.

Horne, R., Pearson, S., Leake, H., Fisher, M. and Weinman, J. (1999c) 'Do patients' beliefs about HAART influence adherence?' in *Proceedings of the British HIV Association Annual Conference*, Cambridge, UK.

Horne, R., Sumner, S., Jubraj, B., Weinman, J. and Taube, D. (2001c) 'Haemodialysis patients' beliefs about treatment: implications for adherence to medication and dietary/fluid restrictions', *International Journal of Pharmacy Practice* **9**: 169–175.

James, D. (1999) 'The role of patients' perceptions of illness and treatment in myocardial infarction', unpublished Ph.D. thesis, University of Brighton, UK.

Leventhal, H., Leventhal, E.A. and Contrada, R.J. (1998) 'Self-regulation, health and behavior: a perceptual-cognitive approach', *Psychology and Health* **13**: 717–733.

Leventhal, H., Easterling, D.V., Coons, H.L., Luchterhand, C.M. and Love, R.R. (1986) 'Adaption to chemotherapy treatments', in B.L. Andersen (ed) *Women with Cancer: Psychological Perspectives*, New York: Springer Verlag, pp. 172–203.

Morgan, M. and Watkins, C.J. (1988) 'Managing hypertension: beliefs and responses to medication among cultural groups', *Sociology of Health and Illness* **10**: 561–578.

New, S.J. and Senior, M.L. (1991) ' "I don't believe in needles": qualitative aspects of a study into the uptake of immunisation in two English health authorities', *Social Science and Medicine* **33**: 509–518.

Peters, K.F., Horne, R., Kong, F., Francomano, C.A. and Biesecker, B.B. (2001) 'Living with Marfan Syndrome 2. Medication adherence and physical activity modification', *Clinical Genetics* **60**: 283–292.

Petrie, K.J. and Wessely, S. (2002) 'Modern worries, new technology and medicine', *BMJ* **324**: 690–691.

Petrie, K.J., Sivertsen, B., Hysing, M., Broadbent, E., Moss-Morris, R., Eriksen, H.R. and Ursin, H. (2001) 'Thoroughly modern worries: the relationship of worries about modernity to reported symptoms, health and medical care utilization', *Journal of Psychosomatic Research* **51**: 395–401.

Prochaska, J.O. and DiClemente, C.C. (1984) *The Transtheoretical Approach: Crossing Traditional Boundaries of Change*, Homewood, IL: Irwin.

Richardson, P. (1995) 'Placebos: their effectiveness and modes of action', in A. Broome and S. Llewellyn (eds) *Health Psychology: Processes and Applications*, London: Chapman Hall, pp. 75–98.

Rosenstock, I. (1974) 'The health belief model and preventative health behaviour', *Health Education Monographs* **2**: 354–386.

Siegel, K. and Gorey, E. (1997) 'HIV infected women: barriers to AZT use', *Social Science Medicine* **45**: 15–22.

Siegel, K., Dean, L. and Schrimshaw, E.W. (1999) 'Symptom ambiguity among late-middle-aged and older adults with HIV', *Research on Ageing* **21**: 595–618.

Siegel, K., Schrimshaw, E.W. and Raveis, V.H. (2000) 'Accounts for non-adherence to antiviral combination therapies among older HIV-infected adults', *Psychology, Health and Medicine* **5**: 29–42.

Waller, J. and Weinman, J. (2001) *Patients' Illness and Treatment Beliefs and their Relation to Treatment Compliance in Asthma*, report for the NHS R&D Programme on Asthma Management, Department of Health.

Webb, D.G., Horne, R. and Pinching, A.J. (2001) 'Treatment-related empowerment: preliminary evaluation of a new measure in patients with advanced HIV disease', *International Journal of STD and AIDS* **12**: 103–107.

Part III
Emotional processes

8 Anxiety, cognition, and responses to health threats

Linda D. Cameron[1]

Illness represents a fundamental threat to survival and well-being, and few life events are more capable of eliciting anxiety and fear. Other affective experiences such as depression, anger, and even joy also occur over the course of many illness experiences, but anxiety generally plays a predominant role. This chapter focuses on how anxiety arousal shapes and directs the cognitions and behavioral responses involved in health and illness self-regulation.

There is a tendency to regard anxiety as responsible for inducing irrational and maladaptive responses in health threat situations. Yet this orientation is at odds with the general understanding that the emotional system evolved as an adaptive set of mechanisms for promoting survival. Anxiety plays a crucial role in motivating goal-related behaviors, delegating physiological and psychological resources for action, and providing feedback regarding our progress in attaining goals (Carver and Scheier, 1998; Mayne, 1999). Anxiety alters perceptual, cognitive, and behavioral tendencies to achieve these tasks, and whether or not these effects are conducive to well-being will depend on both the situation and the individual's abilities to regulate them. Understanding anxiety's effects on cognitive and behavioral responses to health threats will facilitate efforts to develop intervention techniques for shaping arousal responses in ways that promote health and well-being.

I will consider anxiety's influence on illness cognition and behavior from a perspective that integrates the emotion regulation principles identified by Leventhal's common-sense model (CSM) of health threat regulation (Leventhal *et al.*, this volume, Chapter 3) with those delineated in Scheier and Carver's general model of behavioral self-regulation (Scheier and Carver, this volume, Chapter 2; Carver and Scheier, 1998). In particular, I focus on how anxiety arousal, construed by Scheier and Carver as reflecting the activation of a behavioral avoidance system, alters the cognitive and behavioral processes identified in the CSM. Following a brief overview of anxiety and self-regulation theory, I discuss how anxious states shape the development of illness representations, coping responses, and health habits by activating specific perceptual, cognitive, and behavioral processes. Next, I consider the role of trait anxiety in illness cognition and self-regulation. Trait anxiety is

associated with distinctive qualities arising from psychophysiological characteristics and lifelong experiences of anxiety proneness, and so it is not
surprising that state and trait effects of anxiety often have distinctive self-
regulatory influences (Eysenck, 1997). Finally, I discuss intervention techniques aimed at facilitating anxiety regulation as a means of promoting adjustment and physical health.

Anxiety and cognition: self-regulation theory and physiology

Empirical developments on the distinctive, yet highly interactive nature of
the cognition and emotion systems underscore the need for models that
capture the reciprocal influences of cognitions and affects (Forgas, 2000b;
Leventhal, 1984). The CSM highlights the interactive nature of illness cognitions and anxious distress with its delineation of two parallel and partially
independent processes: cognitive processes for regulating the objective health
threat, and emotion-focused processes for regulating anxiety and fear.
According to the CSM, illness-relevant stimuli (e.g., bodily symptoms and
diagnoses) elicit both the development of a cognitive representation of the
health threat and an emotional representation of anxiety and fear. These
representations guide the formation of coping procedures, and appraisals of
coping outcomes are used to modify representations and further coping
efforts. Both cognitive (problem-focused) and emotion-focused processes
operate at an abstract, conceptual level and a concrete, perceptual level. For
example, illness representations and emotion representations will incorporate both abstract knowledge and concrete imagery. These cognitive and
emotional processes are highly interactive, with bi-directional links.
Representations and threat appraisals can shape anxiety and fear responses;
in turn, anxiety can affect perceptions of threat cues, representation development, selection of coping strategies, and selection of criteria for outcome
appraisals.

The proposed dual-process nature of cognitive and emotional processes is
consistent with evidence that cognition and emotion involve distinct, yet highly
interactive neural substrates (see Leventhal, 1984; Zajonc, 2000). The neural
structures underlying emotion processing and memory involve amygdala-based
circuits that are tuned to biologically significant triggers, whereas the neural
structures involving semantic memory, abstract thinking, problem-solving, and
related cognitive processes are hippocampus-centered, with circuits involving
frontal and other cortical areas (Metcalfe and Jacobs, 1998). These systems are
in constant interaction as they simultaneously process information regarding
emotionally evocative stimuli.

Further insights into the nature of anxiety influences on cognitive behavioral processes are provided by theoretical models of behavioral avoidance
and approach motivational systems. Carver and Scheier's (1998) model
represents a modification of the motivational systems theory developed by
Gray (1987), and it integrates ideas from other researchers as well (see

Carver *et al.*, 2000). According to the Carver and Scheier (1998) model, the behavioral avoidance system responds to cues of threat or punishment with the activation of anxiety and associated psychophysiological processes that facilitate actions for avoiding the feared states. These processes include a narrowing of attention, increased scanning for and attention to threat-relevant stimuli, and preparedness of the hypothalamic motor system for sudden action to move oneself away from a feared outcome or state. Low activation, on the other hand, corresponds with the experience of relief. The behavioral approach system, in contrast, is oriented to activating and coordinating approach tendencies. Triggered by cues of reward, this system is associated with elation (at high activation levels) and depression (at low activation levels). These motivational systems have distinctive neurophysiological substrates, with the avoidance system involving activity in the septo-hippocampal system and areas in the right anterior cortex, and the activation system involving positive emotion processing in the left anterior cortex (Gray, 1987; Sutton and Davidson, 1997). Threat appraisals also elicit patterns of cardiovascular responses that differ from those elicited by challenge appraisals, further demonstrating that threat-induced distress involves a distinctive system of physiological responding (Blascovich and Mendes, 2000).

The emotional process arm of the CSM reflects activation of the behavioral avoidance system in response to health threat cues. Considering the perceptual, cognitive, goal activation, and behavioral readiness patterns associated with this behavioral avoidance system within the context of the CSM framework enables us to further delineate how these processes influence the contents of illness representations and the selection of coping strategies. To the extent that individuals experience different levels of anxiety arousal in health threat situations, their representations and coping decisions will be shaped to varying degrees by these behavioral avoidance processes.

Influences of anxiety on the construction of illness representations

Anxiety arousal is likely to influence the formation of the key attributes of illness representations: beliefs about identity (particularly symptoms), timeline (illness duration), consequences (severity of outcomes), cause, and control (potential for disease cure or control). There are several routes by which anxiety can influence these representational attributes. First, anxiety-related changes in perceptual processes may enhance detection of and attention to illness-related cues. Anxiety may also elicit more subtle information processing effects, such as priming anxiety-related memories and concepts and amplifying concrete-experiential processing. Additionally, anxious distress may play an informational role in evaluating illness-related experiences. For example, someone who feels anxious about a physical therapy regimen may interpret the anxiety as a gut-level indicator that she can't do it. These attention, processing, and informational effects of anxious distress on representation development are considered in the following sections.

Anxiety influences on perception and attention

Evidence substantiates the hypothesis that anxiety increases perceptual sensitivity and attention to threatening stimuli (Öehman *et al.*, 2001), suggesting that anxiety arousal could enhance attention to health threat cues such as symptoms. Such attentiveness would increase the amount of information available for representation development; for example, attention to symptoms would provide input for developing and refining identity (symptom) beliefs. Interestingly, there is strong evidence that experimentally-induced sad and depressed moods (compared to induced happy moods) increase reports of physical symptoms (Croyle and Uretsky, 1987; Salovey and Birnbaum, 1989), but there is little evidence that induced anxiety has these effects. State anxiety is correlated with higher levels of reported symptoms in field studies (Leventhal *et al.*, 1996; Watson and Pennebaker, 1989), but these increments in symptom reports may reflect anxiety-induced symptoms or increased susceptibility to illnesses (Cohen *et al.*, 1995). Although evidence confirms that trait anxiety is associated with greater symptom sensitivity (as discussed in a later section), we lack evidence confirming that state anxiety promotes sensitivity to symptoms and other illness cues.

If anxiety about a health threat does enhance monitoring for associated symptoms, then there are likely to be beneficial consequences in terms of increased accuracy in reports of symptom characteristics used for diagnosis and disease monitoring. These effects seem particularly favorable in light of evidence that ill patients typically under-report symptoms (Mayne, 1999). On the other hand, anxiety arousal may undermine the accuracy of identity beliefs if anxiety-induced sensations add confusion to symptom interpretation efforts. Anxiety can induce gastrointestinal disturbances, heart rate awareness (Katkin, 1985), and other visceral changes, and these sensations may make it difficult to determine which symptoms are illness-related and which are not. Heightened anxiety can also have the detrimental effect of exacerbating the painfulness of symptoms (Ahles *et al.*, 1983; Plaghaus *et al.*, 2001), although extreme anxiety experienced during traumatic events (e.g., surgery) can induce analgesic effects through the release of beta-endorphins (deBruin *et al.*, 2001).

Anxiety can further enhance the perceptual processing of threat cues by inhibiting the disengagement of attention. Supporting evidence reveals that individuals who are induced to feel anxious are less able than non-anxious individuals to withdraw their attention from threatening cues in order to attend to non-threatening cues (Fox *et al.*, 2001). When faced with a health threat, sustained attention can enhance the amount of information integrated into illness representations. However, by reducing one's ability to disengage from threatening health information (such as worrying symptoms), anxiety can provoke rumination and intrusive thoughts that undermine functioning and well-being (Lerman *et al.*, 1993).

Anxiety influences on information processing strategies

Anxiety can also influence illness representations through its automatic, subconscious effects on a variety of information processing strategies. Anxiety promotes the in-depth, systematic processing of relevant information, including the systematic strategies of directed processing and substantive processing (Clore *et al.*, 1994; Forgas, 2000a). Directed processing involves biased evaluations of information in ways that support favored positions. In the context of health threat situations, anxiety is likely to direct information processing in a self-protective manner. For example, individuals with metastatic cancer may tend to process information about alternative treatments in ways that support their curative potentials. Directed processing of health information often involves the engagement of various defensive bias mechanisms for protecting one's sense of security, as discussed by Wiebe and Korbel (this volume, Chapter 9).

Yet individuals facing health threats want to act in the most optimal, health-protective manner, and so they are motivated to engage in substantive processing – that is, open and effortful reasoning aimed at developing accurate evaluations of information. Forgas (2000a) proposes that affective states 'infuse' substantive processing by facilitating the retrieval of affect-consistent memories through priming. As his research demonstrates, these effects lead to the counter-intuitive phenomenon whereby the more an emotionally aroused individual attempts to formulate accurate evaluations through careful consideration of information, the greater the affective influence on the evaluations (see Forgas, 2000b). Through these substantive processing effects, anxiety arousal can increase the emotional, threatening contents integrated into an illness representation. For example, anxiety may lead to more symptoms being associated with the illness identity and more catastrophic consequence beliefs.

Substantive processing and directed processing are likely to operate simultaneously when individuals confront health threat information, as they must balance the motivation to act in the most optimal manner with motivations to reduce distress. The former motivation prompts open, extensive evaluation of information, whereas the latter can prompt biases to interpret information as indicative that one will be safe. These simultaneous processes can explain some complex and seemingly contradictory patterns of cognitions and appraisals. For example, worried individuals may develop more threatening beliefs about illness consequences and timeline, yet they may develop greater faith in potential treatments or cures.

The simultaneous effects of worry-induced directed processing and worry-infused substantive processing on the formation of illness-related beliefs were observed in a study of responses to information about genetic testing for breast cancer risk by women who were unfamiliar with this test (Cameron and Diefenbach, 2001). These women, after completing a cancer-worry measure, read one of several messages about the genetic test and its psychosocial advantages (e.g., positive test results can promote protective action, normal test results can provide reassurance) and disadvantages (e.g., positive test results can be traumatic for individuals and their families). Regardless of the message contents, women with high (versus low) cancer worry responded to the messages with stronger consequence beliefs that testing would induce emotional distress. Worry appears to have infused substantive considerations so as to enhance beliefs that the procedure would be traumatic. Yet women with high (versus low) worry also expressed greater interest in obtaining testing and more positive beliefs that testing would lead to better health protection. Worry appears to have motivated directed processing to generate beliefs that this new procedure will help to control cancer progression. These information processing effects may partially account for the observed associations between cancer worry and the uptake of genetic testing among at-risk individuals (Lerman *et al.*, 1997).

In addition to influencing substantive processing of new information, anxiety can also infuse elaborations of recalled material so that distressing memories become more extreme over time. Representations of symptoms, consequences, and other illness attributes may evolve through substantive processing as prior illness episodes are recalled and evaluated. In a study by Kent (1985), patients attending a dental appointment completed an anxiety measure and then rated their experience of pain during the dental procedure. Three months later, they were asked to indicate how much pain they had experienced during the appointment. Although low-anxious patients gave reports that were similar to their original reports, high-anxious patients reported much greater pain than they had reported at the appointment. High-anxious patients apparently continued to revise and elaborate their memories of symptom pain following the event.

By promoting systematic and in-depth information processing, anxiety and worry foster the development of more extensive and detailed representations (Cameron, 1997). These extensive representations may have many effects, including the development of a strong resistance to attitude-discrepant material. For example, a woman with high cancer worry may develop an intricate causal model of cancer and associated control beliefs regarding methods for reducing its development (e.g., through vitamins). Because of her extensive representation ('expertise'), she may be particularly adept at developing counter-arguments about the potential veracity of messages that question or refute her beliefs (e.g., messages refuting the association of vitamins with cancer development). Extensive representations can also enhance one's propensity to take protective action, such as seeking care for atypical symptoms (Cameron *et al.*, 1993) and using disease detection procedures (Cameron, 1997).

Anxiety influences on concrete processing

Another anxiety-induced shift in information processing is an enhanced focus on concrete-perceptual information. Evidence suggests that anxious, avoidance-oriented states promote concrete, spatial processing and inhibit the verbal processing of information; in contrast, approach-oriented states (positive affects) induce the opposite pattern (Gray, 2001). Anxiety may facilitate the integration of concrete and imagery-laden information into illness representations, but it may also cause difficulties in integrating the abstract-conceptual content of informational presentations. During a clinic visit, for example, an anxious patient may absorb many concrete images (pictorial information, non-verbal cues from her doctor, etc.) but process and retain little of the doctor's explanations of the condition and its treatment. The enhanced integration of concrete images into representations may have some beneficial effects, as concrete images can be powerful prompts to take protective action. For example, the mental image of one's doctor holding out a bottle of red pills can be a more powerful prompt to take the medication than the abstract knowledge about the need to take it. Of course, vivid images of threatening consequences can elicit avoidance responses that undermine protective actions. Yet the associated difficulties in integrating conceptual information such as verbal instructions can undermine adherence and well-being. These effects can be further exacerbated by anxiety-induced impairment of working memory (Oaksford *et al.*, 1996) and by memory impairments resulting from efforts to suppress displays of distress (Richards and Gross, 1999). With impoverished conceptual processing, information recall may be poor and susceptible to biases and confabulations.

Anxiety as information about health threat attributes

Anxiety can shape the development of illness representations by virtue of the information it provides about the health threat experience (Martin, 2000; Schwartz and Clore, 1988). These influences involve more controlled strategies compared to the involuntary influences of anxiety on perception, attention, directed and substantive processing, and concrete-emotional processing. Individuals make inferences about their health status and illness attributes by observing their affective states and the contexts in which they occur. Inferences can be based on a 'feeling heuristic' (Schwartz and Clore, 1988), whereby a mood state is regarded as reflecting one's affective evaluation of an issue. Anxiety and relief experiences provide concrete cues of danger and safety that are used to evaluate one's status in health threat situations. For example, anxious individuals who are asked to estimate the risk of contracting various diseases and their personal control over disease occurrence may give relatively high risk estimates and low control evaluations based on their feelings of threat (Johnson and Tversky, 1983; Lerner and Keltner, 2001). More effortful evaluations of anxious states may shape illness cognitions, as people carefully consider the meaning of their feelings within the particular context (Martin, 2000). Anxious affect can have different implications depending on its relation within the configuration of the personal and environmental factors of a situation.

The meaning ascribed to anxious affect within the context of a situation is often used to inform the interpretations of symptoms. Evidence for the informational role of anxious mood is provided by a study of stress effects on symptom attributions (Baumann *et al.*, 1989). Undergraduates participated in the study either the day before an examination or on a Friday early in the semester. They were induced to experience either a happy mood or an anxious mood and then asked to imagine experiencing a set of symptoms on the following day. When asked about the likely causes of the symptoms, students facing an examination were more likely to attribute ambiguous or unfamiliar symptoms to stress rather than to illness, whereas students in the other condition exhibited the opposite pattern of attributions. The mood manipulation was successful, but induced mood had no effect on symptom interpretations. These symptom interpretations were influenced by the information that the following day would or would not be stressful, not by the directed or substantive processing effects of stressed mood. This use of stress information in the symptom interpretation process reflects a 'stress-illness' rule for the configurations of symptoms and environmental features for stress conditions and illness conditions (Leventhal *et al.*, 2001). Further support for the use of this cognitive rule is provided by findings that community residents undergoing stressful experiences were more likely to attribute ambiguous symptoms to stress than to illness, and they were less likely to seek care for these symptoms when the stressors had started recently (Cameron *et al.*, 1995).

Individuals also rely on information about their distress experiences when forming causal attributions for illness. Individuals frequently identify stress as a primary cause of their illnesses, including chronic conditions such as heart disease and diabetes (French *et al.*, 2001; Hampson, 1997). In a study of hospitalized myocardial infarction patients (Cameron *et al.*, in review (a)), it was found that tendencies to attribute the myocardial infarction to stress were associated with high anxiety levels and experiences of post-infarction symptoms that are commonly associated with stress (e.g., fatigue and breathlessness). These causal attributions remained highly stable over the following months, suggesting that any effects of anxiety and stress-like symptoms on attributions persisted well into the future.

These informational effects of anxiety have important clinical implications, as understanding how individuals evaluate emotional distress to determine identity, causal, and other beliefs can be useful in developing strategies for promoting adaptive representations. Because these informational effects on representational beliefs result from reasoned evaluations, they may be particularly amenable to change through education concerning the role of stress in symptom generation and illness development.

This overview of evidence regarding anxiety's influence on perceptual and cognitive processes underscores the potential for anxiety to shape illness representations in important ways. Individuals who experience high anxiety at key points during health threat experiences are likely to develop representations that differ both qualitatively (in terms of contents) and quantitatively (in terms of extensiveness) from those that might have developed under low anxiety arousal. These representational effects may be beneficial or detrimental, depending in large part on the kinds of coping responses they motivate.

Illness-related anxiety and coping responses

Anxiety can influence coping responses both through its impact on representations and through more direct effects. Anxiety, reflecting activation of the behavioral avoidance system, motivates efforts to increase discrepancies between one's current status and a feared status (e.g., disability or death). In response to a health threat, it fuels the planning and use of problem-focused strategies (to manage the objective threat) as well as emotion-focused strategies (to reduce distress), as guided by the representations. This energizing nature of anxiety has characteristic effects on coping responses at both problem-focused and emotion-focused levels of self-regulation. First, anxiety provokes more impulsive, dominant, and well-learned responses such as automatic searches of the body for related symptoms, swift use of familiar medications in response to symptoms, and impulsive searches for disease-related information on the Internet or in books. Moreover, anxiety can foster sustained, vigilant coping over time by enhancing accessibility to representations and coping plans. These effects can promote protective behavior such as seeking medical care for atypical symptoms (Cameron *et al.*, 1993) and getting vaccinations (Leventhal *et al.*, 1965), particularly when individuals have a clear script or plan for enacting the procedure. In addition to these general effects on coping, anxiety induces changes that are distinctive to problem-focused regulation, emotion regulation, and efforts to maintain new health habits.

Anxiety and problem-focused regulation

In problem-focused coping, anxiety can impair reasoned decision-making processes involved in selecting procedures for managing a health problem. For example, anxious individuals exhibit difficulties with identifying alternative strategies and considering multiple criteria when making decisions, and so they may be less effective in choosing among alternative health measures (Aspinwall and Taylor, 1997; Luce *et al.*, 1997). Anxiety also influences implicit (subconscious) learning in temporally extended choice situations; that is, in situations in which one makes a behavioral choice repeatedly, such as decisions to exercise or to take medication. Anxiety arousal increases preferences for choices offering short-term benefits at the expense of long-term gains, and these choices appear to involve learning processes occurring at preconscious stages (Gray, 1999). This research suggests that anxiety may impede efforts to make choices that promote long-term health benefits. For example, a post-surgery patient experiencing distress may end up relying on pain relievers and rest rather than attempting to regain strength and resuming activities. Similarly, a cardiac patient may acknowledge the importance of physical activity and yet forego exercise in favour of short-term gains afforded by concentrating on work responsibilities. Although many patients may face these temptations, anxiety may exacerbate these non-optimal tendencies.

Anxiety and emotion regulation

Anxiety arousal activates the use of procedures for controlling the experience of distress. Gross (1999) identifies five emotion regulation strategies elicited by distress: (1) situation selection, or placing oneself in particular settings to alter mood; (2) situation modification, or changing features of the situation; (3) attentional deployment, such as focusing closely on or distracting attention away from the distress; (4) cognitive change, or altering the meaning of the situation through reappraisal; and (5) response modulation, or altering the experience or expression of moods through relaxation, substance use, or other strategies. Interesting patterns and effects of strategy use are likely to arise in anxiety-arousing health situations. For example, cognitive change is commonly employed during illness experiences and it can significantly alter psychological and physical outcomes. Patients often engage in positive reappraisal by finding meaning in and identifying personal benefits arising from traumatic illnesses (see Aspinwall, 2001). The identification of benefits (e.g., improved personal relationships, personal growth) has been found to predict lower distress and improved health outcomes (Affleck and Tennen, 1996; Bower *et al.*, 1998).

Emotion regulation procedures may be used in synchrony with procedures for managing the objective health threat, but when they conflict then emotion regulation motivations will have the dominating influence on behavior (Leowenstein *et al.*, 2001; Leventhal, 1970). For example, situation avoidance and distraction may be used when distress is extreme, with one's attention turning to more problem-focused coping efforts as arousal levels are brought under control (Cameron and Leventhal, 1995; Wiebe and Korbel, this volume, Chapter 9).

Disease detection behaviors represent cases where danger control and emotion control motivations are likely to clash. Although screening procedures (e.g., mammograms and cholesterol tests) are recognized as important aids in disease control, they present individuals with the anxious prospect of revealing the presence of disease. Detection behaviors differ from health protection behaviors (e.g., exercise and sunscreen use) in that they elicit more negative cognitions and distressed moods (Millar and Millar, 1995). Consideration of detection behaviors appears to activate behavioral avoidance motivations, and so detection behavior decisions are particularly likely to be influenced by the associated perceptual, cognitive, and behavioral processes.

Disease-related worry can amplify ambivalence toward disease detection procedures: it can enhance the motivation to use these procedures while at the same time exacerbate anxiety and test avoidance. Evidence supports this hypothesis. Worry appears to sustain the motivation to obtain screening, so that over time it promotes screening use (Diefenbach *et al.*, 1999). Yet extreme worry can reduce use of screening techniques such as mammograms (Lerman et al.,1993) and lung X-rays (Leventhal and Watts, 1966) because of the strong fear of a disease being found.

As a final consideration of emotion regulation, it is important to consider that people vary in their abilities and predilections to regulate their emotions (Salovey and Mayer, 1990). An intriguing research issue concerns whether emotion regulation abilities influence illness representations and the selection and appraisal of coping efforts, and whether these capabilities lead to better adaptation and outcomes (see Goldman *et al.*, 1996). For example, individuals who are adept at repairing their mood states using positive reappraisals may be inclined to develop illness representations with high control beliefs and non-catastrophic consequence beliefs, effects that may promote adaptive behaviors and outcomes. They may also be relatively adherent to recommendations for disease detection techniques, medical check-ups, and aversive procedures as they are better able to control anxiety-induced avoidance tendencies.

Anxiety and sustained health habits

Habits such as eating healthy foods, exercising regularly, and moderating alcohol intake are critical for preventing and controlling many illnesses. Yet adopting and maintaining these lifestyle habits can be challenging, as they typically require sustained will-power, both to abstain from indulging in gratifying substances or activities, and also to engage in uncomfortable or inconvenient activities. Anxiety typically lowers one's resistance to temptation when it comes to partaking in soothing and mood-altering behaviors such as drinking alcohol or eating high-fat foods (Mayne, 1999). Indeed, anxiety is a risk factor in substance abuse (Merikangas and Angst, 1995), binge eating (Stice *et al.*, 2001), and other destructive habits. Experimental evidence further confirms that people experiencing emotional distress exhibit poorer self-control and a depletion of will-power (Baumeister and Heatherton, 1996).

Mischel *et al.* (1972), in a study using their delay-of-gratification paradigm, demonstrated the disruptive effects of distress on will-power. Children were shown two treats (a marshmallow and a pretzel) and asked to indicate which one they preferred. They were then told that they could either wait a designated time and get their preferred treat, or they could opt instead to eat the other treat before the designated time. Compared to children induced to think about positive things (e.g., doing fun activities), children who were induced to think about negative things (e.g., falling down, crying) exhibited substantially poorer delay of gratification: a higher proportion chose to eat the less-preferred treat instead of waiting the allotted time for their preferred treat.

Metcalfe and Mischel (1999) interpret these findings within the context of their 'hot/cool' theory of self-regulation, a theory that corresponds well with the parallel-process CSM (see also Epstein, 1994). It identifies a 'cool' cognitive system, which directs active self-regulation and control efforts, and a 'hot' emotional system, which primes impulsive reactions in response to emotionally evocative stimuli. The cognitive system can become dysfunctional when the emotional system becomes activated and takes dominance. Distress activates the emotional system and amplifies the propensity for exposure to a 'hot' (emotionally rewarding or aversive) stimulus to elicit an automatic, impulsive response.

This self-regulatory perspective elucidates the potentially disruptive effects of emotional distress on self-control efforts required for sustaining many health behavior changes. It also points to several strategies for reducing anxiety's disruptive effects on efforts to maintain new health habits. As Metcalfe and Mischel note, physically or mentally obscuring the tempting object will reduce hot-system responding and thus facilitate will-power. Simple efforts to remove the objects from sight, mentally 'cool' the object (e.g., imagining a picture frame around a tempting dessert) or distract one's attention from the tempting activity can facilitate will-power, at least in the short term. Developing alternative means of self-soothing when distressed is another common strategy. Finally, self-monitoring techniques can be helpful in maintaining a self-regulatory focus on health goals during times when stressful events distract attention (Kirschenbaum, 1987).

Overall, theory and research point to the distinctive ways in which anxiety directly influences behavioral impulses, decision-making processes, attention to problem-focused and emotion regulation goals, and the will-power to sustain challenging habits. Given the variability in anxiety arousal during health threat experiences, it is clear that illness-related behaviors can only be fully understood if we take into account anxiety's influences on representations and behavioral decisions.

Trait anxiety and self-regulation in response to health threats

In this section, I focus on trait anxiety as representing a stable proneness to apprehension, worry, and heightened autonomic activity and associated neuroendocrine changes – in effect, a proneness to the activation of the behavioral avoidance system – and its role in the self-regulation of illness-related behavior. Trait anxiety is generally regarded as synonymous with negative affectivity and neuroticism (although the constructs of the latter include depression, anger, and other affects), and as representing a primary dimension of personality (Digman, 1990). Trait-anxious individuals are prone to experience more intense distress in response to health threats and, in turn, greater arousal influences on cognitive processes that shape illness representations and coping strategies. Moreover, their repeated experiences of anxiety can have cumulative effects on cognitive structures and self-regulation propensities. Through repeated evocations of anxiety, cognitive contents of representations become linked with fearful emotion so that they are more likely to resonate to related cues (e.g., symptoms). Autonomic and neuroendocrine patterns associated with trait anxiety can also influence somatic experiences in ways that shape illness representations and self-regulation behaviors. These cumulative effects and physiological responses contribute to distinctive perceptual, cognitive, and coping patterns that influence self-regulatory health behavior.

Trait anxiety: perceptual and cognitive processing of health threat cues

High trait anxiety is associated with three perceptual-cognitive propensities: (1) hypervigilant scanning for and selective attention to threat-related stimuli; (2) a tendency to interpret ambiguous stimuli in a threatening manner; and (3) a tendency to recall threatening information (Eysenck, 1997). In contrast, low trait anxiety is associated with propensities to direct attention away from threat cues, interpret ambiguous stimuli in a non-threatening manner, and exhibit poor recall of threatening information. Anxious mood amplifies these opposing tendencies associated with high and low trait anxiety; that is, state anxiety and trait anxiety have interactive effects on perception, interpretation, and recall of threat-related stimuli (Eysenck, 1997). For example, high trait-anxious participants exhibit greater sensitivity to threatening stimuli when under high stress than when under low stress, whereas low trait-anxious participants exhibit poorer sensitivity to the threatening stimuli when under high stress than when under low stress (MacLeod and Rutherford, 1992).

These findings on general processing tendencies associated with trait anxiety are consistent with evidence regarding trait anxiety's more specific associations with perceptions, attributions, and recall of symptoms (moreover, the interactive effects of trait and state anxiety may explain the lack of evidence for the main effects of state anxiety on symptom reports noted earlier). Substantial evidence links trait anxiety with heightened symptom reports, and this phenomenon is believed to arise because trait anxious individuals search vigilantly for bodily cues of illness (Watson and Pennebaker, 1989). Although some expect that this hypervigilance leads to exaggerated symptom reports, evidence suggests that this is not so. Instead, trait anxiety appears to accurately enhance sensitivity in detecting symptoms. Trait anxiety was associated with heightened symptom sensitivity in a toxicity study of tamoxifen therapy in which postmenopausal women with breast cancer in remission were randomly assigned to take either tamoxifen or placebo pills for two years (Cameron *et al.*, 1998). It was not known at the trial's onset that tamoxifen induces hot flushes and vaginal irritation, and so the women did not expect to experience these symptoms. Trait anxiety predicted greater increases in reported hot flushes and vaginal irritation among tamoxifen users, but it was unrelated to these symptom reports among placebo users. Moreover, trait anxiety did not predict increases in reports of symptoms that are unaffected by tamoxifen (e.g., fatigue, joint pain).

These findings indicate that trait anxiety is associated with greater sensitivity in symptom detection. Yet further analyses suggest that these effects may have arisen in part because trait anxiety corresponds with greater physiological reactivity to tamoxifen. Trait anxiety predicted greater retention of lumbar bone mineral density and muted increases in sex hormone-binding globulin in response to tamoxifen (Cameron *et al.*, 2002). Given that physiological mechanisms underlying trait anxiety interact with these endocrine-related effects of tamoxifen, it is possible that anxiety-related physiological processes may also influence the endocrine changes producing hot flushes and vaginal irritation. These findings underscore the potential role of trait anxiety as an indicator of distinctive neuroendocrine processes that may influence both symptomatology and physical health (see Rabin *et al.* (2001) for additional evidence that associations between trait anxiety and symptom reports are due to veridical differences in symptom detection sensitivity, physiological activity, or both processes).

Although trait anxiety is associated with accuracy in symptom detection, it is clearly linked with a propensity to misattribute symptoms to threatening conditions. In the placebo condition of the tamoxifen trial, for example, high anxious women were more likely than low anxious women to misattribute their symptom experiences to their pill use. Similarly, trait anxiety predicts greater misattributions of symptoms to blood glucose levels among diabetic adolescents (Wiebe *et al.*, 1994). These findings are consistent with evidence linking trait anxiety with general tendencies to interpret situations in a threatening manner (Eysenck, 1997), and they may reflect the outcomes of anxiety-infused substantive processing.

A predisposition to anxiety-infused substantive processing of symptom information may have additional effects on symptom responses, such as presentations of symptoms to others. In a study by Ellington and Wiebe

(1999), participants were asked to play the role of a patient with specific symptoms in a mock consultation with a medical student. High (compared to low) neuroticism participants gave more elaborate presentations of symptoms and their psychosocial concerns; moreover, those presenting severe symptoms disclosed more information about stress and other psychological issues. Medical residents who watched the videotaped role-plays rated these high neuroticism participants as less credible, less in need of treatment, and more in need of psychological services than the low neuroticism participants. These findings suggest that trait-anxious individuals may engage in symptom presentation behaviors that could undermine their medical care.

Trait anxiety and problem-focused coping

Given that trait anxiety represents a stable sensitivity of the behavioral avoidance system, it is likely to correspond with amplified propensities for coping responses that are linked with state anxiety, such as vigilant coping and impulsive reactions (Cameron *et al.*, 1998). Yet evidence suggests that trait anxiety is also associated with coping reactions that are distinctive from those observed in association with state anxiety. For example, trait anxiety is associated with unique behavioral patterns when facing uncertain conditions – situations in which decisions are shaped by confidence in and doubt about potential outcomes. In many instances, it is not clear which medical treatment is superior; sometimes, it is unclear whether any treatment will be effective. Trait-anxious patients may be more likely to make conservative treatment choices in these situations, as suggested by evidence that dispositional fear is associated with heightened tendencies to make risk-aversive choices in uncertain conditions (Lerner and Keltner, 2001). Moreover, trait-anxious individuals may be particularly inclined to give up coping attempts when there is doubt that the efforts will be effective. In a study of women with early-stage breast cancer, high threat sensitivity (synonymous with trait anxiety) predicted higher levels of behavioral disengagement and of 'giving up' when confidence of remaining cancer-free was low, although not when confidence was high (Carver *et al.*, 2000). As Carver and colleagues note, these effects take on particular significance in light of evidence that giving-up tendencies are associated with cancer recurrence (Greer *et al.*, 1990).

Trait anxiety and emotion regulation

Trait-anxious individuals experience high distress when confronted with illness threats, and so they are particularly challenged by the need for effective emotion regulation. Whether trait anxiety promotes adaptive coping or maladaptive coping will depend on how effectively this anxiety arousal is managed. Of the emotion regulation strategies identified by Gross (1999), response modulation through emotional suppression has received particular attention in terms of its relationship with trait anxiety. Managing distress through expressing one's feelings has been found to promote coping and well-being (Pennebaker, 1995), and it is a necessary step in eliciting support and assistance. Individuals who actively suppress negative emotions in order to 'put on a brave face' and maintain composure may therefore experience difficulties in adaptation over time. Emotional constraint has been linked with various psychological and physical costs. In laboratory studies, emotional suppression has been found to impair memory and increase cardiorespiratory activity (Richards and Gross, 1999). Similarly, longitudinal research suggests that links exist between anger inhibition and cardiac disease progression (Graves *et al.*, 1994), and between emotional inhibition and cancer progression (McKenna *et al.*, 1999).

Recent studies suggest that the combination of high trait anxiety and high constraint may have particularly detrimental effects on health and well-being. The personality configuration of high negative affectivity and high social inhibition has been found to predict higher levels of distress, morbidity, and mortality among heart disease patients (Denollet, 2000). Moreover, a study of women with recurrent breast cancer found that the combination of low trait anxiety and low constraint was associated with longer survival (Weihs *et al.*, 2000). These findings are limited, however, by a small sample and the assessment of constraint as tendencies to repress emotions rather than as conscious suppression efforts.

In a survey of women with newly diagnosed breast cancer (Cameron *et al.*, 2002), it was found that the combination of trait anxiety and emotional constraint (i.e., the conscious effort to inhibit expressions of negative emotions) predicted poor coping and adjustment in the early stages of treatment. This personality configuration was associated with self-reports of high distress, poor coping efficacy, and poor illness adjustment. The women also wrote essays about 'their deepest thoughts and feelings' regarding their cancer experiences, and textual analyses revealed that the high anxiety/high constraint configuration was associated with a linguistic pattern involving the use of fewer words about negative emotions (particularly anxiety). These women, who reported the highest emotional distress in the questionnaires, avoided expressing distress even in confidential essays. Trained staff who evaluated the essays rated high constraint women as exhibiting poor adjustment and low self-awareness, providing further support for the idea that these constraint attempts are maladaptive. Finally, women with high trait anxiety and high constraint reported relatively low levels of support from family and friends during treatment. This personality configuration may create friction or difficulties in eliciting support from others (see Aspinwall, 2001), although it is also possible that poor support (e.g., indications that distress will not be tolerated) exacerbates anxiety and emotional constraint.

In summary, emerging evidence suggests that trait anxiety processes underlie unique coping patterns in health threat situations. These processes may promote protective action and impulsive reactions, but they may discourage higher-risk or persistent actions under conditions of uncertainty. Trait anxious individuals are in particular need of emotion regulation strategies, and their adjustment to illness experiences will depend on how well their strategies manage distress in an adaptive manner.

Emotion-focused interventions, anxiety regulation, and health

Illness-related anxiety is not only a quality of life concern; its influences on the cognitive and behavioral processes involved in managing illness underscore its potential health consequences and further justify the development of interventions that facilitate anxiety regulation for ill or at-risk individuals. Many psychosocial interventions for patients focus on improving emotion regulation through the implementation of relaxation techniques, group support, meditation, cognitive behavioral therapy, and other such methods. There is substantial evidence that these emotion-focused interventions provide psychological and health benefits. A review of this extensive literature is beyond the scope of this chapter, but a compelling example of the potential benefits of these interventions is provided by research on stress management programs for cardiac patients. These programs, which typically include relaxation training and group support or counseling, have been found to promote beneficial changes in mood, health, and behaviors, and to reduce cardiac morbidity and mortality (Dusseldorp *et al.*, 1999).

There is considerable variance in the responses to these emotion-focused interventions, and no one technique works well for everyone. As expected, some evidence indicates that these interventions can be particularly effective for individuals experiencing high anxiety. Some stress management programs for cardiac patients have been found to enhance psychological well-being (Engretson *et al.*, 1999) and improve survival rates (Frasure-Smith, 1991), primarily for high anxious patients. Similarly, relaxation therapy may provide greater psychological and health benefits for high trait-anxious individuals than for low trait-anxious individuals (Gray and Cameron, 2002; Lane *et al.*, 1993).

Further research on how these techniques influence self-regulation processes will accelerate their improvement and enhance our abilities to target individuals who can benefit from them. Presented here are three examples of therapeutic tools for facilitating anxiety self-regulation processes: strategies for concentrating one's focus on the objective attributes of a stressor; emotional disclosure writing techniques; and mental simulation techniques. These techniques share an emphasis on developing an adaptive integration of objective processing with emotion processing within the context of the situation.

Objective processing strategies

Objective processing techniques utilize the strategy of drawing attention away from emotional distress by increasing one's focus on the abstract features of stimuli. One example is the pain management technique of focusing on objective aspects of sensations experienced during a painful procedure. This strategy was designed to weaken the link between pain-inducing stimuli and emotional activation by fostering a more abstract interpretation of the experience, and evidence confirms that it significantly improves pain tolerance (Ahles *et al.*, 1983; Johnson *et al.*, 1973). An objective-focused approach also underlies some cognitive behavioral practices that promote a reasoned focus and reduced attention to emotional distress.

Objective processing strategies may be particularly effective in certain conditions, such as those requiring short-term tolerance of aversive procedures. These strategies may not be useful in conditions involving prolonged distress, however, as they may block emotion processing and resolution. Suggestive evidence was provided by a trial of a psychoeducational intervention with myocardial infarction patients (Petrie *et al.*, 2002). The intervention focused on changing maladaptive illness representations (e.g., catastrophic consequence beliefs) and developing objective coping strategies while providing information in a reassuring manner. Although the intervention accelerated the patients' return to work and reduced angina levels, it improved cardiac rehabilitation attendance and functional status only for those patients with low negative affectivity (i.e., low trait anxiety). Not only did the intervention have negligible effects on rehabilitation attendance and functional status for highly anxious patients, but over time it led to poorer rates of exercise and dietary fat intake for these patients relative to standard-care patients (Cameron *et al.*, in review (b)).

Why was this intervention less beneficial for anxious patients? It is possible that both the objective attentional focus and the reassurance of a good recovery suppressed emotional processing. Reassurance provided by medical staff often increases distress over time, particularly for patients with high health anxiety (Coia and Morley, 1998). Reassurance and an objective-focused orientation may convey to the patient that distress is unwarranted and inappropriate, thereby inducing emotional suppression. Moreover, the message that 'everything is all right' may be inconsistent with their illness representations and symptom experiences (Coia and Morley, 1998). For the anxious cardiac patients, their continuing experiences of distress, weakness, and other symptoms may have conflicted with the intervention-induced expectations that they would feel better soon. These discrepancies may have elicited appraisals that they were in relatively poor condition, which led them to cut back or give up on activities, exercise, and dietary change efforts. Objective-focused strategies may be effective when short-term tolerance is required and with low-anxious individuals, but they may impair self-regulation when extended emotion regulation is needed (e.g., with anxious individuals experiencing prolonged illness).

Emotional disclosure techniques

Disclosure writing techniques are designed to promote adaptation to stressful experiences through the expression and processing of strong emotions (Pennebaker, 1995). These techniques can facilitate self-regulation by fostering the development of meaningful representations of distressing experiences and effective coping strategies, particularly through the integration of conceptual-level information with concrete-emotional aspects of experiences. Brief writing interventions have been found to increase adaptive coping, reduce health clinic visits, and enhance immunocompetence in healthy populations (see Smyth, 1998); they have also been found to promote functional status in patients with rheumatoid arthritis and asthma (Smyth *et al.*, 1999).

Yet there is considerable variation in the benefits arising from disclosure writing. From a self-regulation perspective, adaptive responses should occur when writing fosters the development of effective representations and coping strategies. With this perspective in mind, a modified disclosure task was developed in which the writer focuses on current problems and then identifies coping strategies and appraises their effectiveness. In a study of adults entering university, it was found that this self-regulation writing task was more effective than the traditional disclosure task in minimizing anxiety and fostering adjustment. Moreover, this task reduced health visits for both optimistic and pessimistic participants, whereas the disclosure task reduced health visits only for optimistic participants (Cameron and Nicholls, 1998). The self-regulation writing task may be particularly beneficial for pessimistic individuals who may dwell on negative aspects in ways that inhibit coping efforts, as it compels them to formulate and appraise coping plans. Whereas optimistic individuals may spontaneously generate coping plans using the traditional disclosure task, pessimistic individuals may not. Whether or not the self-regulation writing task can promote adaptation to illness experiences remains to be explored.

Interventions that encourage emotional expression through writing or talking may facilitate emotion regulation for patients in part by promoting post-traumatic growth through finding benefits in their illness experiences. In research with breast cancer patients, Cordova *et al.* (2001) found that experiencing high trauma (perceiving the illness as severe and experiencing intense fear) and talking with others about the experience predicted greater post-traumatic growth. Fear may be a catalyst for adaptive shifts in priorities, self-concepts, and goals, and talking with others may facilitate the development of these adaptive representations and shifts in goals and actions.

Mental simulation

A final strategy to be considered is a mental simulation technique for facilitating self-regulation in challenging situations that require sustained effort

(Taylor *et al.*, 1998). This imagery technique focuses on the mental rehearsal of steps needed to achieve one's goals. Mental rehearsal helps one to develop action plans, and to anticipate emotional reactions and identify ways to control them. Moreover, it activates concrete-experiential processing so that action plans are bolstered with vivid imagery and concrete information. Taylor *et al.* have found that mental simulation improves performance on challenging tasks (e.g., academic examinations), and mediational analyses indicate that the effects are due to both reductions of anxiety and increases in planning. They also found that the mental simulation of coping with ongoing stressors increased the use of problem-focused efforts and emotion regulation strategies (e.g., eliciting emotional support from others and employing positive reappraisals; Taylor *et al.*, 1998). Mental simulation techniques of this nature are used in smoking cessation programs and other programs promoting abstinence from detrimental behaviors (Brownwell *et al.*, 1986). These techniques may also be effective in promoting sustained behaviors such as adherence to medications, dietary changes, and exercise.

Objective-focus strategies, emotional disclosure techniques, and mental simulation have considerable promise as intervention tools for promoting anxiety regulation during illness-related experiences. They focus on developing adaptive representations, emotion processing, and appraisals that are consistent with internal and external experiences that facilitate adaptive behavior. Assessments of how anxiety-related individual characteristics are associated with differential responses to these interventions will enhance our efforts to tailor these interventions and target them to those individuals who are most likely to benefit from them.

Concluding remarks

Anxiety is a pervasive aspect of illness and, as this selective review demonstrates, it can affect virtually all aspects of behavioral self-regulation. Although this chapter focuses primarily on anxiety's interactions with illness-related cognitive and behavioral processes, it is also important to appreciate anxiety's direct influence on physiological processes and health (for a review see Mayne, 1999), and how these effects feed into the dynamic process of illness experience and regulation.

Anxious states and anxious traits can be adaptive or maladaptive, depending on the particular context. Anxiety-induced enhancement of attention to health threats, elaborated representations, and vigilance in protective action can promote swift and effective treatment of illness in many situations. Yet anxiety effects such as symptom misattributions, anxiety-infused substantive processing, focus on short-term benefits, and depletion of will-power may undermine health-protective action. Optimal health behavior necessitates the regulation of anxiety to appropriate levels in relation to the health threat, a feat that requires accurate understanding of the health threat as well as effective problem-focused and emotion regulation strategies.

The CSM, with the integration of behavioral avoidance processes into the emotion regulation arm, provides a useful framework for understanding the complex array of findings on anxiety processes and their effects on illness cognitions and behaviors, and for guiding further research on anxiety, avoidance motivations, and health. Significant gaps remain in our understanding of the self-regulatory dynamics involving anxiety, illness cognition, and behavior, particularly in terms of how general effects vary according to individual, social, illness, and contextual characteristics. More research is also needed to further discriminate the differential effects of state anxiety and trait anxiety on self-regulation processes, with greater attention paid to the physiological processes underlying both forms of anxiety and how they influence perceptual experiences, cognitions, and behaviors.

Psychosocial interventions for improving psychological and physical well-being in ill and at-risk populations will be most effective if they foster effective self-regulation of emotional distress. More efforts are needed to develop interventions that are sensitive to the dynamics of illness cognitions and emotions as delineated by self-regulation theory. The well-placed use of strategies such as objective-focused processing, therapeutic writing techniques, and mental simulation show promise in being able to achieve these goals. Such empirical efforts will further our understanding of self-regulation and advance our abilities to promote health and well-being.

Note

1   Correspondence concerning this chapter should be addressed to Linda D. Cameron, Department of Psychology (Tamaki Campus), The University of Auckland, Private Bag 92019, Auckland, New Zealand. E-mail: L.cameron@auckland.ac.nz

References

Affleck, G. and Tennen, H. (1996) 'Construing benefits from adversity: adaptational significance and dispositional underpinnings,' *Journal of Personality* 64: 899–922.

Ahles, T.A., Blanchard, E.B. and Leventhal, H. (1983) 'Cognitive control of pain: attention to the sensory aspects of the cold pressor stimulus,' *Cognitive Therapy and Research* 7: 159–178.

Aspinwall, L.G. (2001) 'Dealing with adversity: self-regulation, coping, adaptation and health,' in A. Tesser and N. Schwartz (eds) *Blackwell Handbook of Social Psychology: Intraindividual Processes*, Malden, MA: Blackwell Publishers, pp. 591–614.

Aspinwall, L.G. and Taylor, S.E. (1997) 'A stitch in time: self-regulation and proactive coping,' *Psychological Bulletin* 121: 417–436.

Baumann, L.J., Cameron, L.D., Zimmerman, R. and Leventhal, H. (1989) 'Illness representations and matching labels with symptoms,' *Health Psychology* 8: 449–470.

Baumeister, R.F. and Heatherton, T.F. (1996) 'Self-regulation failure: an overview,' *Psychological Inquiry* **7**: 1–15.

Blascovich, J. and Mendes, W.B. (2000) 'Challenge and threat appraisals: the role of affective cues,' in J.P. Forgas (ed) *Feeling and Thinking: The Role of Affect in Social Cognition*, Cambridge: Cambridge University Press, pp. 59–82.

Bower, J.E., Kemeny, M.E., Taylor, S.E. and Fahey, J.L. (1998) 'Cognitive processing, discovery of meaning, CD4 decline and AIDS-related mortality among bereaved HIV-seropositive men,' *Journal of Consulting and Clinical Psychology* **66**: 979–986.

Brownwell, K.D., Marlatt, G.A., Lichtenstein, E. and Wilson, G.T. (1986) 'Understanding and preventing relapse,' *American Psychologist* **41**: 765–782.

Cameron, L.D. (1997) 'Screening for cancer: illness worry and illness perceptions,' in K.J. Petrie and J. Weinman (eds) *Perceptions of Health and Illness: Current Research and Applications*, Amsterdam: Harwood Academic, pp. 291–322.

Cameron, L.D. and Diefenbach, M.A. (2001) 'Responses to information about psychosocial consequences of genetic testing for breast cancer susceptibility: influences of cancer worry and risk perceptions,' *Journal of Health Psychology* **6**: 47–59.

Cameron, L.D. and Leventhal, H. (1995) 'Vulnerability beliefs, symptom experiences and the processing of health threat information,' *Journal of Applied Social Psychology* **25**: 1859–1883.

Cameron, L.D. and Nicholls, G. (1998) 'Disclosure of stressful experiences through writing: effects of a self-regulation manipulation for pessimists and optimists,' *Health Psychology* **17**: 84–92.

Cameron, L.D., Leventhal, E.A. and Leventhal, H. (1993) 'Symptom representations and affect as determinants of care seeking in a community-dwelling, adult sample population,' *Health Psychology* **12**: 171–179.

Cameron, L.D., Leventhal, H. and Leventhal, E.A. (1995) 'Seeking medical care in response to symptoms and life stress', *Psychosomatic Medicine* **57**: 37–47.

Cameron, L.D., Leventhal, H. and Love, R.R. (1998) 'Trait anxiety, symptom perceptions and illness-related responses among women with breast cancer in remission during a tamoxifen clinical trial,' *Health Psychology* **17**: 459–469.

Cameron, L.D., Leventhal, H., Love, R.R. and Patrick-Miller, L. (2002) 'Trait anxiety and tamoxifen effects on bone mineral density and sex hormone binding globulin,' *Psychosomatic Medicine* **64**: 612–620.

Cameron, L.D., Booth, R.J., Schlatter, M., Ziginskas, D. and Harman, J. (2002) 'Trait anxiety, emotional constraint and psychological responses to newly diagnosed breast cancer,' paper presented at the Annual Meeting of the Society of Behavioral Medicine, Washington, DC.

Cameron, L.D., Petrie, K.J., Ellis, C., Buick, D. and Weinman, J. (in review (a)) 'Symptom experiences, symptom attributions and causal attributions in patients following first-time myocardial infarction.'

—— (in review (b)) 'Trait negative affectivity and responses to a psychoeducational intervention for myocardial infarction patients.'

Carver, C.S. and Scheier, M.F. (1998) *On the Self-Regulation of Behavior*, New York: Cambridge University Press.

Carver, C.S., Meyer, B. and Antoni, M.H. (2000) 'Responsiveness to threats and incentives, expectancy of recurrence and distress and disengagement: moderator effects in women with early stage breast cancer,' *Journal of Consulting and Clinical Psychology* **68**: 965–975.

Carver, C.S., Sutton, S.K. and Scheier, M.F. (2000) 'Action, emotion and personality: emerging conceptual integration,' *Personality and Social Psychology Bulletin* **26**: 741–751.

Clore, G.L., Schwarz, N. and Conway, M. (1994) 'Affective causes and consequences of social information processing,' in R.S. Wyer and K. Srull (eds) *Handbook of Social Cognition* 2nd edn, Hillsdale, NJ: Lawrence Erlbaum Associates, pp. 323–417.

Cohen, S., Doyle, W.J., Skoner, D.P., Fireman, P., Gwaltney, J.M. and Newsom, J.T. (1995) 'State and trait negative affect as predictors of objective and subjective symptoms of respiratory viral infections,' *Journal of Personality and Social Psychology* **68**: 159–169.

Coia, P. and Morley, S. (1998) 'Medical reassurance and patients' responses,' *Journal of Psychosomatic Research* **45**: 377–386.

Cordova, M.J, Cunningham, L.C, Carlson, C.R and Andrykowski, M.A. (2001) 'Posttraumatic growth following breast cancer: a controlled comparison study,' *Health Psychology* **20**: 176–185.

Croyle, R.T. and Uretsky, M.B. (1987) 'Effects of mood on self-appraisal of health status,' *Health Psychology* **6**: 239–253.

deBruin, J.T., Schaefer, M.K., Krohne, H.W. and Dreyer, A. (2001) 'Preoperative anxiety, coping and intra-operative adjustment: are there mediating effects of stress-induced analgesia?' *Psychology and Health* **16**: 253–271.

Denollet, J. (2000) 'Type D personality: a potential risk factor refined,' *Journal of Psychosomatic Research* **49**: 255–266.

Diefenbach, M.A., Miller, S. and Daly, M. (1999) 'Specific worry about breast cancer predicts mammography use in women at risk for breast and ovarian cancer,' *Health Psychology* **18**: 532–536.

Digman, J.M. (1990) 'Personality structure: emergence of the five-factor model,' *Annual Review of Psychology* **41**: 417–440.

Dusseldorp, E., van Elderen, T., Maes, S. and Kraaij, V. (1999) 'A meta-analysis of psychoeducational programs for coronary heart disease patients,' *Health Psychology* **18**: 506–519.

Ellington, L. and Wiebe, D.J. (1999) 'Neuroticism, symptom presentation and medical decision-making,' *Health Psychology* **18**: 634–643.

Engebretson, T.O., Clark, M.M., Niaura, R.S., Phillips, T., Albrecht, A. and Tilke-meier, P. (1999) 'Quality of life and anxiety in a phase II cardiac rehabilitation program,' *Medicine and Science in Sports and Exercise* **6**: 216–223.

Epstein, S. (1994) 'Integration of the cognitive and the psychodynamic unconscious,' *American Psychologist* **49**: 709–724.

Eysenck, M.W. (1997) *Anxiety and Cognition: A Unified Theory*, Brighton, UK: Psychology Press.

Forgas, J.P. (2000a) 'Affect and information processing strategies: an interactive relationship,' in J.P. Forgas (ed) *Feeling and Thinking: The Role of Affect in Social Cognition*, Cambridge: Cambridge University Press, pp. 253–282.

—— (ed.) (2000b) *Feeling and Thinking: The Role of Affect in Social Cognition*, Cambridge: Cambridge University Press.

Fox, E., Russo, R., Bowles, R. and Dutton, K. (2001) 'Do threatening stimuli draw or hold visual attention in subclinical anxiety?' *Journal of Experimental Psychology: General* **130**: 681–700.

Frasure-Smith, N. (1991) 'In-hospital symptoms of psychological stress as predictors of long-term outcome after acute myocardial infarction in men,' *American Journal of Cardiology* **67**: 21–27.

French, D.P., Senior, V., Weinman, J. and Marteau, T. (2001) 'Causal attributions for heart disease: a systematic review,' *Psychology and Health* **16**: 77–98.

Goldman, S.L., Kraemer, D.T. and Salovey, P. (1996) 'Beliefs about mood moderate the relationship of stress to illness and symptom reporting,' *Journal of Psychosomatic Research* **41**: 115–128.

Graves, P.L., Mead, L.A., Wang, N.Y., Liang, K. and Klag, M.J. (1994) 'Temperament as a potential predictor of mortality: evidence from a 41-year prospective study,' *Journal of Behavioral Medicine* **17**: 111–126.

Gray, J.A. (1987) *The Psychology of Fear and Stress*, Cambridge: Cambridge University Press.

Gray, J.R. (1999) 'A bias toward short-term thinking in threat-related negative emotional states,' *Personality and Social Psychology Bulletin* **25**: 65–75.

—— (2001) 'Emotional modulation of cognitive control: approach-withdrawal states double-dissociate spatial from verbal two-back task performance,' *Journal of Experimental Psychology: General* **130**: 436–452.

Gray, T. and Cameron, L.D. (2002) 'Relaxation therapy effects on health care use,' unpublished manuscript.

Greer, S., Morris, T., Pettingdale, K.W. and Haybittle, J.L. (1990) 'Psychological responses to breast cancer and 15-year outcome,' *Lancet* **335**: 49–50.

Gross, J.J. (1999) 'Emotion and emotion regulation,' in L.A. Pervin (ed) *Handbook of Personality: Theory and Research*, 2nd edn, New York: Guilford Press, pp. 525–552.

Hampson, S.E. (1997) 'Illness representations and the self-management of diabetes,' in K.J. Petrie and J.A. Weinman (eds) *Perceptions of Health and Illness: Current Research and Applications*, Amsterdam: Harwood Academic.

Johnson, E.J. and Tversky, A. (1983) 'Affect, generalization and the perception of risk,' *Journal of Personality and Social Psychology* **45**: 20–33.

Johnson, J.E., Morrissey, J.F. and Leventhal, H. (1973) 'Psychological preparation for an endoscopic examination,' *Gastrointestinal Endoscopy* **19**: 180–182.

Katkin, E.S. (1985) 'Blood, sweat and tears: individual differences in autonomic self-perception,' *Psychophysiology* **22**: 125–137.

Kent, G. (1985) 'Cognitive processes in dental anxiety,' *British Journal of Clinical Psychology* **24**: 259–264.

Kirschenbaum, D.S. (1987) 'Self-regulatory failure: a review with clinical implications,' *Clinical Psychology Review* **7**: 77–104.

Lane, J.D., McCaskill, C.C., Ross, S.L., Feinglos, M.N. and Surwit, R.S. (1993) 'Relaxation training for NIDDM: predicting who may benefit,' *Diabetes Care* **16**: 1087–1094.

Leowenstein, G.F., Weber, E.U., Hsee, C.K. and Welch, N. (2001) 'Risk as feelings,' *Psychological Bulletin* **127**: 267–286.

Lerman, C., Schwartz, M.D., Lin, T.H., Hughes, C., Narod, S. and Lynch, H.T. (1997) 'The influence of psychological distress on use of genetic testing for cancer risk,' *Journal of Consulting and Clinical Psychology* **65**: 414–420.

Lerman, C., Daly, M., Sands, C., Balshem, A., Lustbader, E., Heggan, T., Goldstein, L., James, J. and Engrstrom, P. (1993) 'Mammography adherence and psychological distress among women at risk for breast cancer,' *Journal of the National Cancer Institute* **85**: 1074–1080.

Lerner, J.S. and Keltner, D. (2001) 'Fear, anger and risk,' *Journal of Personality and Social Psychology* **81**: 146–159.

Leventhal, E.A, Hansell, S., Diefenbach, M., Leventhal, H. and Glass, D.C. (1996) 'Negative affect and self-report of physical symptoms: two longitudinal studies of older adults,' *Health Psychology* **15**: 193–199.

Leventhal, H. (1970) 'Findings and theory in the study of fear communication,' in L. Berkowitz (ed) *Advances in Experimental Social Psychology*, vol. 5, New York: Academic Press, pp. 119–186.

—— (1984) 'A perceptual-motor theory of emotion,' in L. Berkowitz (ed) *Advances in Experimental Social Psychology*, vol. 17, Orlando, FL: Academic Press, pp.117–182.

Leventhal, H. and Watts, J. (1966) 'Sources of resistence to fear-arousing communications on smoking and lung cancer,' *Journal of Personality* **34**: 155–175.

Leventhal, H., Leventhal, E. and Cameron, L.D. (2001) 'Representations, procedures and affect in illness self-regulation: a perceptual-cognitive approach,' in A. Baum, T. Revenson and J. Singer (eds) *Handbook of Health Psychology*, Hillsdale, NJ: Lawrence Erlbaum Associates, pp. 19–48.

Leventhal, H., Singer, R. and Jones, S. (1965) 'Effects of fear and specificity of recommendations upon attitudes and behavior,' *Journal of Personality and Social Psychology* **2**: 20–29.

Luce, M.F., Bettman, J.R. and Payne, J.W. (1997) 'Choice processing in emotionally difficult decisions,' *Journal of Experimental Psychology: Learning, Memory and Cognition* **23**: 384–405.

MacLeod, C. and Rutherford, E.M. (1992) 'Anxiety and the selective processing of emotional information: mediating roles of awareness, trait and state variables and personal relevance of stimulus materials,' *Behaviour Research and Therapy* **30**: 479–491.

Martin, L.L. (2000) 'Moods do not convey information: moods in context do,' in J.P. Forgas (ed) *Feeling and Thinking: The Role of Affect in Social Cognition*, Cambridge: Cambridge University Press pp. 153–177.

Mayne, T.J. (1999) 'Negative affect and health: the importance of being earnest,' *Cognition and Emotion* **13**: 601–635.

McKenna, M.C., Zevon, M. and Corn, B. (1999) 'Psychosocial factors and the development of breast cancer: a meta-analysis,' *Health Psychology* **18**: 520–531.

Merikangas, K.R. and Angst, J. (1995) 'Comorbidity and social phobia: evidence from clinical, epidemiologic and genetic studies,' *European Archives of Psychiatry and Clinical Neuroscience* **244**: 197–203.

Metcalfe, J. and Jacobs, W.J. (1998) 'Emotional memory: the effects of stress on "cool" and "hot" memory systems,' in D.L. Medin (ed) *The Psychology of Learning and Motivation*, vol. 38, San Diego, CA: Academic Press, pp. 187–222.

Metcalfe, J. and Mischel, W. (1999) 'A hot/cool-system analysis of delay of gratification: dynamics of willpower,' *Psychological Review* **106**: 3–19.

Millar, M.G. and Millar, K. (1995) 'Negative affective consequences of thinking about disease detection behaviors,' *Health Psychology* **14**: 141–6.

Mischel, W., Ebbeson, E.B. and Zeiss, A.R. (1972) 'Cognitive and attentional mechanisms in delay of gratification,' *Journal of Personality and Social Psychology* **21**: 204–218.

Oaksford, M., Morris, F., Grainger, B. and Williams, J.M.G. (1996) 'Mood, reasoning and central executive processes,' *Journal of Experimental Psychology: Learning, Memory and Cognition* **22**: 476–492.

Öehman, A., Flykt, A. and Esteves, F. (2001) 'Emotion drives attention: detecting the snake in the grass,' *Journal of Experimental Psychology: General* **130**: 466–478.

Pennebaker, J.W. (1995) *Emotion, Disclosure and Health*, Washington, DC: American Psychological Association.

Petrie, K.J., Cameron, L.D., Ellis, C., Buick, D. and Weinman, J. (2002) 'Changing illness perceptions following myocardial infarction: an early intervention randomized controlled trial,' *Psychosomatic Medicine* **64**: 580–586.

Ploghous, A., Narain, C., Beckmann, C.F., Clare, S., Bantick, S., Wise, R., Matthews, P.M., Rawlins, J., Nicholas, P. and Tracey, I. (2001) 'Exacerbation of pain by anxiety is associated with activity in a hippocampal network,' *Journal of Neuroscience* **21**: 9896–9903.

Rabin, C., Ward, S., Leventhal, H. and Schmitz, M. (2001) 'Explaining retrospective reports of symptoms in patients undergoing chemotherapy: anxiety, initial symptom experience and posttreatment symptoms,' *Health Psychology* **20**: 91–98.

Richards, J.M. and Gross, J.J. (1999) 'Composure at any cost? The cognitive consequences of emotion suppression,' *Personality and Social Psychology Bulletin* **25**: 1033–1044.

Salovey, P. and Birnbaum, D. (1989) 'Influence of mood on health-relevant cognitions,' *Journal of Personality and Social Psychology* **57**: 539–551.

Salovey, P. and Mayer, J.D. (1990) 'Emotional intelligence,' *Imagination, Cognition and Personality* **9**: 185–211.

Schwartz, N. and Clore, G.L. (1988) 'How do I feel about it? Informative functions of affective states,' in K. Fiedler and J.P. Forgas (eds) *Affect, Cognition and Social Behavior*, Toronto: Hogrefe International, pp. 44–62.

Smyth, J.M. (1998) 'Written emotional expression: effect sizes, outcome types and moderating variables,' *Journal of Consulting and Clinical Psychology* **66**: 174–184.

Smyth, J.M, Stone, AA, Hurewitz, A. and Kaell, A. (1999) 'Effects of writing about stressful experiences on symptom reduction in patients with asthma or rheumatoid arthritis: a randomized trial,' *Journal of the American Medical Association* **281**: 1304–1309.

Stice, E., Agras, W.S., Telch, C.F., Halmi, K.A., Mitchell, J.E. and Wilson, T. (2001) 'Subtyping binge eating-disordered women along dieting and negative affect dimensions,' *International Journal of Eating Disorders* **30**: 11–27.

Sutton, S.K. and Davidson, R.J. (1997) 'Prefrontal brain symmetry: a biological substrate of the behavioral approach and inhibition systems,' *Psychological Science* **8**: 204–210.

Taylor, S.E., Pham, L.B., Rivkin, I.D. and Armor, D.A. (1998) 'Harnessing the imagination: mental simulation, self-regulation and coping,' *American Psychologist* **53**: 429–439.

Watson, D. and Pennebaker, J.W. (1989) 'Health complaints, stress and distress: exploring the central role of negative affectivity,' *Psychological Review* **96**: 234–254.

Weihs, K.L., Enright, T.M., Simmens, S.J. and Reiss, D. (2000) 'Negative affectivity, restriction of emotions and site of metastases predict mortality in recurrent breast cancer,' *Journal of Psychosomatic Research* **49**: 59–68.

Wiebe, D.J., Alderfer, M.A., Palmer, S.C., Lindsay, R. and Jarrett, L. (1994) 'Behavioral self-regulation in adolescents with Type I diabetes: negative affectivity and blood glucose symptom perception,' *Journal of Counseling and Clinical Psychology* **62**: 1204–1212.

Zajonc, R.B. (2000) 'Feeling and thinking: closing the debate over the independence of affect,' in J.P. Forgas (ed) *Feeling and Thinking: The Role of Affect in Social Cognition*, Cambridge: Cambridge University Press, pp. 31–58.

9   Defensive denial, affect, and the self-regulation of health threats

Deborah J. Wiebe and Carolyn Korbel[1]

Upon becoming aware that one's health is in danger, people face a 'self-control dilemma' (Trope and Pomerantz, 1998) – a trade-off between engaging in long-term management of the threat at the cost of immediate emotional distress. How do people accomplish the dual tasks of managing sometimes extreme distress while simultaneously taking action to reduce the objective danger? The purpose of this chapter is to examine the role of defensive denial in how people respond to health threats. We focus specifically on understanding whether and how defensive processes work to regulate negative affect, and whether this comes at the cost of reduced motivation to behaviorally manage the threat. We will suggest that subtle defensive processes often enhance the effectiveness of a dynamic system designed to manage health threats because they efficiently keep negative emotional arousal at adaptive levels so that health protective actions can be identified, implemented, and maintained.

Leventhal's self-regulation model of illness cognition (Leventhal, 1970; Leventhal *et al.*, 1992) provides a useful framework for considering the role of denial and affect in responses to health threats. According to this model, health threats activate a self-regulatory process where we initially develop a coherent, common-sense understanding of the problem. Consistent with evidence that cognition involves two distinct but interacting processing systems (Epstein, 1994; Miller *et al.*, 1996), Leventhal proposes that health threats are represented at two levels: at an abstract, rational, long-term, and 'cool' level (e.g., 'I have high cholesterol which may increase my risk of heart disease'); and at a more concrete, emotional, impulsive, and 'hot' level (e.g., emotional memories of a father's heart attack, feeling afraid and helpless as you recall recent symptoms of fatigue). This bi-level representation of the threat guides efforts to manage both the objective health risk and the associated emotional distress. Attempts to manage the objective threat often work in parallel or converge with attempts to regulate negative emotions (e.g., medication and exercise reduce cholesterol and ease anxiety). However, if negative emotional arousal is too high or the objective threat is perceived as unmanageable, affect regulation is presumed to become primary (Cameron and Leventhal, 1995).

In the following sections, we will argue that reality-based defensive denial processes work to cool the health threat representation, thereby diminishing the need for affect to become a primary target of self-regulation, and facilitating active attempts to manage the objective danger. After defining the defensive denial construct, we review the affective and behavioral features of several forms of defensive denial, and then provide a theoretical discussion of the processes that may be involved. We end the chapter by discussing how defensive responses to both acute and chronic health threats emerge out of and interface with the complex workings of the self-system.

Defining defensive denial

Weisman (1972) made an important distinction between first-order 'denial of facts' – denial that is difficult to maintain in the face of data – and the more subtle, second-order 'denial of implications.' Although first-order denial exists, we suspect it is relatively infrequent and qualitatively different from the processes examined here. The defensive processes we will discuss are best interpreted as specific instantiations of the vast number of procedures people have for neutralizing negative self-relevant information. These often take the form of subtle cognitive distortions that are systematically made in a self-protective direction.

These defensive processes are also dynamic. People are continually trying to understand what is happening to them in order to make the best choices for their ongoing lives. Defensive denial can be viewed as a set of processes that are activated as we construct tentative understandings of threatening information. These 'tentative constructions' (Lazarus, 1983) may be positively biased, but we will demonstrate that they are responsive to reality and are continually updated to incorporate new information. The dynamic, reality-based nature of these processes is crucial for long-term adaptation (Schneider, 2001; Taylor *et al.*, 1989). It should also be noted that, because these defensive processes seem to be elicited automatically, they should not be viewed as active self-regulation mechanisms per se, but rather as having ongoing influences on the various inputs into our self-regulation efforts (e.g., health threat representations, or the presence of an affect-regulation goal).

It is also important to distinguish defensive denial from avoidance (Lazarus, 1983). People sometimes avoid being fully informed of health threats, and avoidance can be defensively motivated (e.g., Conley *et al.*, 1999; Croyle and Lerman, 1999; Reed and Aspinwall, 1998). However, in contrast to the defensive processes reviewed below, avoidance-based self-protection consistently appears ineffective at regulating distress and precautionary behaviors (Avants *et al.*, 2001; Conley *et al.*, 1999; Lerman *et al.*, 1998; Suls and Fletcher, 1985). The reality-denying nature of avoidance seems to allow fears and vulnerability beliefs to remain active, but does not direct actions to alter the source of those fears.

Defensive denial, affect regulation, and precautionary behavior

In the following sections, we review data regarding several forms of defensive denial to determine whether these processes function to regulate negative affect, and whether they are ultimately adaptive. Toward this end, each section is organized to examine: (a) whether the process is 'motivated' to regulate negative affect/self-views or whether more rational models can explain the data; (b) whether the process is effective at regulating affect; (c) whether the process undermines motivation to alter the threat; and (d) whether the process is responsive to reality constraints. This is not intended to be a thorough review. People are extremely creative in their ability to neutralize health threats (Weinstein and Klein, 1995), making it inevitable that our defensive arsenal is much larger than that described below. We focus here on three processes for which an informative literature exists. In each case, both experimental and correlational data are available, and the emotional and behavioral consequences of the presumed defensive process have been at least indirectly examined.

Minimization of health threats

When people first learn their health is at risk, they commonly play down the seriousness of the threat. In both correlational and experimental studies of health threat responses, individuals acknowledge that they are at risk, but deny the adverse implications of that risk. For example, when individuals are diagnosed with potentially dangerous health risks (e.g., as having high cholesterol levels, or as HIV-seropositive), they rate the risk as less serious than those who are not (Croyle *et al.*, 1993; Taylor *et al.*, 1992). From a different but related perspective, smokers who attempt to quit but then relapse report subsequent declines in the negative consequences of smoking; such risk perception changes are not seen among those who remain non-smokers (Gibbons *et al.*, 1991; Gibbons *et al.*, 1997). Finally, in experimental studies, people who *randomly* receive information that they are at risk of suffering from health problems routinely state the health risk is less serious than those who receive low risk information (for a review see Ditto and Croyle, 1995). Overall, there is strong and consistent evidence that, when personally relevant health threats are encountered, the implications of those threats are minimized.

Can such evidence be interpreted as reflecting rational processes? In laboratory studies, it is relatively healthy people who are sometimes falsely informed that they have a health threat. Being good common-sense lay scientists (Baumann *et al.*, 1989), these individuals may respond by searching for symptoms that are consistent with the risk information, and then assume that the threat is not serious when they find few or minor confirmatory signs. People do consider such rational issues when forming their perceptions, but this cannot explain laboratory evidence of defensive minimization. Individuals who are randomly told that they are at risk from a bogus health threat actually report more confirmatory symptoms and do not show reduced seriousness ratings when minor symptoms are found (Croyle and Sande, 1988; McCaul *et al.*, 1991).

Overall, then, the minimization of health threats appears to be defensive. Decreased seriousness ratings occur only after the individual is personally threatened (i.e., after relapse, or after receiving threatening test results), and minimization is reduced when participants believe that the threat can be altered (e.g., Ditto *et al.*, 1988; Rimes *et al.*, 1999). This latter point is important. If minimization is a rational, non-motivated process, one would expect a condition that is treatable to be viewed as less serious than one that is not. However, threatened participants show less minimization (i.e., *higher* severity ratings) when they are aware of potential treatments than when they are not.

There is also evidence that minimization is effective at repairing mood and maintaining positive self-perceptions. Gibbons *et al.* (1997) found that smokers who relapsed showed a decline in their positive self-conceptions if they did not minimize the risks of smoking, but maintained positive self-conceptions if they did minimize the risk; the level of minimization was correlated with the level of self-protection. Similarly, individuals report reduced worries about health threats when they (Croyle and Sande, 1988) or even a peer (Croyle and Hunt, 1991) minimize the risks.

Do these affective benefits undermine one's motivation to alter the risk? There are few data directly examining the behavioral consequences of defensive minimization. Those who try but fail to quit smoking, and who appear to mend their threatened self-conceptions by playing down smoking risks, do report reduced commitment to make another attempt at giving up; however, they also reinvest in their commitment to quit over time (Gibbons *et al.*, 1997). Thus, minimization may have immediate but not prolonged inhibitory effects on health behaviors. Rimes *et al.* (1999) found that minimization which occurred with unfavorable results of bone density screening was unrelated to subsequent prevention behaviors. Laboratory studies also indicate that individuals who are told that they have a health risk actively seek out information (Croyle and Hunt, 1991; Croyle *et al.*, 1993; Jemmott *et al.*, 1986) and plan to make lifestyle changes to manage the risk (Croyle *et al.*, 1993) while simultaneously playing down its severity.

It is important to remember that defensive minimization takes place in the context of ongoing attempts to understand the threat. The need to develop a representation of the health threat that is congruent with available information (Leventhal *et al.*, 1992) is likely to keep minimization 'in check' and responsive to reality. For example, Croyle (1990) measured illness timeline beliefs among participants who had randomly received either high or normal blood pressure test results. Those in the high blood pressure condition minimized the seriousness of hypertension only if they also viewed hypertension as an acute or cyclical health condition; individuals who had reason to believe hypertension is chronic did not delude themselves into thinking this was not serious. There is also some evidence that minimization softens with time (Croyle *et al.*, 1993; McCaul *et al.*, 1991), presumably because people continue to seek out information, talk to important others, and alter their risk perceptions to be less positively biased in response to new information (e.g., Gerrard *et al.*, 1996; Wiebe and Black, 1997). Thus, there is reason to believe that minimization is an initial defensive process which blunts distress, but does not prevent one from actively understanding and managing the health threat over time.

Self-serving social comparisons

People gain important self-knowledge by comparing themselves to others, but often use these comparisons in a self-serving manner. In the context of health threats, people commonly construct false consensus beliefs by increasing their perceptions of how common the threat is in order to support their own attitudes and behaviors. Across a range of risky behaviors, individuals who engage in the behavior report it as more prevalent than those who do not (Sherman *et al.*, 1983; Suls *et al.*, 1988), and individuals who increase their risky behaviors show simultaneous increases in prevalence perceptions (Gerrard *et al.*, 1996).

Presumably, such perceptions are defensively motivated because they normalize and justify one's risk behaviors, and contribute to the process of minimization. However, they could also be explained via rational processes. Individuals who engage in risky behaviors often interact with similar others, so increased exposure to the risk could account for increased prevalence estimates. Although such rational processes contribute to prevalence estimates, they cannot account for all findings. Sherman *et al.* (1983) found smoking prevalence biases were more extreme among groups with more reason to defend themselves (e.g., adolescents for whom smoking is illegal versus adults; smokers from non-tobacco-growing versus tobacco-growing states). In addition, experimental manipulations of health threats – which obviously control for peer-group experience – demonstrate individuals randomly told they were at risk, display heightened prevalence ratings compared to those told they are not at risk (Croyle and Hunt, 1991; Croyle and Sande, 1988; Croyle *et al.*, 1993; Ditto and Lopez, 1992; McCaul *et al.*, 1991). It thus appears that false consensus biases are at least partially motivated attempts at defending against health threats.

There are limited data regarding the affective or behavioral consequences of false consensus biases. Manipulations of the prevalence of bogus health threats suggest that increased prevalence perceptions are comforting (Croyle and Hunt, 1991; Ditto and Jemmott, 1989; Jemmott *et al.*, 1986). With regard to behavior, Gerrard *et al.* (1996) found adolescents who shifted their prevalence estimates upward after adopting risky health behaviors were at risk of subsequent increases in these behaviors compared to those who did not. Similarly, individuals manipulated to believe that they have a common health risk express less interest in obtaining additional information (Ditto and Jemmott, 1989) and lower intentions to adopt risk-reducing behaviors (Croyle and Hunt, 1991) than those told that they have a rare health risk. Such data suggest that the defense of believing one's health risk is common could undermine motivation to reduce the risk. However, in the experimental studies, individuals assigned to the rare condition (i.e., those with higher intentions to change risk behaviors) were also the ones to demonstrate other forms of defensiveness (e.g., minimization, denigrating test accuracy). Thus, low prevalence manipulations appeared to generate defensiveness without interfering with active coping. Because manipulated high prevalence perceptions may activate a process that is quite different from defensively-generated high prevalence perceptions, data are currently too limited to determine whether false consensus biases have emotional benefits or behavioral costs.

Self-serving social comparisons do appear to be responsive to new information and to occur within the constraints of reality. Klein and Kunda (1993) asked participants to report the frequency of their own and their peers' risk behaviors (e.g., dietary fat intake, alcohol use). Consistent with false consensus biases, participants reported that their peers' risk behaviors were more frequent than their own. In a later session, this belief was countered by telling participants that their peers' risk behaviors were less frequent than their own. Participants responded to this information by reducing the recalled frequency of their own risk behaviors. Thus, participants appeared to accept this new information, but quickly substituted an alternative form of self-protection by biasing recollections of their own risk behaviors (see also Croyle and Hunt, 1991; Ditto and Jemmott, 1989). Importantly, these biased recollections were subtle and reality-based. When manipulated to believe that their peers' risk behaviors were only slightly less frequent than their own, participants displayed a small but detectable recollection bias. However, when manipulated to believe that their peers' behaviors were much less frequent than their own, participants did not display an incrementally larger bias in their recollections.

Overall, then, self-serving social comparisons appear to be fairly common, defensively motivated, and yet reality-based responses to health threats. Although there is some evidence that increased prevalence perceptions can be comforting without clearly undermining behavioral intentions, data are currently too limited to make strong conclusions regarding affective or behavioral consequences.

Denigrating validity and the biased processing of health threat information

The information people want to believe is often perceived as more valid or accurate than information they do not want to believe (Ditto *et al.*, 1998). Although people may readily accept the accuracy of health threat information if it is highly consistent with prior experiences (e.g., accepting a positive genetic test when you have an extensive family history of the associated disease), the validity of unwanted health threat information is often questioned upon initial exposure. For example, individuals who test positive for bogus or real health risks question the accuracy of the test results more than those who test negative (Croyle and Sande, 1988; Croyle *et al.*, 1993; Ditto *et al.*, 1988; Ditto and Lopez, 1992; Jemmott *et al.*, 1986). In fact, Croyle and Sande (1988) found personal relevance to have stronger effects on perceived test accuracy than did the experimental manipulation of accuracy, leading them to argue for the primacy of ego-defense motives in response to health threats.

In a similar vein, individuals exposed to information linking their own behavior to health problems appear facile at identifying weaknesses and discrediting the validity of the data (Liberman and Chaiken, 1992; Reed and Aspinwall, 1998). These effects occur primarily when the individual is personally threatened (Freeman *et al.*, 2001), and are minimized when the motivation to self-protect is experimentally reduced. For example, Reed and Aspinwall (1998) exposed participants to information regarding the link between caffeine and fibrocystic disease. Half of the subjects affirmed their positive self-conceptions (i.e., by focusing on their kindness) prior to viewing the risk information. Coffee drinkers who had self-affirmed were less likely to discount the risk-confirming information than those who had not. Thus, there is reason to believe that these biases are activated by self-protection or affect-regulation motives.

It is possible, however, that decreased perceptions of accuracy are partially the unintended consequence of a deeper processing of the threat information, rather than of motivated attempts to repair negative affect and self-perceptions (Ditto *et al.*, 1998). Negative affect generally produces more systematic processing and less heuristic processing than positive affect, presumably because negative affect provides information of a threat that needs to be fully understood (Bless and Schwarz, 1999; Clore *et al.*, 1994). Careful scrutiny of threatening information could increase one's chances of detecting weaknesses in the data, leading to reduced perceptions of validity. In a test of this 'quantity-of-processing' hypothesis, Ditto *et al.* (1998) found that individuals who randomly received threatening health information were more sensitive to the quality of the information than those who received favorable information. If there was a bias, it was that people seemed surprisingly willing to accept favorable feedback as valid even when told such information may be inaccurate. Although this explanation cannot completely account for findings reported above, reduced accuracy and validity perceptions in response to health threats may partially reflect increased processing of threat information.

What are the affective consequences of defensive processing? There are several ways by which processing biases could mute negative emotions. Careful and detailed processing may lead to a sense of comfort and relief if

risk-disconfirming information is found, and may instill a sense of controllability or self-efficacy regarding the risk if not (c.f., Reed and Aspinwall,
1998). Given the absence of direct data, however, further research will be
necessary to elucidate the role of affect in both the mechanisms and the
outcomes of biased processing. Does defensive processing undermine motivation to alter the objective threat? Individuals who denigrate the validity of
health threat information nevertheless continue to request further information (e.g., Jemmott *et al.*, 1986; Croyle and Sande, 1988) and to report
intentions to change behavior (Croyle *et al.*, 1993; Liberman and Chaiken,
1992; Reed and Aspinwall,1998). To the extent that such indices are related
to actual health behaviors, defensive processing does not necessarily impair
behavioral outcomes.

The defense of denigrating the validity of health threats does appear
responsive to new information. Ditto and Lopez (1992) demonstrated this
by manipulating the outcome of a self-administered diagnostic test for a
bogus health risk. Individuals who randomly received threatening test
results took more time to be convinced that the test was completed, viewed
the initial test as less accurate, and were more likely to conduct additional
tests to confirm the results than those who had received favorable results.
Eventually, however, they accepted the validity of the results. Thus, although
individuals may set a higher standard for accepting the accuracy of threatening information, they appear eventually to do so.

Summary

This limited review supports early speculation that defensive self-protection
is a widespread, normative response to health threats. Individually, these
defensive biases are subtle and malleable – they are less common when
active coping alternatives are available, they are responsive to new information, and they occur within the fuzzy constraints of reality. As a system,
however, defensive processes are very difficult to eliminate, as the disarming
of one process results in the quick substitution of another. Such over-deter-
mination in our ability to defend against the negative implications of health
threats creates a self-protective system that is stable and resilient.

Is this affect regulation?

It is hard to demonstrate that these processes are motivated to regulate negative affect. There are often rational alternatives, and it is quite difficult to
measure affect regulation directly. Emotions are highly reactive to the extent
that focusing one's attention on negative emotions or self-esteem generates a
variety of processes that alter the very phenomenon being studied (Steele,
1988; Pysczynski and Greenberg, 1987). This is also a fluid and bi-directional
process where defensive biases are hypothesized to be elicited by negative
affect (i.e., resulting in a positive association between negative affect and

biases), but then to quickly dispel negative affect (i.e., resulting in a negative association between affect and biases). Thus, results are often open to alternative interpretations. Finally, the sheer number and substitutability of defensive processes make it difficult to link specific biases to emotional outcomes.

Despite such difficulties, these processes appear to be defensive and to have the effect of minimizing distress or maintaining positive self-conceptions. First, exposure to information that one's health is even mildly at risk generates emotional distress (e.g., Cameron and Leventhal, 1995; Croyle *et al.*, 1993; Ditto and Lopez, 1992; Liberman and Chaiken, 1992; Wiebe and Black, 1997) and accompanying defenses. Second, defensive processes occur more often when an individual is personally threatened and has not self-enhanced, suggesting that they are motivated. Finally, the weight of evidence suggests that reality-based defenses function to minimize distress and/or enhance self-perceptions.

Are there behavioral costs?

The effectiveness of these defensive processes in neutralizing health threats raises concerns that short-term emotional benefits come at the very high cost of long-term health problems due to an individual's reduced motivation to engage in protective behaviors. There is surprisingly little research carefully evaluating the relationship between defensive processes and subsequent health behaviors. A major problem is that the full model has rarely been tested. Although many studies show that the presumed outcomes of defensive biases (e.g., reduced risk perceptions) are related to health behaviors, few of these demonstrate that defensiveness was part of the process. This is problematic because perceptions that emerge out of defensiveness differ from those that reflect rational processes. Wiebe and Black (1997) distinguished between individuals with 'unrealistic' (i.e., defensive) and 'realistic' (i.e., rational) low-risk perceptions of contracting sexually transmitted diseases. Compared to individuals identified as having 'realistic' high-risk perceptions, individuals in both low-risk groups reported less interest in viewing risk information (i.e., information on contraception and risky sexual behaviors) and claimed such information was not personally relevant. Interestingly, however, these denial-like variables were associated with reduced negative affect only in the defensive group. Analogously, studies linking low-risk perceptions to poor health behaviors do not clearly address the question of whether defensive denial is maladaptive unless they distinguish between rationally and defensively generated perceptions (see also Leventhal *et al.*, 1999; McCaul and Tulloch, 1999).

Studies that do carefully document defensiveness are also problematic because they often use behavioral measures that are weakly associated with actual health behaviors and outcomes (e.g., information seeking and intentions). Requesting additional information may demonstrate the development of an action plan, but it may also provide an additional defensive resource via biased processing. Similarly, although intentions predict behavior, unhealthy behaviors can be unintentional reflections of impulsive lapses in self-control (Gibbons *et al.*, 1998; Leith and Baumeister, 1996). The self-regulatory processes that form risk perceptions and good intentions are simply quite different from those necessary to generate and maintain healthy behaviors over time (Leventhal *et al.*, 1999; Miller *et al.*, 1996). Given such complexities, it is premature to conclude that defensively generated cognitive distortions compromise the performance of precautionary behaviors over time.

There is, of course, reason to be concerned about adverse behavioral consequences. Most health behavior models view perceived vulnerability as a primary motivator of precautionary behaviors (see Gerrard *et al.*, 1996). Thus, any process that minimizes risk perceptions could theoretically inhibit behavior. Perceived vulnerability is related to a variety of precautionary behaviors (McCaul and Tulloch, 1999), but this association is weak and breaks down in the presence of high emotional arousal such as when the health problem is very threatening and self-relevant, or when the options for managing the threat are complex (Gerrard *et al.*, 1996; Miller *et al.*, 1996). In these situations, unregulated negative affect may disrupt rational influences on behavior. In the following sections, we suggest that defensive processes may serve to keep negative emotions at an optimal level which activates protective behaviors without disrupting the complex set of self-regulatory tasks necessary to maintain such behaviors over time. That is, subtle reality-based defensive processes may be part of a system that calibrates negative affect at adaptive levels so that limited resources do not become dedicated solely to working toward affect-regulation goals.

Rethinking the roles of defensive denial and affect regulation

The benefits and costs of negative affect

Negative emotions are essential features of a well-functioning self-regulation system as they focus attention toward threats, arouse action, and provide feedback on progress toward important goals (Aspinwall and Taylor, 1997; Bless and Schwarz, 1999; Carver and Scheier, 1998; Miller *et al.*, 1996; Ochsner and Lieberman, 2001). Extreme distress, however, can compromise one's ability to fully evaluate the threat or the available coping options (Schwarz and Clore, 1996; Wegener and Petty, 1994), and can undermine resources for mobilizing a response (Baumeister *et al.*, 1998; Salovey and Birnbaum, 1989). Thus, although crucial to effective self-regulation, negative affect left unchecked can disrupt the ongoing regulation of health and illness (see Cameron, this volume, Chapter 8).

Affect-regulating systems and affect-regulation goals

Given the benefits and costs of negative affect, it seems clear that adaptive responses to health threats involve being sensitively attuned to negative emotions while simultaneously being able to mute the experience and check their escalation. We believe the subtle defensive processes that occur in response to health threats are part of a system that efficiently allows individuals to maintain a 'cool' focus on the danger, while periodically or simultaneously benefitting from doses of 'warm' motivation. As Miller *et al.* (1996) argued, effective management of health threats requires individuals 'to cool and abstract the situation to create the necessary psychological distance to tune out the aversiveness and anxiety of the situation, while concentrating on the task contingencies and encouraging performance and progress at each step' (p. 82). Although avoidance and extreme forms of denial may not serve this function, the reality-based second-order denial processes are likely to do so.

Importantly, this perspective could mean that affect-regulation is not the final objective; rather, affect is regulated because doing so maximizes survival. That is, the system that responds to health threats may include a finely calibrated affect-regulating component, without necessarily being directed toward affect-regulation goals. It is often implied that the defensive processes reviewed above reflect a maladaptive situation where affect regulation goals have become primary at the expense of managing the objective threat. We suggest instead that reality-based defenses reflect a system that is working, and it is when these processes fail that disruptive levels of emotional distress occur and resources become temporarily oriented around affect-regulation goals.

The role of the self in defensive responses to health threats

Although we have suggested that defensive denial functions to regulate emotional distress, these processes are inseparable from 'self' regulation – the system by which stable and positive images of the self are maintained. Greenberg *et al.* (1997) posit that the need for self-esteem and the mechanisms used to maintain positive self-views exist specifically to defend against the paralyzing terror of acknowledging our mortality. Threats to health are salient reminders of our mortal status and, thus, may ultimately engage the self-system. In this section, we suggest that a broader understanding of defensive denial can be obtained by considering how it interfaces with the complex workings of the self-system. We specifically explore how the self-system may influence: (a) when defensive denial occurs; (b) the form that defensive denial takes; and, ultimately, (c) the effects of defensive self-protection on ongoing self-regulation efforts.

Self-system influences on the generation of defensive denial

Consistent with emerging theory that the self-system underlies the regulation of health and illness (Brownlee *et al.*, 2000; Contrada and Ashmore,

1999; Hooker, 1999), the self is certainly integral to the generation of defensive responses. Freeman *et al.* (2001) found that defensive processing of anti-smoking messages was predicted less by the current relevance of threat (i.e., smokers' current levels of smoking) than by the extent to which smoking was viewed as a stable component of the self (i.e., having a smoking 'possible self'). Furthermore, when positive self-perceptions are bolstered prior to or during the experience of health threats, participants display less defensive denial (Croyle and Williams, 1991; Reed and Aspinwall, 1998). That is, in response to objectively identical threats, those who have focused on positive self-images display less defensiveness than those who have not – even when those images are unrelated to the threat. Such data suggest defensive denial is primarily about maintaining positive self-perceptions.

Self-system influences on the form and adaptiveness of defensive processes

Self-system influences on the form and adaptiveness of defensive processes can be demonstrated by considering how people cope with chronic health threats. In response to a diagnosis of chronic illness, people are likely initially to experience the defensive procedures discussed above as they develop an illness representation that fits existing self-conceptions (i.e., assimilation). For example, people initially view chronic illness as an acute episode, but eventually shift to view their illness as chronic (Nerenz and Leventhal, 1983). The initial representation is likely to be somewhat defensive, as manipulated chronic illness threats have been found to induce acute timeline perceptions (Croyle, 1990).

As people come to recognize the permanence of their condition and experience its ongoing disruptions, they may engage in very different forms of defensive self-protection. For example, as these initial assimilation processes conflict with the stark realities of chronic disease, people may move toward altering aspects of the self (i.e., accommodation) in order to mend or preserve positive self-images. Heidrich *et al.* (1994) found that patients who viewed their cancer as a permanent part of their lives reported larger discrepancies between their current actual self and their desired ideal self than did patients who viewed cancer as an acute disruption. This suggests that important self-images are threatened once one accepts the permanence of chronic illness. Furthermore, larger actual–ideal self-discrepancies mediated the association between perceptions of chronicity and poorer psychological adjustment. Although preliminary, these data suggest that the manner in which the self-system accommodates health threat information influences adjustment. Specifically, people may be able to regulate a more positive self-image in the face of chronic disease if they reformulate their future self-conceptions to be compatible with the limitations of illness. Ironically, then, maintaining the phenomenology of a stable and positive self in response to chronic health threats may actually involve changing the self (cf., Brownlee *et al.*, 2000; Charmaz, 1999; Nerenz and Leventhal, 1983).

One way to do this involves developing compensatory identities (Gollwitzer and Wicklund, 1985) by increasing the importance of positive self-conceptions that are compatible with illness, and decreasing the importance of positive conceptions that are threatened by illness or of negative conceptions that are caused by illness. This possibility was studied recently among adolescents with diabetes (Wiebe *et al.*, 2002). Participants described themselves in the context of their diabetes, and rated the valence and importance of the descriptors as well as the extent to which diabetes is generally important to their identity. Consistent with the possibility that chronic health threats activate the self-system's ability to generate compensatory identities, negative diabetes self-conceptions (e.g., 'disabled,' 'sick,' 'weird') were rated as less important, and positive diabetes self-conceptions (e.g., 'responsible,' 'mature,' 'compassionate') were rated as more important to participants' self-identities. In addition, participants with negative diabetes self-conceptions displayed better adherence and lower depression when they viewed diabetes as peripheral, rather than central, to their identity. In contrast, participants who described diabetes as having positive consequences for the self displayed better adjustment when they viewed the illness as central. Such data suggest illness experiences create new self-images that can be negative *or* positive, and that the structural features of the self-system influence whether these illness-related self-conceptions are adaptive.

The self-protective processes discussed thus far may partially reflect the 'bottom-up' workings of the self-system (Brownlee *et al.*, 2000). That is, defensive biases and compensatory identities may develop somewhat automatically as we rapidly attend to self-relevant information, efficiently process self-congruent information, and readily recruit self-affirming images into our working self-concept when threatened (Markus and Wurf, 1987). However, personal accounts of coping with chronic illness suggest this also occurs through ongoing struggles to find meaning in one's illness experiences, to foster alternative sources of self-worth, and to construct a new life plan that is optimistically compatible with one's illness (e.g., Charmaz, 1999). These more effortful, 'top-down' processes for regulating a positive self in the face of chronic health threats may account for the fact that patients often find benefits and an improved quality of life in debilitating illness (Taylor, 1983; Tedeschi *et al.*, 1998). Emerging evidence on the adaptiveness of benefit-finding in response to illness suggests that research on the automatic and effortful processes involved in regulating a positive self may enhance our understanding of how people regulate acute and chronic health threats.

Negative and positive affect as feedback on the self

If defensive responses to health threats are specific items in our 'self-zoo' (i.e., our large and diverse collection of self-esteem-enhancing strategies;

Tesser *et al.*, 1996), what is the role of affect? As others have suggested (e.g., Carver and Scheier, 1998; Tesser *et al.*, 1996), negative affect may mediate self-regulatory procedures by providing salient information regarding the status of one's current and future self. As such, threats to the self may arouse negative affect, signaling danger and activating a cascade of self-protective strategies, which remain active until negative arousal is returned to its steady state (cf. Wiebe and Black, 1997).

Positive affect may also influence defensive responses to health threats. A growing literature reveals that positive affect brings a variety of immediate and long-term coping benefits, as it is associated with increased cognitive flexibility, more creative problem-solving, and enhanced self-efficacy, all of which can build on each other to create an upward spiral of health and well-being (Aspinwall, 1998; Frederickson, 2001; Isen, 1999). In the context of health threats, elevated levels of positive affect may generate resources and signal that one is able to confront the threat directly, thus minimizing the need for defensive denial (Reed and Aspinwall, 1998). Deficits in positive affect, on the other hand, may activate self-defensive procedures.

Once activated, reality-based defensive processes are likely, both rapidly and potentially, unconsciously, to return affect to its steady state, creating a tightly calibrated affect-regulating system. These 'bottom-up' defenses may smooth the path toward the broader goal of achieving positive hedonic balance in one's emotional life (i.e., being happy), but should not be equated with more effortful 'top-down' attempts to regulate affect. Affect-regulation as a conscious goal is likely to be fairly common (Larsen, 2000), and skill at being able to maintain a positive hedonic balance is likely to have wide-ranging effects (cf. Frederickson, 2001). We are not convinced, however, that defensive denial is the lead actor in these more effortful affect-regulation procedures.

Summary and conclusions

In this chapter, we have suggested that people's responses to acute and chronic health threats may ultimately entail maintaining a continuous and positive conception of the self, while preserving the integrity of the body. Even minor threats to health can be potent reminders of our mortality. If the need for self-esteem exists to defend against existential paralysis (Greenberg *et al.*, 1997), health threats could directly activate the protective features of the self-system.

Many of the defensive denial processes we have reviewed may represent an almost automatic, front line of defense that is relied on as we encounter and attempt to understand health threats. As long as this understanding is consistent with internal and external information – particularly information about the self – it remains a stable guide to coping efforts. If there is inco-herence, however, something must change to stabilize the system (cf. Leventhal *et al.*, 1992). Such changes may involve turning to alternative subtle defensive denials, refining illness perceptions to be compatible with existing information, or even changing the self. Permanent alterations of the self-system are unlikely in response to acute health threats, but may be fairly common as individuals face or anticipate cycles of debilitation often associated with serious chronic illnesses.

We have also argued that – with the exception of avoidance – defensive procedures for maintaining positive self-images are potentially adaptive because they diminish the experience of disruptive distress and/or enhance the experience of resource-generating positive affect, but do not clearly demobilize action. It may not be surprising, therefore, that interventions designed to alter behavior by breaking down defensive biases are sometimes less than successful (e.g., Weinstein and Klein, 1995; Weinstein *et al.*, 1991), as these interventions could be working against a highly stable and generally adaptive system. These processes may be adaptive because they are reality-based, dynamic, and contextualized. Lazarus (1983) has argued that the impact of denial is context-dependent, being beneficial when denial happens early in the threat process, when direct action is not possible, and when resources to mobilize a response are minimal. The defensive processes we have reviewed are most prominent in each of these situations: they appear early and tend to diminish over time, presumably because they are continually responsive to new information; they are less extreme when participants are aware of direct actions to eliminate the threat; and they are less common when positive resources are enhanced via self-affirmation. It is even possible that the benefits of defensive denial go beyond this static interactional model to reflect a transactional system where self-regulation creates more favorable contexts. For example, by diminishing distress and maintaining or enhancing positive affect, defensive denial may allow one to take a longer-term perspective on the threat (Gray, 1999), and mobilize resources to generate novel ideas for addressing the threat (Aspinwall, 1998).

Although we have suggested that defensive processes do not generally inhibit precautionary behavior, our understanding of the mechanisms and timing of the behavioral effects of defensive denial remains extremely limited. Few studies have actually tested the full model linking defensively generated biases to precautionary behaviors over time. Given the importance of behavior in preventing the development and progression of disease, research that clarifies these associations is a high priority. As this research proceeds, it will be necessary to move beyond static, rational models of precautionary behavior to examine the dynamic transactions between affect, cognition, and behavior as people engage in the ongoing task of regulating health and well-being. For example, we know very little about the bi-directional associations between defensive self-protection in response to health threats and the ongoing development of a coherent health threat representation. Yet information presented in this chapter suggests that the real 'action' of defensive denial is in this ongoing transaction. Careful examination of these transactional dynamics will improve our understanding of when and why defensive self-protection is or is not adaptive (e.g., defenses may be maladaptive if they motivate avoidance, if immediate action is highly beneficial, and so on). Such research may also point to novel interventions to capitalize on the adaptive features or deactivate the maladaptive features of defensive denial (e.g., by coupling the provision of risk information with self-enhancement procedures; Reed and Aspinwall, 1998).

In closing, we return to the role of affect and its regulation in defensive responses to health threats. Although affect appears to be regulated by defensive self-protection, the specific role of affect in how people respond to health threats remains elusive. At one level, affect may provide feedback in a system that is directed toward maintaining self-worth and the integrity of the physical self. Specifically, negative affect may indicate that the self is threatened and in need of defense, while positive affect may indicate that one has resources to spend to confront the threat. In this context, affect would be regulated to the extent that it effectively guides self-enhancement and active threat reduction, but affect regulation would not be the intended goal. Affect and its regulation appears integral to the ongoing dynamics of managing health threats, but the specific role of affect in these responses awaits further explication. We look forward to the emerging story.

Note

1   Correspondence should be addressed to Deborah J. Wiebe, Department of Psychology, 380 South 1530 East, Rm. 502, University of Utah, Salt Lake City, UT 84112, USA. E-mail: Deborah.wiebe@psych.utah.edu

References

Aspinwall, L.G. (1998) 'Rethinking the role of positive affect in self-regulation,' *Motivation and Emotion* **22**: 1–32.

Aspinwall, L.G. and Taylor, S.E. (1997) 'A stitch in time: self-regulation and proactive coping,' *Psychological Bulletin* **121**: 417–436.

Avants, S.K., Warburton, L.A. and Margolin, A. (2001) 'How injection drug users coped with testing HIV-seropositive: implications for subsequent health-related behaviors,' *AIDS Education and Prevention* **13**: 207–218.

Baumann, L.J., Cameron, L.D., Zimmerman, R.S. and Levanthal, H. (1989) 'Illness representations and matching labels with symptons,' *Health Psychology* **8**: 449–469.

Baumeister, R.F., Bratslavsky, E., Muraven, M. and Tice, D.M. (1998) 'Ego-depletion: is the active self a limited resource?' *Journal of Personality and Social Psychology* **74**: 1252–1265.

Bless, H. and Schwarz, N. (1999) 'Sufficient and necessary conditions in dual-process models: the case of mood and information processing,' in S. Chaiken and Y. Trope (eds) *Dual-Process Theories in Social Psychology*, New York: Guilford Press, pp. 423–440.

Brownlee, S., Leventhal, H. and Leventhal, E.A. (2000) 'Regulation, self-regulation, and construction of the self in the maintenance of physical health,' in M.

Boekaerts, P.R. Pintrich and M. Zeidner (eds) *Handbook of Self-Regulation*, San Diego, CA: Academic Press, pp. 369–416.

Cameron, L.D. and Leventhal, H. (1995) 'Vulnerability beliefs, symptom experiences, and the processing of health threat information: a self-regulatory perspective,' *Journal of Applied Social Psychology* **25**: 1859–1883.

Carver, C.S. and Scheier, M.F. (1998) *On the Self-Regulation of Behavior*, New York: Cambridge University Press.

Charmaz, K. (1999) 'From the "sick role" to stories of self: understanding the self in illness,' in R.J. Contrada and R.D. Ashmore (eds) *Self, Social Identity, and Physical Health*, New York: Oxford University Press, pp.209–239.

Clore, G.L., Schwarz, N. and Conway, M. (1994) 'Affective causes and consequences of social information processing,' in R.S. Wyer and K. Srull (eds) *Handbook of Social Cognition*, 2nd edn, Hillsdale, NJ: Lawrence Erlbaum Associates, pp. 323–417.

Conley, T.D., Taylor, S.E., Kemeny, M.E., Cole, S.W. and Visscher, B. (1999) 'Psychological sequelae of avoiding HIV-serostatus information,' *Basic and Applied Social Psychology* **21**: 81–90.

Contrada, R.J. and Ashmore, R.D. (eds) (1999) '*Self and Social Identity. Vol. 2: Self, Social Identity, and Physical Health* New York: Oxford University Press.

Croyle, R.T. (1990) 'Biased appraisal of high blood pressure,' *Preventive Medicine* **19**: 40–44.

Croyle, R.T. and Hunt, J.R. (1991) 'Coping with health threat: social influence processes in reactions to medical test results,' *Journal of Personality and Social Psychology* **60**: 382–389.

Croyle, R.T. and Lerman, C. (1999) 'Risk communication in genetic testing for cancer susceptibility,' *Journal of the National Cancer Institute* **25**: 59–66.

Croyle, R.T. and Sande, G.N. (1988) 'Denial and confirmatory search: paradoxical consequences of medical diagnoses,' *Journal of Applied Social Psychology* **18**: 473–490.

Croyle, R.T. and Williams, K.D. (1991) 'Reactions to medical diagnosis: the role of illness stereotypes,' *Basic and Applied Social Psychology* **12**: 227–241.

Croyle, R.T., Sun, Y. and Louie, D.H. (1993) 'Psychological minimization of cholesterol test results: moderators of appraisal in college students and community residents,' *Health Psychology* **12**: 503–507.

Ditto, P.H. and Croyle, R.T. (1995) 'Understanding the impact of risk factor test results: insights from a basic research program,' in R.T. Croyle (ed.) *Psychosocial Effects of Screening for Disease Prevention and Detection*, New York: Oxford University Press, pp.144–181.

Ditto, P.H. and Jemmott, J.B., III (1989) 'From rarity to evaluative extremity: effects of prevalence information on evaluations of positive and negative characteristics,' *Journal of Personality and Social Psychology* **57**: 16–26.

Ditto, P.H. and Lopez, D.F. (1992) 'Motivated skepticism: use of differential decision criteria for preferred and nonpreferred conclusions,' *Journal of Personality and Social Psychology* **63**: 568–584.

Ditto, P.H., Jemmott, J.B., III and Darley, J.M. (1988) 'Appraising the threat of illness: a mental representational approach,' *Health Psychology* **7**: 183–200.

Ditto, P.H., Scepansky, J.A., Munro, G.D., Apanovitch, M. and Lockhart, L.K. (1998) 'Motivated sensitivity to preference-inconsistent information,' *Journal of Personality and Social Psychology* **75**: 53–69.

Epstein, S. (1994) 'Integration of the cognitive and the psychodynamic unconscious,' *American Psychologist* **49**: 709–724.

Fredrickson, B.L. (2001) 'The role of positive emotions in positive psychology: the broaden-and-build theory of positive emotions,' *American Psychologist* **56**: 218–226.

Freeman, M.A., Hennessy, E.V. and Marzullo, M. (2001) 'Defensive evaluation of antismoking messages among college-age smokers: the role of possible selves,' *Health Psychology* **20**: 424–433.

Gerrard, M., Gibbons, F.X. and Bushman, B.J. (1996) 'Relation between perceived vulnerability to HIV and precautionary sexual behavior,' *Psychological Bulletin* **119**: 390–409.

Gerrard, M., Gibbons, F.X., Benthin, A.C. and Hessling, R.M. (1996) 'A longitudinal study of the reciprocal nature of risk behaviors and cognitions in adolescents: what you do shapes what you think, and vice versa,' *Health Psychology* **15**: 344–354.

Gibbons, F.X., Eggleston, T.J. and Benthin, A.C. (1997) 'Cognitive reactions to smoking relapse: the reciprocal relation between dissonance and self-esteem,' *Journal of Personality and Social Psychology* **72**: 184–195

Gibbons, F.X., McGovern, P.G. and Lando, H.A. (1991) 'Relapse and risk perception among members of a smoking cessation clinic,' *Health Psychology* **10**: 42–45.

Gibbons, F.X., Gerrard, M., Blanton, H. and Russell, D.W. (1998) 'Reasoned action and social reaction: willingness and intention as independent predictors of health risk,' *Journal of Personality and Social Psychology* **74**: 1164–1180.

Gollwitzer, P.M. and Wicklund, R.A. (1985) 'The pursuit of self-defining goals,' in J. Kahl and J. Beckmann (eds) *Action Control: From Cognitions to Behavior*, New York: Springer, pp. 61–85.

Gray, J.R. (1999) 'A bias toward short-term thinking in threat-related negative emotional states,' *Personality and Social Psychology Bulletin* **25**: 65–75.

Greenberg, J., Solomon, S. and Pyszczynski, T. (1997) 'Terror management theory of self-esteem and cultural worldviews: empirical assessments and conceptual refinements,' *Advances in Experimental Social Psychology* **29**: 61–136.

Heidrich, S.M., Forsthoff, C.A. and Ward, S.E. (1994) 'Psychological adjustment in adults with cancer: the self as mediator,' *Health Psychology* **13**: 346–353.

Hooker, K. (1999) 'Possible selves in adulthood: incorporating teleonomic relevance into studies of the self,' in T.M. Hess and F. Blanchard-Fields (eds) *Social Cognition and Aging*, San Diego, CA: Academic Press, pp. 97–122.

Isen, A.M. (1999) 'Positive affect,' in T. Dagleish and M. Power (eds) *Handbook of Cognition and Emotion*, New York: Wiley & Sons Ltd, pp. 521–539.

Jemmott, J.B., III, Ditto, P.H. and Croyle, R.T. (1986) 'Judging health status: effects of perceived prevalence and personal relevance,' *Journal of Personality and Social Psychology* **50**: 899–905.

Klein, W.M. and Kunda, Z. (1993) 'Maintaining self-serving social comparisons: biased reconstruction of one's past behaviors,' *Personality and Social Psychology Bulletin* **19**: 732–739.

Larsen, R.J. (2000) 'Toward a science of mood regulation,' *Psychological Inquiry* **11**: 129–141.

Lazarus, R.S. (1983) 'The costs and benefits of denial,' in S. Brznitz (ed.) *The Denial of Stress*, New York: International Universities Press, pp. 1–30.

Leith, K.P. and Baumeister, R.F. (1996) 'Why do bad moods increase self-defeating behavior? Emotion, risk-taking, and self-regulation,' *Journal of Personality and Social Psychology* **71**: 1250–1267.

Lerman, C., Hughes, C., Main, D., Snyder, C., Durham, C., Narod, S. Lemon, S.J., and Lynch, H.T. (1998) 'What you don't know can hurt you: adverse psychologic effects in members of BRCA1-linked and BRCA2-linked families who decline genetic testing,' *Journal of Clinical Oncology* **16**: 1650–1654.

Leventhal, H. (1970) 'Findings and theory in the study of fear communications,' in L. Berkowitz (ed.) *Advances in Experimental Social Psychology*, vol. 5, New York: Academic Press, pp. 119–186.

Leventhal, H., Diefenbach, M. and Leventhal, E.A. (1992) 'Illness cognition: using common sense to understand treatment adherence and affect cognition interactions,' *Cognitive Therapy and Research* **16**: 143–163.

Leventhal, H., Kelly, K. and Leventhal, E.A. (1999) 'Population risk, actual risk, perceived risk, and cancer control: a discussion,' *Journal of the National Cancer Institute Monographs* **25**: 81–85.

Liberman, A. and Chaiken, S. (1992) 'Defensive processing of personally relevant health messages,' *Personality and Social Psychology Bulletin* **18**: 669–679.

Markus, H. and Nurius, P. (1986) 'Possible selves,' *American Psychologist* **41**: 954–968.

Markus, H. and Wurf, E. (1987) 'The dynamic self-concept: a social and psychological perspective,' *Annual Review of Psychology* **38**: 299–337.

McCaul, K.D. and Tulloch, H.E. (1999) 'Cancer screening decisions,' *Monograph of the National Cancer Institute* **58**: 52–58.

McCaul, K.D., Thiesse-Duffy, E. and Wilson, P. (1991) 'Coping with medical diagnosis: the effects of at-risk versus disease labels over time,' *Journal of Applied Social Psychology* **22**: 1340–1355.

Miller, S.M., Shoda, Y. and Hurley, K. (1996) 'Applying cognitive-social theory to health-protective behavior: breast self-examination in cancer screening,' *Psychological Bulletin* **118**: 70–94.

Nerenz, D.R. and Leventhal, H. (1983) 'Self-regulation theory in chronic illness,' in T.G. Burish and L.A. Bradley (eds) *Coping with Chronic Disease: Research and Applications*, New York: Academic Press, pp. 13–37

Ochsner, K.N. and Lieberman, M.D. (2001) 'The emergence of social cognitive neuroscience,' *American Psychologist* **56**: 717–734.

Pyszczynski, T. and Greenberg, J. (1987) 'Toward an integration of cognitive and motivational perspectives on inferential bias: a biased hypothesis-testing model,' in L. Berkowitz (ed.) *Advances in Experimental Social Psychology*, vol. 20, New York: Academic Press, pp. 297–340.

Reed, M.B. and Aspinwall, L.G. (1998) 'Self-affirmation reduces biased processing of health-risk information,' *Motivation and Emotion* **22**: 99–132.

Rimes, K.A., Salkovskis, P.M. and Shipman, A.J. (1999) 'Psychological and behavioural effects of bone density screening for osteoporosis,' *Psychology and Health* **14**: 585–608.

Salovey, P. and Birnbaum, D. (1989) 'Influence of mood on health-relevant cognitions,' *Journal of Personality and Social Psychology* **57**: 539–551.

Schneider, S. (2001) 'In search of realistic optimism: meaning, knowledge, and warm fuzziness,' *American Psychologist* **56**: 250–263.

Schwarz, N. and Clore, G.L. (1996) 'Feelings and phenomenal experiences,' in E.T. Higgins and A.W. Kruglanski (eds) *Social Psychology: Handbook of Basic Principles*, New York: Guilford, pp. 433–465.

Sherman, S.J., Presson, C.C., Chassin, L., Corty, E. and Olshavsky, R. (1983) 'The false consensus effect in estimates of smoking prevalence: underlying mechanisms,' *Personality and Social Psychology Bulletin* **9**: 197–207.

Steele, C.M. (1988) 'The psychology of self-affirmation: sustaining the integrity of the self,' in L. Berkowitz (ed.) *Advances in Experimental Social Psychology*, vol. 21, San Diego, CA: Academic Press, pp. 261–302.

Suls, J. and Fletcher, B. (1985) 'The relative efficacy of avoidant and nonavoidant coping strategies: a meta-analysis,' *Health Psychology* **4**: 249–288.

Suls, J., Wan, C.K. and Sanders, G.S. (1988) 'False consensus and false uniqueness in estimating the prevalence of health-protective behaviors,' *Journal of Applied Social Psychology* **18**: 66–879.

Taylor, S.E (1983) 'Adjustment to threatening events: a theory of cognitive adaptation,' *American Psychologist* **25**: 1161–1173.

Taylor, S.E., Collins, R.L., Skokan, L.A. and Aspinwall, L. (1989) 'Maintaining positive illusions in the face of negative information: getting the facts without letting them get to you,' *Journal of Social and Clinical Psychology* **8**: 114–129.

Taylor, S.E., Kemeny, M.E., Aspinwall, L.G., Schneider, S.G., Rodriguez, R. and Herbert, M. (1992) 'Optimism, coping, psychological distress, and high-risk sexual behavior among men at risk for acquired immune deficiency syndrome,' *Journal of Personality and Social Psychology* **63**: 460–473.

Tedeschi, R.G., Park, C.L. and Calhoun, L.G. (1998) *Post-Traumatic Growth: Positive Change in the Aftermath of Crisis* Mahwah, NJ: Lawrence Erlbaum Associates.

Tesser, A., Martin, L. and Cornell, D. (1996) 'On the substitutability of self-protective mechanisms,' in P.M. Gollwitzer and J.A. Bargh (eds) *The Psychology of Action: Linking Motivation and Cognition in Behavior*, New York: Guilford, pp. 48–68.

Trope, Y. and Pomerantz, E.M. (1998) 'Resolving conflicts among self-evaluative motives: positive experiences as a resource for overcoming defensiveness,' *Motivation and Emotion* **22**: 53–72.

Wegener, D.T. and Petty, R.E. (1994) 'Mood management across affective states: the hedonic contingency hypothesis,' *Journal of Personality and Social Psychology* **66**: 1034–1048.

Weinstein, N.D. and Klein, W.M. (1995) 'Resistance of personal risk perceptions to debiasing interventions,' *Health Psychology* **14**: 132–140.

Weinstein, N.D., Sandman, P.M. and Roberts, N.E. (1991) 'Perceived susceptibility and self-protective behavior: a field experiment to encourage home radon testing,' *Health Psychology* **10**: 25–33.

Weisman, Avery D. (1972) *On Dying and Denying: A Psychiatric Study of Terminality*, New York: Behavioral Publications.

Wiebe, D.J. and Black, D. (1997) 'Illusional beliefs in the context of risky sexual behaviors,' *Journal of Applied Social Psychology* **27**: 1727–1749.

Wiebe, D.J., Berg, C., Palmer, D., Korbel, C., Beveridge, R., Lindsay, R., Swinyard, M.T., and Donaldson, D. (2002) 'Illness and the self: examining adjustment among adolescents with diabetes,' paper presented at the Annual Meeting of the Society of Behavioral Medicine, Washington, DC.

Part IV

The social and cultural context

10 Carer perceptions of chronic illness

John Weinman, Monique Heijmans and Maria Joao Figueiras[1]

Illness takes place within the family and has reciprocal effects on those who are close to the patient. Studies on the effects of social support in illness adaptation have shown clearly that those who are close to the patient can have a significant influence on the process and outcome of the illness (e.g., Berkman *et al.*, 1992; Schwarzer and Schulz, in press). Although we know that there is considerable variation in the pattern of carers' responses, we know far less about the reasons underlying this variation. Why are some individuals extremely responsive to the needs of their ill relatives whereas others may be indifferent, avoidant or even critical? Part of this variation may stem from pre-existing relationships but there is now an emerging research literature showing that the carers' perceptions of their relatives' illness are not only a key determinant of their own behaviour but also have broader effects on their own well-being as well as that of the patient.

In this chapter we will begin with an introduction to the family context in illness and then provide a selective overview of recent studies that have examined carer illness perceptions, their congruence with patients' perceptions and their effects on outcome. Although the primary focus will be on carers within the family setting, one section will also describe recent research examining the nature and effects of differences between professional health carers' and patients' perceptions of illness. All the evidence reviewed will be restricted to those studies where the patient is an adult because we feel that, although there are parallel issues for understanding carer responses to children with illness, these merit separate consideration.

The family context in illness

The family and broader social context play a crucial role in chronic disease. A chronic disease often brings a profound disruption of normal life: patients have to preserve a reasonable emotional balance and a satisfactory self-image, maintain a sense of competence and mastery, sustain relationships with family and friends, and prepare themselves for an uncertain future (Moos and Tsu, 1977). For the patient coping with these threats and challenges, the family setting provides the central context. As Leventhal *et al.*

(1986) have noted, 'every component of the illness control system from the representation of disease through the development and execution of coping to appraisal is heavily influenced by interaction with the family and by its impact on the family unit' (p.116). This is particularly true now as most chronic illness is managed within the home environment and inevitably involves other family members.

The quality of close relationships can therefore play a vital role for people undergoing the difficult experience of a chronic disease and its subsequent treatment. The relationship between the patient and his or her spouse has been shown to be an important determinant of the patient's well-being. Research on cancer patients and patients with arthritis indicates that emotional support provided by spouses are associated with better psychological adjustment (Manne *et al.*, 1997). Generally, spouses appear to be the most important source of emotional and instrumental support for most patients suffering from chronic illness (Thompson and Pitts, 1992). Unfortunately, spouses as well as other family and friends may also respond in unsupportive ways, which may be intentional (e.g., criticising how the patient is coping with the disease), unintentional (e.g., providing unwanted advice or help), or insensitive (e.g., behaving as if the patient is not ill).

Within the context of recovery from myocardial infarction (MI), a range of studies have shown that the spouse's ability to deal with the ill partner has a significant impact not only on the health and functioning of the family, but also on the patient's physical and emotional adjustment to the illness (Nyamathi, 1987). Research has suggested that a wife's perceptions of her husband's physical capabilities can either assist or impede the recovery process (Rudy, 1980; Taylor *et al.*, 1985). The congruence between a patient's and spouse's causal attributions has been found to be related to better convalescence in the short term (Bar-On, 1987). In contrast, Waltz *et al.* (1988) have shown that depressive symptoms were at their highest and subjective well-being at its lowest among patients who rated their marriages as low in marital intimacy.

Spouse/carer perceptions

The ways in which spouses and other family members cope with a chronic disease and the ways in which they behave towards the patient will be influenced by their own ideas about that specific disease. However, the family context has been rather neglected in illness representation research. Little is known about how other people influence the representation of a health threat and the planning and performance of procedures to cope with it (Leventhal *et al.*, 1997). Until recently, the main focus of illness representation research has been the individual. The representation of an illness and the performance of coping procedures for coping with that illness have been viewed from an intra-psychic perspective (i.e., by concentrating on the mental operations of the individual as problem-solver). Criticism of self-regulation theory such as Ogden's (1995) contention that self-regulation models stay within the head of the individual and ignore the social context, while correct with regard to the empirical findings available at the time, is incorrect with regard to the conceptual structure of self-regulatory models. Linkages to the social context were recognized early on (Leventhal *et al.*, 1986) and more recent presentations have articulated a multi-level approach with three levels of social factors involved, such as the influence of the 'neighbourhood' (Leventhal *et al.*, 2001). Nevertheless, we still know relatively little about how the representations of spouses or other carers differ from those of patients and how a difference would influence a patient's representation of a health threat and the planning and performance of procedures to cope with it.

Heijmans and colleagues have conducted a number of studies in which they have explored the illness perceptions of significant others as a factor influencing the coping responses and adaptive outcomes of chronic disease patients. In a study conducted in 1998, the illness representations of patients suffering from chronic fatigue syndrome (CFS) and Addison's disease (AD) and those of their spouses were compared (Heijmans *et al.*, 1999). The main question under investigation was how a difference in the illness representations of patients and their spouses would affect the patients' coping behaviour and adaptive outcomes. Although spouses generally are the most important source of emotional and instrumental support for many patients, it is obvious that patients' and spouses' ideas about an illness may diverge. For example, the spouse may feel that the consequences of an illness are not as serious as the patient claims, which is expressed as problem minimization (Cohen Silver *et al.*, 1990; Wortman and Lehman, 1985). The opposite may also occur: the spouse may judge the consequences of an illness as far more serious than does the patient. This expresses itself as problem maximization or exaggeration.

From the literature on social support and chronic disease, it is known that spouses try to establish a balance both in their marital relationship and in the patient's functioning. Minimization or maximization by the spouse may serve the function of establishing this balance: when patients minimize their illness, spouses will tend to maximize and become overprotective and vice versa (Thompson and Pitts, 1992). In general, expression of maximization or overprotective behaviour by the spouse has been found to have a negative effect the patient's well-being. This will serve to support sick-role behaviour on the part of the patient and results in such negative consequences as increased dependency, lowered competence and greater depression (Evans and Miller, 1984; Thompson and Pitts, 1992).

Researchers have explored the effects of minimization and maximization in a group of forty-nine patients meeting research criteria for CFS (Fukuda *et al.*, 1994) and in a group of fifty-two patients with AD (Heijmans *et al.*, 1999). Because of their ambiguous nature, both diseases are of interest when studying the effects of social cognition and interaction. AD is characterized by an adrenal insufficiency resulting in symptoms of weakness, fatigue, weight loss and gastrointestinal complaints (Burke, 1992). Although not curable, AD can be managed quite adequately by medication. Given the right dosage, most AD patients function rather well and they have been found to generally minimize the seriousness of their illness (Knapen and Puts, 1993). Moreover, as AD patients generally look healthy, many people believe they are not really ill. In many ways CFS patients resemble AD patients in terms of their most important complaints – fatigue and weakness – but, in contrast to AD patients, they typically experience their illness as extremely disabling. For CFS, no diagnostic tests are available and patients are often confronted with sceptical reactions from families and friends.

The Illness Perception Questionnaire (IPQ; Weinman *et al.*, 1996) was used to assess illness perceptions in both patient groups. The central question being asked was how differences in the illness representations of the spouse and the patient (expressed as either minimization or maximization by the spouse) would influence the patient's coping behaviour and adaptive functioning. By comparing patients' and spouses' illness representations, the researchers were looking for possible differences in the five dimensions of illness representation: identity, timeline, cure, causes and consequences. The results showed considerable differences between the illness perceptions of the patients and those of the spouses. In the case of CFS, partners tended to minimize the seriousness of the illness: they were less convinced that CFS had a biological basis, a strong identity or serious consequences. In contrast, partners of AD sufferers tended to maximize the seriousness of the illness: they perceived more negative consequences, were less optimistic about the possibilities for cure and believed more in a chronic timeline than did the patients. From the spouse questionnaires it became clear that this minimization in the case of CFS and maximization in the case of AD served a balancing function: the spouses of AD patients felt a need to curb the enthusiasm of their sick partners for undertaking activities whereas the spouses of CFS patients tried to motivate their partners to fight the illness to a greater degree and to become more active. However, this balance-seeking by the spouse was not automatically beneficial.

In general, minimization appeared to be more detrimental to the patient's well-being than maximization, although the actual impact depended on the nature of the disease and the particular dimension of the illness perception. In the case of AD, minimization of the seriousness of the symptoms and consequences by the spouse, combined with more optimistic beliefs about timeline, had a negative impact on the well-being of the sick partner. Those AD patients with minimizing spouses reported more problems, especially in mental and social functioning. In the case of CFS, minimization of the consequences and of the role of biological factors by the spouse was particularly associated with patients having more problems in social functioning and less vitality. Minimizing the seriousness of being chronically ill may give the patient the impression of not being taken seriously. However, it should be noted that this study was cross-sectional in design and the directionality and possible reciprocal nature of these effects needs to be confirmed in prospective studies.

In the literature on social support and chronic illness, problem minimization is commonly seen by the patient as unhelpful (Wortman and Lehman, 1985). Spouses who acknowledge the illness and are realistic about its possible future course and treatment seem to be most beneficial in the case of chronic illness. The contrasting effects of convergence or divergence of spouse and patient perceptions of AD and CFS are striking, but it is possible that these might reflect the ambiguities inherent in the nature of these two conditions. It is possible that the degree of congruence in patient and spouse illness perception may be of much less relevance in more clear-cut medical conditions such as MI.

Spouse perceptions and recovery from MI

Although many studies have emphasized the importance of the role of the spouse in the recovery of patients following MI, they have generally failed to assess the ways in which individuals and their families make sense of and cope with the illness. Some studies have focused on the attributions for MI in patients and spouses and how these change from the acute to the convalescence phases after MI (Bar-On, 1987; Rudy, 1980), but they neglect the possible influence of these attributions on the rehabilitation process. Petrie and Weinman (1997) found that the attributions of patients and spouses for MI showed a high degree of agreement, and predicted changes in diet, exercise and other health behaviours following MI.

Figueiras and Weinman (in press) have completed a prospective study exploring the extent to which the perceptions of MI in patients and their partners are similar and whether the degree of similarity in their illness perceptions might be related to the recovery process following MI. We assessed patients' and spouses' illness perceptions and then developed a comparative patient/partner score which attempted to take account not only of the degree of similarity of their perceptions but also the relative level of the scores (i.e. high/low) on each illness perception component. For this purpose a conservative and simple method was developed to compare patient/partner scores on each IPQ sub-scale. This provided a clear classification of the three possible combinations of perceptions that a couple may hold about the MI – namely, similar positive, similar negative and conflicting.

Despite the fact that MI is a much more clear-cut condition than AD or CFS, considerable differences in illness perception were found between patients as well as within couples. The results showed that, with regard to the degree of overlap between the illness perceptions of patients and partners, the most prevalent similar, positive perceptions were in identity, timeline and consequences. The most prevalent similar, negative and conflicting perceptions were in control/cure. Not surprisingly, patient recovery was better in couples with similar positive perceptions of identity and perceived consequences, compared with couples with similar negative or conflicting perceptions. The patients from couples with similar positive perceptions of identity and perceived consequences reported lower levels of disability and fewer sexual problems, greater vitality, less health distress, better psychological adjustment, and less impact of MI on recreational activities and social interaction.

Although similar negative perceptions of MI were associated with poorer outcomes at six and twelve months post-MI, we found little difference in outcome between patients from couples with a similar positive and those with a conflicting representation of MI. This unexpected finding suggests the need to further explore the role of conflicting views in outcome after MI. One possibility would be to investigate whether it makes a difference as to which person (patient/spouse) has the positive (or negative) view and in what ways that perception is associated with outcome.

In interpreting these findings, it did occur to the authors that a congruent positive perception of the MI within a couple might just be a reflection of the quality of the marital relationship. For example, good marital functioning would promote better communication and, hence, possibly similar perceptions of the illness. However, the quality of marital functioning was not found to be associated with the extent to which these couples had similar or conflicting views about the MI, suggesting that similar or conflicting views are not necessarily an indicator of the quality of marital functioning. The experience of illness is different for each member of the couple, and this fact may influence their representations. Studies with other illness groups (e.g. Ben-Zur *et al.*, 2001; Northouse *et al.*, 2000) have also demonstrated that couples can vary in their pattern of adjustment to illness, and this approach may provide helpful insights. Given the accumulating evidence of the importance of dyadic illness perceptions in illness outcome, it is very likely that intervention and rehabilitation approaches could be enhanced by including a focus on couples' perceptions and their degree of consonance. Further prospective studies are needed to investigate the role of the spouse's perceptions of MI, particularly to evaluate the extent to which these can override or influence outcomes which have been found to be strongly related to the patient's own perceptions (Petrie *et al.*, 1996).

Professional health care and patient perceptions

So far we have only discussed the comparative illness perceptions of patients and family carers. Another central dyad in the health care process is that between the patient and the health care provider, and there are good reasons for investigating the degree of match or mismatch between these two parties. One of the present authors (MH) has compared the illness cognitions of chronic disease patients and those of their general practitioner (GP). The

GP–patient relationship is often a central one in chronic disease, as the management of a chronic illness often requires long-term treatment and adequate health care is a joint responsibility of both provider and patient. Given such a partnership, it is very important that the problems of patients with chronic diseases are recognized and addressed by a health care provider. Despite the importance that is assigned to the recognition of patients' problems, there has been little attempt to systematically compare patients' and providers' perceptions of illness. For example, there has been little systematic study of the extent to which the provider's ideas about a chronic disease match those of the patient, or how incongruence between the patient's and the provider's perception of a chronic disease affects the patient's well-being or use of health care facilities. The study by Heijmans *et al.* (2001) was designed to address these issues in a GP setting. A group of 392 diabetes patients, 188 patients suffering from osteo-arthritis and their GPs completed questionnaires to assess the stressors accompanying the patient's illness. Both patient and GP were asked about the extent to which they felt that the illness was life-threatening, progressive, changeable, controllable by medical or self-care, painful, fatiguing, and accompanied by physical, social and mental impairments.

The perceptions of patients and their GPs were compared and the results showed that the two parties differ in the way they think about the patient's illness. Incongruence was greater in the osteo-arthritis group, osteo-arthritis being a disease with a less clear treatment policy than diabetes. Despite the medical evidence that it is a chronic, progressive and incurable condition that causes pain, disability and distress, the patients tended to view it as stable, controllable and with only moderate impairments. Compared with their GPs, patients with diabetes viewed their condition as more changeable, less controllable by medical care, more painful, less life-threatening but more progressive. Although the patterns of incongruence were different across the two conditions, the overall results indicate that GPs' perceptions are linked more to medical factors, as they attach more weight to the medical severity of the condition. For both conditions, differences in perceptions were associated with a patient's poor health status and an increase in health care use; that is, where patients used more non-prescribed drugs and paid more visits to paramedical and alternative healers.

For doctors, medical knowledge is the main source of information on which perceptions and ideas about a certain disease are based. These perceptions are relatively enduring cognitive schemas that stimulate and guide action. For patients, however, illness perceptions are dynamic entities that fluctuate over time in ways that allow them to be meaningfully incorporated into the mesh of ongoing life circumstances. Patients live with their illness every day and, in the case of a chronic illness, for a very long time. Interactions with health care providers are only one of many social situations that influence the nature and evolution of their illness perceptions. Their own day-to-day experiences with their disease and its symptoms are the main source of information on which perceptions are based. In health care communication, a recommended practice is for the provider to elicit the patients' own beliefs about the nature and cause of their condition, as a basis for an effective consultation (e.g., Kinmonth *et al.*, 1998). A potential danger of this approach is that, instead of using the patient's beliefs as a way of understanding more about their situation and needs, the provider may rush into attempting to replace the patient's beliefs with his or her own medically 'correct' version. Yet it is unlikely that the provider's explanations of symptoms and diseases will be readily accepted by patients as replacements for their own ideas or perceptions (Leventhal *et al.*, 1992).

Carer perceptions and patient outcomes: possible mechanisms

There are various ways of explaining how family carer perceptions might influence patient outcome. As Leventhal and colleagues have pointed out, one important moderating variable here is the stage of illness at which carers respond (Leventhal *et al.*, 1986). During the early appraisal stage, in which patients are first experiencing symptoms (e.g., chest pain) that may indicate serious disease, carers can play a crucial role in preventing patient delay in seeking help. Just as the patient's perceptions of these early symptoms can influence the speed with which help is sought (Horne *et al.*, 2000), those spouses or relatives who perceive the person's symptoms as serious are very likely to be instrumental in activating help-seeking and minimizing delay (Hackett and Cassem, 1969; see also Martin and Suls, this volume, Chapter 11).

Once illness is confirmed, carer perceptions will have direct effects on their behavioural and emotional coping procedures, and on how they interact with the patient. Levels of carer support are likely to vary with the degree to which the disease is perceived as controllable and the extent to which carers believe that they can help the patient. Control beliefs may well arise from causal beliefs (French *et al.*, 2001), and evidence indicates that a spouse's causal beliefs have clear links with lifestyle changes following MI (Weinman *et al.*, 2000). Patients whose spouses held a strong belief that the MI was caused by lifestyle factors subsequently engaged in higher levels of dietary and other lifestyle change. This may be particularly important in MI, where the majority of patients are male and where successful dietary change may crucially depend on the involvement of the spouse.

The extent to which carers offer different types of support may also depend on their perceptions of their relative's condition, and there is evidence to suggest that a mismatch between the patient's and carer's perceptions can be problematic. For example, if the carer believes that their relative has little control over their condition, they may well try to help by providing higher levels of assistance. This will be greatly valued by many patients, but carer assistance is not inevitably perceived as helpful by all recipients (Clark and Stephens, 1996), in which case the result can be poorer emotional and physical outcomes (Martire and Schulz, 2001). Studies of women with osteo-arthritis have shown that those patients for whom functional independence is of greatest importance react more negatively to higher levels of spousal support (Martire *et al.*, 2002). These women showed greater depressive symptomatology and less self-care behaviour, and the authors describe a number of ways in which carer perceptions and consequent unwanted assistance can serve to harm the patient by affecting self-evaluations, perceived competence and control. Unwanted assistance could result in adverse changes in the patient's perceptions of illness controllability and consequences.

Carer causal beliefs could also have potentially damaging effects if they involve blame or criticism of the patient. Evidence from studies of carers of people with schizophrenia indicate that blame, criticism and expressed negative emotion can have very detrimental effects on patient recovery (Barrowclough and Parle, 1997). There is now evidence to show that the carer's perceptions of their relative's illness may directly underlie these critical emotional responses. Barrowclough *et al.* (2001) investigated the illness perceptions of those caring for schizophrenics and, using an adapted version of the IPQ, found clear associations between negative carer perceptions and greater experience and expression of negative feelings in the patients. Carers who saw their relative's illness as less amenable to control engaged in higher levels of criticism which, in turn, was linked with higher levels of negative emotion in the patients. Those carers who perceived the illness as having a more chronic timeline expressed less negative emotion. From their study, Barrowclough *et al.* conclude that 'making sense of relatives' perceptions and evaluations of the illness experience is likely to increase understanding of factors mediating problematic responses in carers'. Similar negative effects of family members' hostile or critical comments have been observed in older adults (e.g. Clark and Stephens, 1996), and there may well be key moments in one's life when such effects can have their most negative consequences.

Finally, the evidence on the congruence of carer and patient perceptions outlined earlier indicates that, in dyads with a shared view of the illness, improved patient outcomes might arise from better communication and a shared approach to problem-solving and coping. Although there is surprisingly little evidence from the coping literature, using a dyadic level of analysis one recent study of the combined and separate effects of couples' coping in response to breast cancer does provide confirmatory evidence (Ben-Zur *et al.*, 2001). The findings revealed that a high level of disparity in emotion-focused coping within the dyad was associated with increased patient distress. More specifically, it was found that the patient's distress was greater when one member of the couple coped by denial and the other did not, and a similar effect was found for coping by emotional venting. Surprisingly, incongruence in patterns of problem-focused coping in couples was not linked to patient distress. Nevertheless, studies of this type provide evidence of another way in which carer perceptions can serve to influence patient outcomes through their separate and dyadic effects on coping in the context of illness.

Conclusions and implications

In this chapter, we have provided an overview of the small but growing body of studies investigating carer/relative perceptions of illness in a range of clinical conditions. The findings from these studies identify a number of common themes that add to our understanding of carers' responses to illness and also raise a number of methodological and theoretical issues.

The studies reported here show that carer perceptions can be investigated using the same five components of illness perception that have provided the foundation for the more extensive research on patients' illness perceptions. All these studies used versions of the IPQ that were reworded and adapted for use with carers. Where psychometric evaluations have been conducted, the evidence indicates that the data are usually acceptable but not as robust as those found with the original, patient-focused versions. There is certainly scope for methodological development and refinement of existing measures, as well as for the development of new measures for assessing carer perceptions. Nevertheless, the data do show that the five components of carers' illness representations relate to each other in expected ways, indicating that they can be thought of as coherent schemas that are used for the processing of illness-related information as well as for generating coping procedures.

We have seen that carers' illness perceptions are wide-ranging, and that this dispersion accounts for some of the variation in behavioural and emotional responses in both carers and patients. A particularly important finding to emerge from these studies is that the degree of congruence or similarity in patient and carer perceptions has important, independent effects on the patient's well-being and other illness outcomes. Congruence is likely to be particularly influential in diseases that depend on good self-management (e.g. diabetes) since it may serve to enhance self-efficacy, or in those diseases where the symptoms are vague and ambiguous (e.g. CFS) and where patients may have a particular need to be taken seriously by significant others. Future work will need to determine where and how congruence exerts its effects. There will also be considerable scope for developing methodologies for assessing the ways in which patients and their carers differ in their perceptions of illness

Given the generally ubiquitous, positive effects of social support in illness adaptation, the evidence reviewed in this chapter provides some insights into how carer perceptions might be influential in this process. Critical examination of the social support literature shows that there is considerable uncertainty as to how social support exerts its effects on outcome in health and illness. As was discussed above, there are some situations in which high levels of well-intended support are not valued by those patients needing to preserve a sense of personal control, and the lack of fit between the patient's needs and the carer's perceptions and responses can result in unforeseen negative outcomes. In an excellent critical review, Schwarzer *et al.* (in press) conclude that a variety of psychological processes link social support to illness outcomes and that our understanding of these relationships is still limited. It seems likely that some of the variation in patterns of instrumental and emotional support could be traced back to the carer's representation of the patient's health problem. Developing a better understanding of these representations provides a fundamental starting point for identifying the origins of supportive behaviour as well as for developing interventions to facilitate outcome in chronic illness.

Note

1   Correspondence should be addressed to Professor John Weinman, Unit of Psychology, Guy's, Kings and St Thomas's School of Medicine, University of London, Thomas Guy House, London Bridge, London SE1 9RT, UK. E-mail: john.weinman@kcl.ac.uk

References

Bar-On, D. (1987) 'Causal attribution and the rehabilitation of myocardial victims', *Journal of Social and Clinical Psychology* 5: 114–122.

Barrowclough, C. and Parle, M. (1997) 'Appraisal, psychological adjustment and expressed emotion in relatives of patients suffering from schizophrenia', *British Journal of Psychiatry* 171: 26–30.

Barrowclough, C., Lobban, F., Hatton, C. and Quinn, J. (2001) 'Models of illness in carers of schizophrenic patients', *British Journal of Clinical Psychology* 40: 371–385.

Ben-Zur, H., Gilbar, O. and Lev, S. (2001) 'Coping with breast cancer: patient, spouse and dyad models', *Psychosomatic Medicine* 63: 32–39.

Berkman, L.F., Leo-Summers, L. and Horwitz, R.I. (1992) 'Emotional support and survival following myocardial infarction: a prospective population-based study of the elderly', *Annals of Internal Medicine* 117: 1003–1009.

Burke, C.W. (1992) 'Primary adrenocortical failure', in A. Grossman (ed.) *Clinical Endocrinology*, Oxford: Blackwell, pp. 393–404.

Clark, S.L. and Stephens, M.A.P. (1996) 'Stroke patients' well-being as a function of caregiving spouses' helpful and unhelpful actions', *Personal Relationships* 3: 171–184.

Cohen Silver, R., Wortman, C.B. and Crofton, C. (1990) 'The role of coping in social support provision: the self-presentational dilemma of victims of life crises', in B.R. Sarason and I.G. Sarason (eds) *Social Support: An Interactional View*, New York: Wiley, pp. 397–427.

Evans, R.L. and Miller, R.M. (1984) 'Psychosocial implications of treatment of stroke', *Social Casework: The Journal of Contemporary Social Work* 65: 242–257.

Figueiras, M.J. and Weinman, J. (in press) 'Do congruent patient and spouse perceptions of MI predict recovery?' *Psychology and Health*.

French, D.P., Senior, V., Weinman, J. and Marteau, T.M. (2001) 'Causal attributions for heart disease: a systematic review', *Psychology and Health* **16**: 77–98.

Fukuda, K., Straus, S.E., Hickie, I., Sharpe, M.C., Dobbins, J.G. and Komaroff, A. (1994) 'The Chronic Fatigue Syndrome: a comprehensive approach to its definition and study', *Annals of Internal Medicine* **121**: 953–959.

Hackett, T.P. and Cassem, N.H. (1969) 'Factors contributing to the delay in responding to the signs and symptoms of acute myocardial infarction', *The American Journal of Cardiology* **24**: 651–658.

Heijmans, M., de Ridder, D. and Bensing, J. (1999) 'Dissimilarity in patients' and spouses' representations of chronic illness: exploration of relations to patient adaptation', *Psychology and Health* **14**: 451–466.

Heijmans, M., Foets, M., Rijken, M., Schreurs, K., de Ridder, D. and Bensing, J. (2001) 'Stress in chronic disease: do the perceptions of patients and their general practitioners match?' *British Journal of Health Psychology* **6**: 229–242.

Horne R., James D., Petrie K.J., Weinman J. and Vincent R. (2000) 'Patients' interpretation of symptoms as a cause of delay in reaching hospital during acute myocardial infarction', *Heart* **83**: 388–393.

Kinmonth, A.L., Woodcock, A., Griffin, S., Spiegal, N. and Campbell, M.J. (1998) 'Randomised controlled trial of patient centred care of diabetes in general practice: impact on current well-being and future disease risk', *British Journal of General Practice* **317**: 1202–1208.

Knapen, M.H.J.M. and Puts, P.H.M. (1993) *'Addison patienten in Nederland Sociale gegevens van een onderzoek, integrale onderzoeksresultaten',* The Hague: NVACP.

Leventhal, H., Diefenbach, M. and Leventhal, E.A. (1992) 'Illness cognition: using common sense to understand treatment adherence and affect cognition interactions', *Cognitive Therapy and Research* **16**: 143–163

Leventhal, H., Leventhal, E.A. and van Nguyen, T. (1986) 'Reactions of families to illness: theoretical models and perspectives', in D. Turk and R. Kerns (eds) *Health, Illness and Families: A Life-Span Perspective*, New York: Wiley.

Leventhal, H., Rabin, C., Leventhal, E.A. and Burns, E. (2001) 'Health risk behaviours and aging', in R. Birren and W. Schaie (eds) *Handbook of the Psychology of Aging*, 5th edn, San Diego, CA: Academic Press, pp. 186–214.

Leventhal, H., Benyamini, Y., Brownlee, S., Diefenbach, M., Leventhal, E.A. and Patrick-Miller, L. (1997) 'Illness representations: theoretical foundations', in K.J. Petrie and J.A. Weinman (eds) *Perceptions of Health and Illness: Current Research and Applications*, Amsterdam: Harwood Academic, pp. 19–46.

Manne, S.L, Taylor, K.L., Dougherty, J. and Kemeny, M. (1997) 'Supportive and negative responses in the partner relationship: their association with psychological adjustment among individuals with cancer', *Journal of Behavioral Medicine* **20**: 101–125.

Martire, L.M. and Schulz, R. (2001) 'Informal caregiving to older adults: health effects of providing and receiving care', in A. Baum, T. Revenson and J. Singer (eds) *Handbook of Health Psychology*, Mahwah, NJ: Lawrence Erlbaum Associates, pp. 477–493.

Martire, L.M., Stephens, M.A.P., Druley, J.A. and Wojno, W.C. (2002) 'Negative reactions to received spousal care: predictors and consequences of miscarried support', *Health Psychology* **21**: 167–176.

Moos, R.H. and Tsu, W.D. (1977) 'The crisis of physical illness', in R.H. Moos (ed.) *Coping With Physical Illness*, New York: Plenum Press.

Northouse, L.L., Mood, D., Templin, T., Mellon, S. and George, T. (2000) 'Couples patterns of adjustment to colon cancer', *Social Science and Medicine* **50**: 271–284.

Nymathi, A.M. (1987) 'The coping responses of female spouses of patients with myocardial infarction', *Heart and Lung* **16**: 86–92.

Ogden, J. (1995) 'Changing the subject of health psychology', *Psychology and Health* **10**: 257–265.

Petrie, K.J. and Weinman, J.A. (1997) 'Illness representations and recovery from myocardial infarction,' in K.J. Petrie and J.A. Weinman (eds) *Perceptions of Health and Illness*, Amsterdam: Harwood Academic, pp. 441–461.

Petrie, K., Weinman, J. and Sharpe, N. (1996) 'Role of patients' view of their illness in predicting return to work and functioning after myocardial infarction: a longitudinal study', *British Medical Journal* **312**: 1191–1194.

Rudy, E.B. (1980) 'Patients' and spouses' causal explanations of myocardial infarction', *Nursing Research* **29**: 352–356.

Schwarzer, R. and Schulz, U. (in press) 'The role of stressful life events', in A.M. Nezu, C.M. Nezu and P.A. Geller (eds) *Comprehensive Handbook of Psychology. Vol. 9: Health Psychology*, New York: Wiley.

Schwarzer, R., Knoll, N. and Rieckmann, R. (in press) 'Social support', in A. Kaptein and J. Weinman (eds) *Introduction to Health Psychology*, Oxford: Blackwell.

Taylor, C.B., Bandura, A., Ewart, C.K., Miller, N.H. and DeBusk, R.F. (1985) 'Exercise testing to enhance wives' confidence in their husbands' cardiac capability soon after clinically uncomplicated acute myocardial infarction', *American Journal of Cardiology* **55**: 628–636.

Thompson, S.C. and Pitts, J.S. (1992) 'In sickness and in health: chronic illness, marriage, and spousal caregiving', in S. Spacapan and S. Oskamp (eds) *Stress and Anxiety*, vol. 6, Washington: Hemisphere, pp. 291–311.

Waltz, M., Kriegel, W. and van't Pad Bosch, P. (1998) 'The social environment and health in rheumatoid arthritis: marital quality predicts individual variability in pain severity', *Arthritis Care and Research* **11**: 356–374.

Weinman, J., Petrie, K.J., Moss-Morris, R. and Horne, R. (1996) 'The Illness Perception Questionnaire: a new method for assessing the cognitive representation of illness', *Psychology and Health* **11**: 431–445.

Weinman, J., Petrie, K., Sharpe, N. and Walker, S. (2000) 'Causal attributions in patients and spouses following first-time myocardial infarction and subsequent lifestyle changes', *British Journal of Health Psychology* **5**: 263–273.

Wortman, C.B. and Lehman, D.R. (1985) 'Reactions to victims of life crises: support attempts that fail', in I.G. Sarason and B.R. Sarason (eds) *Social Support: Theory, Research and Applications*, Dordrecht, the Netherlands: Martinus Nijhoff, pp. 498–513.

11 How gender stereotypes influence self-regulation of cardiac health care-seeking and adaptation

René Martin and Jerry Suls[1]

This chapter concerns medical care-seeking and adjustment to cardiac disease. Like the other chapters in the present volume, this one conceptualizes humans as active problem-solvers who try to make sense of changes in their somatic states. This ongoing adaptive process involves peoples' naïve theories or common-sense beliefs about symptoms and illness, appraisals of current states and possible action plans, and sociocultural influences (Leventhal *et al.*, 2001). Our topic is distinctive, however, in two ways. First, we focus on cardiovascular disease as the health threat, both in the initial symptom phase and also during recovery. Second, we are concerned with how common-sense beliefs and performance standards regarding gender influence this self-regulatory process. Although gender stereotypes may also have import for other physical conditions (see Martin and Lemos, 2002), a special connection exists between gender stereotypes and heart disease which influences the meaning that people give to cardiac symptoms and the activities they pursue as they adjust to coronary heart disease (CHD). Before considering this special connection, we briefly discuss two general models of self-regulation of health threats to place our work in context. Earlier chapters in this volume describe particular models of self-regulation in greater detail.

A general approach to self-regulation mechanisms

To understand the integral role of self-regulation in coping with health threats, the control systems approach articulated by Carver and Scheier (1981) and the multiple-process model proposed by Leventhal *et al.* (2001) are good places to start. The fundamental construct of the control systems theory (Carver and Scheier, 1981) is the feedback loop. In such a loop, a sensed value is compared to a reference value or standard and adjustments are made in an output function (if a discrepancy is detected) to shift the sensed value in the direction of the standard. The familiar thermostat controlling the household heating system serves as a good mechanical example. These feedback loops are conceptualized as being arranged in parallel and in hierarchies (where the upper-level loops in a hierarchy provide reference level values for lower-level loops), and loops in adjacent hierarchies provide reference values useful for shifting the ongoing process in new directions when obstructions are encountered.

Leventhal *et al.* (2001) also adopt the feedback loop as a central construct but give greater emphasis to the active problem-solving elements that are involved in identifying and reducing discrepancies. Three elements are crucial: the individual's *representation* of the status of a health problem; the actor's plans and tactics (i.e., *procedures*) for controlling the threat; and the actor's *appraisal* of the discrepancy and the consequences of coping efforts. For each element, the specific content is important. Different representations, procedures, and appraisals are associated with different physical symptom constellations, kinds of coping, and assessments of success. In the case of the individual experiencing typical cardiac symptoms – chest pain, labored breathing, sweating – detection of a discrepancy involves an appraisal of present input (e.g., internal and external signs and symptoms) against a standard – in this case, mental representations or standards about normal levels of physical sensation. An appraisal of current symptoms will involve the retrieval of mental representations or common-sense beliefs about symptoms that are benign versus symptoms that have serious implications and require action. A negative appraisal should lead to the adoption of procedures, which are also based on common-sense beliefs about which actions or antecedents will produce which outcomes ('*if-then*' rules). For example, an individual who experiences the symptoms described above may decide to lie down and rest because of the common-sense rule that resting will reduce certain kinds of symptoms (e.g., heavy breathing, chest pain). Then another appraisal will be conducted, and so on, until no discrepancy is detected – signaling a normal and safe state of affairs.

The specific contents of the input (i.e., the symptoms detected) plus common-sense beliefs and standards are very important because certain symptoms might be represented as cardiac in nature in a person's naïve theory of illness, but other symptoms (e.g., lower gastrointestinal distress and fever) may represent something quite different (e.g., the flu). Procedures such as resting or taking nitroglycerin might be seen as appropriate for cardiac symptoms, but taking antacids might be seen as appropriate if the same symptoms are interpreted merely as an upset stomach.

Of course, the self-regulation of health threats is not limited to symptom episodes. For example, patients who are recovering from a coronary event or chronic symptoms must monitor their activity to achieve an appropriate balance between too much and too little activity, medication, etc. Adjustment to chronic illness requires a continuing process of monitoring and calibrating activity and health behaviors. Throughout this process, patients appraise their current status, adopt strategies based on common-sense beliefs, and then assess the success of their efforts, using standards derived from past experience and social influences. In this chapter, we describe how gender stereotypes influence the self-regulation of symptom perception, medical self-referral, and adjustment to cardiac disease.

Gender stereotypes, symptom perception, and medical self-referral

One type of health threat, as given in our example, concerns symptom perception and what the individual does about it. If a person is experiencing cardiac symptoms, they need to seek medical attention promptly. Delays in seeking medical attention for cardiac symptoms contribute to mortality in both men and women, but treatment delay appears to be a more significant problem for women. As we will show, gender stereotypes about cardiac disease may be one important factor responsible for the sex difference in delay time. Stereotypes about which sex is more likely to suffer from cardiac disease, and under what conditions, influence how people interpret and give meaning to cardiac symptoms, which, in turn, influences whether they think that they are experiencing a physical problem requiring medical attention.

Treatment delay and gender

First, let us consider that the elapsed time between the onset of acute symptoms and entry into the emergency medical care system plays an important factor in reducing mortality and preserving cardiac function. Pre-hospital delay takes on special significance given the advent of thrombolytic therapies, which can reduce myocardial infarction (MI) mortality by 50 per cent when administered within one hour of symptom onset (GISSI, 1986). Unfortunately, treatment delay is extremely common among MI victims. Although delay times vary, they range from ninety minutes to greater than twenty-four hours (e.g., Turi *et al.*, 1986). Almost half of MI patients delay for longer than two hours before seeking medical intervention and a large minority delay for longer than four hours. Interestingly, transportation to the hospital represents only a small proportion of total delay time; delay is primarily a function of victim characteristics (Sharkey *et al.*, 1989).

From our perspective, an interesting result of several large-sample, multiple-site studies is that women delay longer than men before seeking medical intervention after the onset of cardiac-related symptoms (Dracup *et al.*, 1997). The sex difference in pre-hospital delay may explain, in part, why women suffer worse post-MI outcomes than do men. This is because extended self-referral delay reduces women's eligibility for thrombolytic therapies. The extended treatment delay among female MI victims is curious in light of the symptom perception and medical referral literatures which consistently show that women in general tend to be more responsive to health threats and report more physical symptoms than do men (Annandale and Hunt, 1990; Pennebaker, 1982). The reverse pattern, however, seems to be occurring in the case of cardiac symptoms.

Gender differences in symptom perception and treatment seeking?

Why should women take longer than men to recognize, interpret, and act upon cardiac-related symptoms? One explanation is that the judgment and decision-making process activated in response to cardiac-related symptoms is different for women than for men. As mentioned above, symptom inter- pretation and medical self-referral are organized and guided by common-sense models of illness (Leventhal *et al.*, 1980). These cognitive representations incorporate information regarding symptom labels, expected timeline, causal attributions, beliefs about symptom control, and perceived consequences. The way that people conceptualize their emerging symptoms influences whether they infer that the symptoms that they are experiencing represent a serious health threat requiring immediate attention.

Studies of lay interpretations of symptoms reveal the operation of certain rules or heuristics. For example, laypeople tend to attribute symptoms that occur during challenging circumstances to stress rather than to disease (Baumann *et al.*, 1989). Such inferences represent the operation of the discounting principle in attribution theory (Kelly, 1967): when two or more plausible causes for an event (in this case, symptoms) are present, it is diffi- cult to confidently attribute causality to any one factor. Another 'decision rule' used in symptom evaluation is to interpret mild, slow-onset symptoms to be a normal consequence of aging, rather than a manifestation of illness (Prohaska*et al.*, 1987). The reader should appreciate that both of these 'rules' or heuristics would delay treatment seeking.

Most importantly for the present discussion, common-sense models of illness also include stereotypes, which in the case of heart disease may lead to an individual using gender as a decision rule. In the context of cardiac- related symptoms (e.g., chest pain, shortness of breath, and sweating), information about gender may be used as a heuristic such that symptoms are more likely to be attributed to angina or a possible heart attack when the victim is male rather than female.

Several factors may contribute to the assumption or stereotype that CHD is a predominately male diagnosis. Although CHD is the leading cause of death among women, CHD is more common among men than women before the age of 65 (Eaker *et al.*, 1999), thus men are over-represented among cardiology patients (Montague *et al.*, 1991). Also, it follows that laypeople are more likely to have visited or known about a male acquain- tance hospitalized for CHD treatment. The image of the typical CHD victim held by laypeople and health care providers may also have been shaped by the well-known characterization of the aggressive, competitive, hard-driving Type A man (Friedman and Rosenman, 1959). Finally, health care providers may convey to laypeople that women are 'protected' from CHD through the effects of reproductive hormones on lipid metabolism.

The fact that CHD is more common among men than women until later in life suggests that two judgment heuristics, availability and representativeness (Tversky and Kahneman, 1973), influence the evaluation of cardiac-related symptoms by laypeople and increase the likelihood that ordinary people will discount the significance of cardiac symptoms experienced by a female victim. According to the availability heuristic, the perceived probability of a target event increases if the decision-maker can easily recall similar events. Based on the differential exposure and attention given to male rather than to female cardiac patients (as described above), laypeople are likely to recall more male than female acquaintances who have suffered from heart disease. As a consequence, laypeople may tend to assume that they will continue to encounter more male than female cardiac victims in the future. Consequently, the symptoms reported by a woman may be less likely to be attributed to CHD causes.

The representativeness heuristic refers to the classification of a target event by comparing it to the defining characteristics of a particular category. Based on the facts presented earlier, laypeople are likely to conceptualize the typical CHD victim as male and therefore be slower to entertain the possibility that a woman might be experiencing an MI.

The availability and representativeness heuristics should not only influence the personal evaluation of cardiac-related symptoms; they should also affect the kind of advice offered to victims suffering such symptoms by family members and friends who also hold similar common-sense models of heart disease. Spouses and other relatives may suggest to the woman reporting cardiac symptoms that she is experiencing indigestion or the flu. The pre-hospital delay found among women cardiac patients is consistent with the operation of the common-sense model described above.

According to the preceding discussion, women and men probably hold common-sense models of cardiac disease as being a 'male disease.' As a consequence, women experiencing cardiac-like symptoms are apt to discount them as indications of stress or some other disorder. This means that symptom labeling is organised in such a way that cardiac causes tend not to be considered. This process is illustrated in Figure 11.1. The male CHD victim experiences symptoms that are consistent with lay stereotypes of heart disease, thus he proceeds efficiently through the processes of symptom attribution and labeling and decides to seek medical intervention. However, because the female CHD victim's symptoms are inconsistent with the lay stereotype, she is likely to encounter uncertainty when interpreting her symptoms and may misattribute them to non-cardiac causes. It also is possible that her uncertainty will prompt her to consult with family members or friends. But these individuals are just as likely to demonstrate a

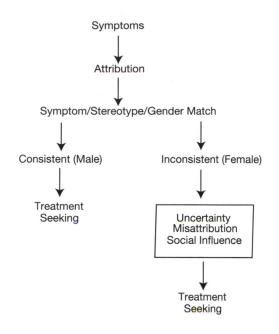

Figure 11.1 The influence of gender and CHD stereotypes on the interpretation of cardiac-related symptoms

Source: Martin *et al.* (1998).

similar stereotypic bias and thus may offer inappropriate advice. The consequence is that the process of symptom perception and interpretation is more complex and time-consuming for female CHD victims.

Empirical evidence

In a series of studies, Martin *et al.* (1998) examined gender disparities in the attribution of cardiac-related symptoms by laypeople. Three hypotheses were tested: (a) laypeople would be more likely to attribute symptoms to cardiac symptoms when the victim was male rather than female; (b) consistent with Baumann *et al.* (1989; see also Leventhal and Diefenbach, 1991), symptoms would be discounted when they were reported in the context of stressful life events; and (c) gender and stressor information might have cumulative effects (of either an additive or interactive nature), so that the symptoms of the female cardiac victim experiencing concurrent life stressors would be most likely to be discounted.

To test these ideas, four studies were conducted in which participants read and responded to a brief vignette, which characterized a victim suffering from symptoms consistent with an evolving MI. Both the gender of the victim and their concurrent life stressors (either low or high) were manipulated as independent variables. After reading the vignette, participants rated the likelihood that the victim's symptoms were due to a cardiac or heart problem.

Laypeople, including two college student samples and a sample of healthy, community-residing adults, were tested in the first three studies. A sample of general practice physicians participated in the fourth study. In all studies, cardiac symptoms were minimized when reported by a woman under stress (see Figure 11.2). In other words, when the victim was a woman who had recently experienced a series of stressful life events, participants were significantly less likely to attribute her symptoms to a heart attack or other cardiac problem, than when the victim was a female without such stressors or a male, regardless of stressor level. The same pattern persisted even when the victim's age (75 years old compared to 45 years old) placed her at a high risk of MI and when she suffered prototypic or classic symptoms of MI (such as crushing chest pain and severe shortness of breath as against jaw pain and indigestion).

In subsequent work, Martin *et al.* (1998) found that subjects were more accurate in recalling information about a male rather than a female MI victim. Furthermore, subjects who received gender-neutral information regarding an MI victim assumed later (erroneously) that they had learned about a male. These findings are consistent with the results of other research which shows that memory for stereotype-consistent information is better

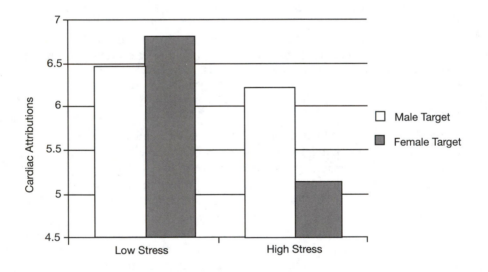

Figure 11.2 Cardiac attributions as a function of information regarding gender and concurrent stressors

Source: Martin *et al.* (1998).

than for stereotype-inconsistent information. Both results support the perspective that laypeople (and physicians) hold stereotypes associating heart disease with male gender.

As mentioned earlier, Martin *et al.* (1998) had subjects make cardiac attributions on rating scales. To ascertain whether symptom discounting would be shown even in spontaneous narrative attributions, Martin and Lemos (2002) had subjects read scenarios about either a woman or a man suffering from cardiac-like symptoms under high stress. Participants were then asked: 'What do you think is most likely to be the cause of Albert/Alice's symptoms?' Analysis of the narrative responses showed consistent evidence that subjects were more likely to attribute identical symptoms to cardiac causes in the case of the male sufferer (85 per cent of responses) than in the case of the female sufferer (15 per cent of responses). Thus, the tendency to discount a woman's cardiac symptoms when she is under high stress is not simply due to a consequence of using rating scales. Participants were also asked: 'What is the first thing Albert/Alice should do?' A higher percentage of subjects recommended seeking medical care in the case of the male sufferer than in the case of the female sufferer.

Taken together, these empirical studies provide consistent evidence to suggest that the greater pre-hospital delay on the part of women with cardiac symptoms may stem from the operation of stereotypes and common-sense models held by the victims and also by their support providers. Parallel evidence emerges from a correlational study with a pilot sample of over 100 male and female MI patients (Martin, 2000). Within a few days after discharge from the hospital, patients were interviewed regarding their symptom perceptions, attributions, and social interactions during the window of time between symptom onset and hospital admission. Although male and female participants were comparable in terms of age, severity of CHD, history of prior MI, and symptom presentation with present MI, women were less likely, during the pre-hospitalization symptomatic period, to realize that their symptoms represented an evolving cardiac event. Men and women were equally likely to engage in lay consultations with support providers regarding their symptoms. However, women were less likely than men to recall that a support provider had spontaneously ascribed symptoms to cardiac causes. Women also were less likely than were men to have been advised by support providers to seek medical care. These findings from MI patients provide additional support for the model described earlier. Stereotypes and common-sense models of heart disease appear to contribute to care-seeking delays among women and their support providers when cardiac symptoms are experienced. Although both women and men are trying actively to understand the meaning of their symptoms, the former are more likely to conclude that they are due to non-cardiac causes that do not require medical attention. Ongoing work with another sample is assessing MI patients' expectations about personal vulnerability, typical MI presentation, and depression, while also collecting data directly from support providers to provide confirmation of patient self-reports and evaluate whether the immediate support network encourages the application of conventional gender stereotypes.

Summary

The above findings suggest how stereotypes and common-sense beliefs can account for differences in care-seeking delays that have important health implications for the CHD patient. This work does not detract from parallel research into gender disparities in medical treatment or diagnosis; it simply indicates that gender disparities also occur earlier in the process, before MI victims ever enter the health care delivery system.[2]

Effects of gender stereotypes on activity post-hospitalization

Gender stereotypes may not only influence how long CHD victims take to seek medical attention for their symptoms, but they may also affect patients' behaviors during recovery. After discharge from the hospital, cardiac patients are asked to gradually assume prior responsibilities, to engage in graded exercise, take medication, etc. For all patients, however, a diagnosis of CHD is a milestone, as is onset of any chronic illness. Moderation during the early weeks after return from the hospital is vital to reduce the possibility of medical complications. The gender stereotypes that patients hold, however, may influence the way in which women compared to men approach the first few weeks of recovery. In particular, domestic responsibilities may be prematurely resumed along sex divisions. Motivated by standards consistent with genders, women may bear undue burdens compared to men during the recovery period. To introduce our argument, we first describe some prior work on the adjustment of male and female post-MI patients and then discuss some of our recent research.

Marriage, social support, and health benefits

Being married is related to lower mortality rates among post-MI patients (e.g., Berkman *et al.*, 1992). This advantage associated with marriage is assumed to be the result of the emotional, informational, and tangible resources received as social support from one's spouse. There have been some indications, however, that women accrue fewer health benefits from social support than do men (e.g., Coombs, 1991; Revenson, 1994). In terms of adjustment and re-infarction, women tend to suffer more post-MI than do men (Schumaker and Czajkowski, 1993). Some studies indicate that women are more likely than men to die during the immediate post-MI period and are also more likely to re-infarct or die within the year following the MI (Weaver *et al.*, 1996). (We should note, however, that too few large-scale studies involving both sexes and controlling for age and severity are available to definitively claim that women's mortality and morbidity post-MI is worse than is men's. Recall that women tend to experience cardiac events at a later age than men.)

Because in traditional marriages women tend to be the domestic and socio-emotional caretakers, the female cardiac patient returning home from the hospital may feel compelled to reassume domestic burdens prematurely instead of obtaining tangible support from their husbands. Ironically, being part of a social network may have a negative effect on them or, at least, not provide the benefits that are provided to male patients (Coombs, 1991; Shumaker and Hill, 1991; Revenson, 1994).

Indirect evidence comes from a report by Hafstrom and Schram (1984) who studied marriages in which either the husband or the wife was a patient of a chronic illness. When the patient was male, his wife assumed many of the tasks previously assumed by her husband. However, husbands of ill wives engaged in no more domestic activities than did healthy husbands whose wives were also healthy. In a sample of MI patients, Young and Kahana (1993) found that women, including those who were married, received less assistance with meals and household tasks than did men. Most significantly, even after adjusting for age, women's relative risk of death compared to men was higher, and women who were married were three times more likely to die than were men. Such results suggest that women with heart disease do not benefit from the social support supposedly provided by marriage.

We are not contending that women who are cardiac patients are 'forced' to reassume domestic responsibilities by other members of the family (i.e., their husbands). Rather, we believe that the division of labor in the traditional marriage reifies the wife as the provider of meals, as laundress, etc. For many wives, foregoing these responsibilities would be a source of stress for them because of the identity crisis that might result from giving up these tasks (Kessler *et al.*, 1985). Stated differently, women in traditional marriages hold standards about the kinds of domestic responsibilities that they are supposed to assume. Several different forms of evidence suggest that women are reluctant to delegate these tasks to others. Interestingly, when men have a heart attack, however, there appears to be a different standard or expectation involved; for them, an extended rest period seems quite appropriate (Conn *et al.*, 1991).

Division of responsibility among female and male cardiac patients

In one of the first studies to compare patterns of activity in male and female post-MI patients, Boogaard and Briody (1985) interviewed twenty patients about the resumption of physical activities in the first week after returning from hospital. Female patients reported resuming many of their prior household responsibilities, such as cooking, cleaning, and laundry, almost immediately upon discharge from the hospital, whereas their male counterparts reported that they were resting and starting cardiac rehabilitation. In addition, even though the women reported performing more high-exertion activities, they felt guilty about their inability to fully resume their usual household responsibilities.

In response to Boogaard and Briody's (1985) findings, Rose and colleagues have conducted three follow-up studies. In the first (Rose *et al.*, 1996) they surveyed twenty-six (50 per cent of whom were female) post-MI patients – matched by age, risk status, and socio-economic status – together with their spouses about the division of labor around the house, both prior to hospitalization and at four, ten, fifteen and twenty-two weeks post-hospitalization. As shown in Figure 11.3, women patients reported a slight reduction in their usual levels of domestic activity (e.g., laundry, cooking, cleaning) during the first few weeks after discharge, while their husbands tended to engage in slightly more domestic activity during this period – *although* women still reported doing somewhat more than their husbands. However, a few weeks later, female patients increased their domestic activity to levels approximating what they had been pre-MI. Meanwhile, their partners returned to their earlier, low levels of activity. In contrast, male patients engaged in low levels

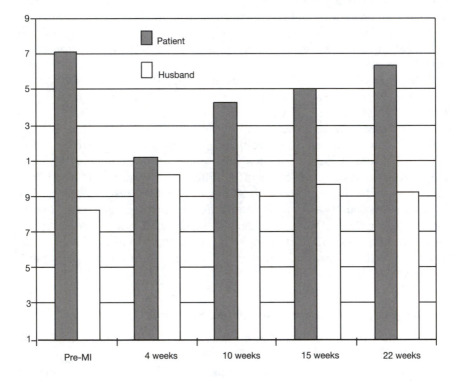

Figure 11.3 Levels of domestic activity undertaken by female post-MI patients and their spouses

Source: Rose *et al.* (1996).

of domestic activity throughout the study period. This does not mean that male patients or caregivers were completely inactive; they did engage in more traditionally masculine activities, such as repairs and home maintenance. However, repairs are more sporadic and can be spread out over days; traditional female domestic tasks, on the other hand, require almost continual attention. Furthermore, cleaning and laundry frequently involve concentrated upper-body movements that create greater cardiac demand.

To summarize, female cardiac patients may be engaging more in potentially risky activities which, in turn, may result in further medical complications, including re-infarction. We believe that women do this because of the gender standards that they hold regarding the appropriate responsibilities of women in the home. As a consequence, they 'overdo' during a period when a gradual return to activity is recommended.

To establish the replicability of these findings, a study with a larger sample of CHD patients was conducted ($N = 63$; Lemos *et al.*, in press) using a similar assessment procedure, although information about typical cardiac symptom levels during the six months post-discharge was also gathered. Again, it was found that female patients assumed more domestic responsibilities than did spouses during recovery. Also, as in the prior study, husbands who were healthy as well as those with heart disease were not completely inactive, but they did little of the conventionally female domestic tasks. They did engage in household repairs, lawn-mowing, and gardening, but these activities tended to be more sporadic.

Of course, an important question is whether women cardiac patients were actually overexerting themselves. An indication that the women patients' domestic activity may be premature would be that they engaged in these activities even when they experienced symptoms indicative of overexertion, such as chest pain and labored breathing. To examine this possibility, we computed correlations between activity and cardiac symptoms separately for male and female patients. For male patients, the correlations tended to be negative, indicating that those males who reported more cardiac symptoms during a given month also reported lower levels of activity that same month. This pattern suggests that men with more symptoms tended to engage in less activity. In contrast, levels of activity and symptoms tended to be less correlated for female patients, consistent with the expectation that symptom levels may play less of a role in determining how much activity the women patients engage in over the month.

In two domains, women showed associations suggesting that they were being active in spite of experiencing symptoms. The correlations between cardiac symptoms and activity in the areas of domestic tasks and outside employment (+0.36 and +0.55) were moderately strong and positive! This suggests that women who engaged in more domestic or outside employment had more symptoms. Overall, then, it seems that women actually seemed to ignore their symptoms when deciding whether to be active, whereas men did not.

In a third study (Jenson *et al.*, in press), eighty CHD patients (fifty-four males and twenty-six females) completed detailed activity diaries for three days at five, ten, fifteen, and twenty weeks post-hospital discharge. These diary entries were then converted to metabolic equivalents (METS; i.e., oxygen cost required to perform a given activity) in accordance with specific guidelines (Ainsworth *et al.*, 1993). The results showed that men and women patients exerted comparable effort in terms of total activity across the day, but women engaged in more domestic activity and tended to consolidate this effort during the morning hours. Men, in contrast, performed household tasks, such as repairs and gardening, but distributed the activity across the day. Stated differently, female patients engaged in more activities with higher energy demands for longer periods. Finally, although it is recommended that patients do not exceed four to six METS in the initial six to eight weeks after hospital discharge (American Association of Cardiovascular and Pulmonary Rehabilitation, 1999), our data indicated that many women exceeded this recommendation when they attended to domestic activities during this time period.

The preceding results are important because they militate against a more positive interpretation of the earlier results: namely, that an early return to previous levels of activity on the part of the woman actually represents progress toward resuming normal activities, and that it may invigorate the cardiac system. Careful examination of the actual activities reported by women in their diaries indicates that many chores, such as vacuuming, require exertion at levels that are explicitly discouraged by physicians and rehabilitation therapists in the early weeks of recovery.

Of course, over-cautiousness also can be a problem during recovery. Some families, fearing that the patient will have another heart attack, assume all of the patient's responsibilities, which leads to cardiac invalidism whereby the patient becomes increasingly dependent and helpless. Our results suggest that this probably occurs more often among male than female patients, although there have been too few studies with appropriate controls comparing men and women cardiac patients during recovery to make a definitive statement. The important issue is that the patient and his/her spouse find ways to make an adaptive resumption of prior activities.

Because women tend to be more socialized into caretaking roles and more responsive to the well-being of others (Gilligan, 1982; Wethington *et al.*, 1987), they may engage in activities that decrease their quality of life and increase their risk of mortality (through risk of re-infarction). The pursuit of these activities, we contend, is not necessarily forced by family members, but is undertaken to meet the patient's internalized standards regarding appropriate domestic responsibilities. Indeed, as implied earlier, a wife returning from the hospital may be reluctant to relinquish tasks that define her identity in the family.

Of course, one limitation of the research described above is the lack of direct evidence to show that premature resumption of activity by women cardiac patients explains the higher morbidity and mortality rates among women after an initial MI, as reported in some studies. Only prospective research assessing activities, symptoms, *and* 'hard' illness outcomes (e.g., death, re-infarction) in a large sample of post-MI men and women will provide a definitive answer. In addition, we should note that gender and sex roles have become less differentiated in recent decades. Thus, the division of domestic labor and expectations seen in the above subject groups (60–70-year-olds who married in the 1950s) may not be exhibited in couples of the future (Revenson, in press).

Although we must wait for the results of prospective research, there is already sufficient evidence for one to concur with Chesney and Darbes (1998) that, 'in the context of women's lives, social relationships are not a proxy for social support. Marriage, rather than being the buffer against adverse health effects that it can be for men, appears to have some detrimental effects for women' (p. 171). In this regard, Orth-Gomer *et al.* (2000) reported that marital stress was associated with nearly three times the normal risk of re-infarction, even after adjustment of traditional risk factors, in a sample of 292 female cardiac patients. Interestingly, work stress did not predict recurrent coronary events. It appears that marital conflict is a more significant risk factor than problems and conflicts at work. One source of marital stress, as suggested above, may be the continuing demands of domestic chores. Just as an initially lower prevalence of CHD in women can contribute to a delay in referring themselves for medical attention, a woman's commitment to their families and to sex-typed responsibilities may have negative consequences as they recover from cardiac events.

Implications

Intervention

This chapter has considered the impact of gender stereotypes about illness and family responsibilities on treatment delay and recovery with respect to cardiac disease. We believe that these phenomena can be understood from a self-regulatory framework where standards and common-sense beliefs serve to direct behavior. This general approach suggests that interventions should be developed to alter maladaptive or incorrect gender stereotypes. In the case of medical referral, public health campaigns already alert women to the risk of heart disease, but little intervention has been concerned with correcting stereotypes and common-sense beliefs so as to short-circuit symptom interpretations that channel attributions to non-cardiac causes. With respect to recovery, in order to increase quality of life and decrease the risk of medical complications, medical staff need to take extra care with female patients and their spouses when explaining the importance of attending closely to physician guidelines regarding the resumption of physical activity, as well as responding meaningfully to cardiac symptoms. In some cases, direct counseling with couples to discuss the need for tangible assistance from spouses or other individuals may be appropriate (Rankin-Esquer *et al.*, 2000).

Emotional support

Our studies of recovery have emphasized the importance of the provision and receipt of tangible support. Partly, this was to provide a counterweight to the emphasis that prior researchers have placed on emotional social support. However, gender stereotypes probably also contribute to the 'costs of caring' (Kessler *et al.*, 1985) in terms of emotional well-being among recovering cardiac patients. Wethington *et al.* (1987) have demonstrated that women more than men show the effects of mental health problems (notably depression) not only as a result of exposure to their own stressors but also to the stressors that occur to others in their social network, especially close family members. We would expect that a wife with heart disease is not only concerned about her own physical condition but that of her husband and other immediate family members. Of course, husbands also exhibit concern about family members, but women who traditionally attend more to the socio-emotional domain as part of their traditional role probably feel this 'weight' more than do men.

There is still another way in which gender stereotypes may affect coping with chronic illness. In marriages where one partner has a chronic illness, coping efforts are not restricted to an individual's physical and emotional needs but also to the integrity of the dyad. This entails managing one's own stress level without creating problems for one's partner. Coyne and Smith (1991) refer to this type of coping as 'relationship-focused.' A particular form of this coping style is protective buffering, which 'involves hiding concerns, denying worries and yielding to the partner to avoid disagreements' (p. 405). Although protective buffering may be intended to protect the relationship, researchers have found that the wives of post-MI patients who engage in more protective buffering tend to be more distressed and depressed (Coyne and Smith, 1991). Presumably, trying to 'bottle-up' and conceal worries has its cost.

There is reason, however, to believe that wives with chronic illness feel a greater need to keep home and family intact and may therefore engage in protective buffering with their healthier husbands. This has not been studied among wives with CHD, but Druley *et al.* (1997) found that a large proportion of women with lupus reported hiding their symptoms and negative feelings about their illness from their spouse. If management of the relationship falls more on the wife, then one would expect that many women with CHD are likely to try to protect their husbands and may, as a consequence, suffer an emotional toll. Ill husbands may also try to keep worries from their wives (Suls *et al.*, 1997), but we would not expect the consequences to be as potentially severe.

Gender-linked traits

From our perspective, gender stereotypes about appropriate activities and illness risk contribute to negative outcomes, such as referral delay and overexertion. We draw these conclusions because the effects appear to fall along sex lines. Not all women, however, may exhibit these behaviors. Helgeson (1993, 1994) has identified a gender-linked personality trait, unmitigated communion orientation, whereby some people are exclusively focused on the welfare of others rather than on themselves. One consequence of an unmitigated communion orientation would be for a patient to return to prior activities or ignore their symptoms because they are so preoccupied with the needs of the other members of the family. Although unmitigated communion is more common among females than males (as noted above, this trait is gender-linked), men can also have this orientation. Fritz (2000) reported that cardiac patients who scored high on a measure of unmitigated communion reported higher levels of cardiac symptoms and increased depression and anxiety four months after hospital discharge. One variable that mediated these relationships was failure to follow an exercise regimen. The other mediator was the perception that network members discouraged the patient's efforts to maintain a healthy lifestyle. Fritz (2000) speculated that the 'unmitigated communion' patient's need to nurture others might cause them to neglect their own condition. Also, family members and friends may fail to recognize the limitations cardiac disease has placed on the patient because the unmitigated communion individual seems to continue serving others' needs despite obvious obstacles.

These findings share elements with results that we presented earlier, but we should emphasize an important difference. Our results suggest that gender stereotypes about cardiac disease and activity level influence most women and most men. (Recall that both men and women think that women who present cardiac-like symptoms under high stress are not experiencing a heart attack. Furthermore, the activities of women recovering from a heart attack seem to be as 'true' to the stereotype as does the activity or inactivity of the men.) Helgeson (1993, 1994) and Fritz (2000), however, identify individuals with an extreme communion orientation as being most vulnerable to problems. Both perspectives may be correct. In general, women holding traditional stereotypes may fall victim to the problems that we observed. Those persons who exhibit an exclusive concern about the welfare of others and neglect themselves may well experience even more invidious outcomes. Of course, we should acknowledge that an unmitigated communion orientation can be viewed from a self-regulatory perspective as contributing to the poor self-regulation of health because other peoples' well-being becomes the salient goal.

Other promising avenues

While the present chapter has focused on the impact of gender stereotypes on responses to CHD, there is considerable potential for taking the same approach with other social stereotypes and health threats. Stereotypes about old age and ethnicity (to name just two salient social dimensions) are likely to shape how people label both their own and others' symptoms. For example, an elderly acquaintance of the authors recently labeled her gradual onset of hip pain as 'arthritis,' an attribution that seemed consistent with her beliefs regarding daily life as an older adult (e.g., 'Aches and pains are a typical part of growing older'). This expectation determined her self-care behaviors (i.e., the use of over-the-counter anti-inflammatories and a heating pad) and her interactions with her health care providers. The fact that the pain in question actually represented bone metastases from an undetected tumor unfortunately went undiscovered for a period of several weeks. It seems very likely that the same symptoms, if experienced by a younger adult with different stereotypes or expectations, would have provoked a different symptom label and response. Along similar lines, a recent study by Martin and Lemos (2002) explored how stereotypes about somatization influence the interpretation of symptoms consistent with gallbladder disease and melanoma.

Conclusion

There is a large amount of literature on sex differences in physical health. Some of the most notable differences are that women tend to report more somatic symptoms, are most apt to refer themselves for medical attention more quickly, and are likely to live on average seven years longer than males. In the domain of cardiac disease, however, women seem to wait longer to seek attention for their symptoms. Cardiac disease is less common among women prior to the age of 65, but incidence, morbidity, and mortality are more severe after that age. Clearly, there is something different about heart disease. The thesis of this chapter is that gender stereotypes formed on the basis of heuristics and traditional conceptions of the role of men and women in traditional marriages provide explanations for these surprising reversals. Although symptom interpretation and activity allocation represent very different domains, hopefully we have persuaded the reader that the common-sense beliefs and standards about men and women are important contributors to the self-regulation of health threats and have significant implications for morbidity and mortality.

Notes

1   This chapter presents two independent lines of research that converge on a single theme. René Martin is responsible for the research on cardiac symptom interpretation and medical referral, which was supported in part by NIH/NIA Grant AG00214-06 and a grant from the American Heart Association (R. Martin, PI). Jerry Suls is responsible for the studies of recovery in CHD patients, which was supported by American Heart Association Grant GS-A-44 (J. Suls, PI). Both authors were assisted by a grant from the National Science Foundation during

the writing of this chapter. Correspondence should be addressed to René Martin, Department of Psychology, E11 Seashore Hall, University of Iowa, Iowa City, IA 52242, USA. E-mail: rene-martin@uiowa.edu

2 Even after taking into account their medical histories and the fact that the onset of MI in women occurs at an older age, CHD is underdiagnosed and under-treated in women (Ayanian and Epstein, 1991; Stone *et al.*, 1996). Women are less likely to undergo angiography, to receive aggressive treatments such as angio-plasty, coronary stenting, or thrombolytic therapies, and are less likely to be referred for exercise rehabilitation following hospitalization (Ayanian and Epstein, 1991; Maynard *et al.*, 1992). Gender disparities in treatment may account partly for women showing greater post-MI mortality and morbidity rates (Gottlieb *et al.*, 1994). However, we contend that gender disparities are apparent *even before* CHD victims have the opportunity to be evaluated by a health care professional.

References

Ahern, D.K., Gorkin, L., Anderson, J.L., Tierney, C., Hallstrom, A., Ewart, C., Capone, R.J., Schron, E., Kornfeld, D., Herd, J.A., Richardson, D.W. and Follick, M.J. (1990) 'Biobehavioral variables and mortality or cardiac arrest in the Cardiac Arrhythmia Polit Study (CAPS),' *American Journal of Cardiology* **66**: 59–62.

Ainsworth, B.E., Haskel, W.L., Leon, A.S., Jacobs, D.R., Montoye, H.J., Sallis, J.F. and Paffenbarger, R.S. (1993) 'Compendium of physical activities: classification of energy costs of human physical activities,' *Medicine and Science in Sports and Exercise* **25**: 71–80.

American Association of Cardiovascular and Pulmonary Rehabilitation (1999) *Guidelines for Cardiac Rehabilitation Programs*, 3rd edn, Champaign, IL: Human Kinetics.

American Heart Association (1987) *1987 Heart Facts*, Dallas, TX: American Heart Association.

Annandale, E. and Hunt, K. (1990) 'Masculinity, femininity and sex: an exploration of their relative contribution to explaining gender differences in health,' *Sociology of Health and Illness* **12**: 24–46.

Ayanian, J.Z. and Epstein, A.M. (1991) 'Differences in the use of procedures between men and women hospitalized for coronary heart disease,' *New England Journal of Medicine* **325**: 221–225.

Baumann, L., Cameron, L.D., Zimmerman, R. and Leventhal, H. (1989) 'Illness representations and matching labels with symptoms,' *Health Psychology* **8**: 449–469.

Berkman, L., Leo-Summers, L. and Horwitz, R. (1992) 'Emotional support and survival after myocardial infarction,' *Annals of Internal Medicine* **117**: 1003–1009.

Berkman, L., Vaccarino, V. and Seeman, T. (1993) 'Gender differences in cardiovascular morbidity and mortality: the contribution of social networks and support,' *Annals of Behavioral Medicine* **15**: 112–123.

Boogaard, M. and Briody, M. (1985) 'Comparison of the rehabilitation of men and women post-myocardial infarction,' *Journal of Cardiopulmonary Rehabilitation* **5**: 379–384.

Burg, M.M., Jain, D., Soufer, R., Kerns, R.D. and Zaret, B.L. (1993) 'Role of behavioral and psychological factors in mental stress-induced silent left ventricular dysfunction in coronary artery disease,' *Journal of the American College of Cardiology* **22**: 440–448.

Carver, C. and Scheier, M. (1981) *Attention and self-regulation: a control-theory approach to human behavior*, New York: Springer-Verlag.

Chesney, M.A. and Darbes, L. (1998) 'Social support and heart disease in women,' in K. Orth-Gomer, M.A. Chesney and Wenger, N.K. (eds) *Women, Stress, and Heart Disease*, Mahwah, NJ: Lawrence Erlbaum Associates, pp. 165–184.

Conn, V.S., Taylor, S.G. and Abele, P.B. (1991) 'Myocardial infarction survivors: age and gender differences in physical health, psychosocial state, and regimen adherence,' *Journal of Advanced Nursing* **16**: 1026–1034.

Coombs, R.H. (1991) 'Marital status and personal well-being: a literature review,' *Family Relations: Journal of Applied Family and Child Studies* **40**: 97–102.

Coyne, J.C. and Smith, D.A. (1991) 'Couples coping with a myocardial infarction: a contextual perspective on wives' distress,' *Journal of Personality and Social Psychology* **61**: 404–412.

Diefenbach, M., Leventhal, E.A., Leventhal, H. and Patrick-Miller, L. (1996) 'Negative affect relates to cross-sectional but not to longitudinal symptom reporting. Data from elderly adults,' *Health Psychology* **15**: 193–199.

Dracup, J., Alonzo, A.A., Atkins, J.M., Bennett, N.M., Braslow, A., Clark, L.T., Eisenberg, M., Ferdinand, K., Frye, R., Green, L., Hill, M.M., Kennedy, J.W., Kline-Rogers, E., Moser, D.K., Ornato, J.P., Pitt, B., Scott, J.D., Selker, H.P., Silva, S.J., Thies, S.J., Weaver, W.D., Wenger, N.K. and White, S.K. (1997) 'The physician's role in minimizing pre-hospital delay in patients at risk of acute myocardial infarction: recommendations for the National Heart Attack Alert Program,' *Annals of Internal Medicine* **126**: 645–651.

Druly, J., Stephens, M. and Coyne, J. (1997) 'Emotional and physical intimacy in coping with lupus: Women's dilemmas of disclosure and approach,' *Health Psychology* **16**: 506–514.

Eaker, E.D., Pinsky, J. and Castelli, W.P. (1992) 'Myocardial infarction and coronary death among women: psychosocial predictors from a 20-year follow-up of women in the Framingham Study,' *American Journal of Epidemiology* **135**: 854–864.

Eaker, E.D., Chesebro, J.H., Sacks, F.M., Wenger, N.K., Whisnant, J.P. and Winston, M. (1999) 'Cardiovascular disease in women,' *Circulation* **88**: 1999–2009.

Fiebach, N.H., Viscoli, C.M. and Horitz, R.I. (1990) 'Differences between women and men in survival after myocardial infarction: biology or methodology?' *Journal of the American Medical Association* **236**: 1092–1096.

Flaherty, J. and Richman, J. (1982) 'Gender differences in the perception and utilization of social support: theoretical perspectives and an empirical test,' *Social Science and Medicine* **28**: 1221–1228.

Forrester, A.W., Lipsey, J.R., Teitlebaum, M.L., DePaulo, J.R. and Andrzejewski, P.L. (1992) 'Depression following myocardial infarction,' *International Journal of Psychiatry in Medicine* **22**: 33–46.

Friedman, M. and Rosenman, R.H. (1974) *Type A Behavior and Your Heart*, New York: Knopf.

Fritz, H. (2000) 'Gender-linked personality traits predict mental health and functional status following a first coronary event,' *Health Psychology* **19**: 420–428.

Gilligan, C. (1982) *In a Different Voice: Psychological Theory and Women's Development*, Cambridge, MA: Harvard University Press.

GISSI (1986) 'Effectiveness of intravenous thrombolytic treatment in acute myocardial infarction,' *Lancet* **8478**: 397–401.

Gottlieb, S., McDermott, M. and Eberly, S. (1994) 'Comparison of posthospital survival after acute myocardial infarction in women and men,' *American Journal of Cardiology* **74**: 727–730.

Hafstrom, J.L. and Schram, V.R. (1984) 'Chronic illness in couples: selected characteristics, including wife's satisfaction with and perception of marital relationships,' *Family Relations* **33**: 195–203.

Helgeson, V.S. (1993) 'The onset of chronic illness: its effect on the patient-spouse relationship,' *Journal of Social and Clinical Psychology* **12**: 406–428.

—— (1994) 'Relation of agency and communion to well-being: evidence and potential explanations,' *Psychological Bulletin* **116**: 429–456.

House, J.S., Landis, K.R. and Umberson, D. (1988) 'Social relationships and health' *Science* **241**: 540–545.

Jenson, M., Suls, J. and Lemos, K. (in press) 'Comparison of physical activity in men and women with cardiac disease: do gender roles create risk for women?' *Women and Health*.

Kelley, H.H. (1967) 'Attribution theory in social psychology,' in D.L. Vine (ed.) *Nebraska Symposium on Motivation*, vol. 15, Lincoln: University of Nebraska Press, pp. 192–241.

Kessler, R., McLeod, J. and Wethington, E. (1985) 'The costs of caring: a perspective on the relationship between sex and psychological distress,' in I.G. Sarason and B.G. Sarason (eds) *Social Support: Theory, Research and Applications*, Boston, MA: Martinus Nijhoff, pp. 491–559.

Lemos, K., Suls, J., Jenson, M., Lounsbury, P. and Gordon, E. (in press) 'How do female and male cardiac patients and their spouses share responsibilities after discharge from the hospital?' *Annals of Behavioral Medicine*.

Leventhal, E.A., Hansell, S., Diefenbach, M., Leventhal, H. and Glass, D.C. (1996) 'Negative affect and self-reports of physical symptoms: two longitudinal studies of older adults,' *Health Psychology* **15**: 193–199.

Leventhal, H. and Diefenbach, M. (1991) 'The active side of illness cognition,' in J.A. Skelton and R.T. Croyle (eds) *Mental Representation in Health and Illness*, New York: Springer-Verlag, pp. 247–272.

Leventhal, H., Leventhal, E. and Cameron, L. (2001) 'Representations, procedures and affect in illness self-regulation: a perceptual-cognitive model,' in A. Baum, T. Revenson and J.E. Singer (eds) *Handbook of Health Psychology*, Mahwah, NJ: Lawrence Erlbaum Associates, pp. 19–48.

Leventhal, H., Meyer, D. and Nerenz, D. (1980) 'The common sense representation of illness danger,' in S. Rachman (ed.) *Medical Psychology*, vol. 2, New York: Pergamon Press, pp. 17–30.

Martin, R. (2000) 'Gender differences on symptom attribution and referral patterns,' paper presented at the Annual Meeting of the Academy of Behavioral Medicine Research, Mont Tremblant, Quebec, Canada.

Martin, R. and Lemos, K. (2002) 'From heart attacks to melanoma: do common-sense models of somatization influence symptom interpretation for female victims?' *Health Psychology* **21**: 25–32.

Martin, R., Gordon, E.I. and Lounsbury, P. (1998) 'Gender disparities in the attribution of cardiac-related symptoms: contributions of common-sense models of illness,' *Health Psychology* **17**: 346–357.

Matthews, K.M., Siegel, J., Kuller, L., Thompson, M. and Varat, M. (1983) 'Determinants of decisions to seek medical treatment by patients with acute myocardial infarction symptoms,' *Journal of Personality and Social Psychology* **44**: 1144–1156.

Maynard, C., Litwin, P.E., Martin, J.S. and Weaver, W.D. (1992) 'Gender differences in the treatment and outcome of acute myocardial infarction. Results from the myocardial infarction triage and intervention registry,' *Archives of Internal Medicine* **152**: 972–976.

Montague, T., Ikuta, R.M., Wong, R.Y., Bay, K.S., Teo, K.K. and Davies, N.J. (1991) 'Comparison of risk and patterns of practice in patients older and younger than 79 years with acute myocardial infarction in a two-year period,' *American Journal of Cardiology* **68**: 843–847.

Moore, S.M (1995) 'A comparison of women's and men's symptoms during home recovery after coronary artery bypass surgery,' *Heart and Lung* **24**: 495–501.

Orth-Gomer, K., Wamala, S., Horsten, M., Schenck-Gustafsson, K., Schneiderman, N. and Mittleman, M. (2000) 'Marital stress worsens prognosis in women with coronary heart disease: the Stockholm Female Coronary Risk Study,' *Journal of the American Medical Association* **284**: 3008–3014.

Pennebaker, J. (1982) *The Psychology of Physical Symptoms*, New York: Springer-Verlag.

Prohaska, T.R., Keller, M.L., Leventhal, E.A. and Leventhal, H. (1987) 'Impact of symptoms and aging attribution on emotions and coping,' *Health Psychology* **6**: 495–514.

Rankin-Esquer, L., Deeter, A. and Taylor, C.B. (2000) 'Coronary heart disease and couples,' in K. Schmaling and T. Sher (eds) *The Psychology of Couples and Illness: Theory, Research and Practice*, Washington, DC: American Psychological Association, pp. 43–70.

Revenson, T. (1994) 'Social support and marital coping with chronic illness,' *Annals of Behavioral Medicine* **16**: 122–130.

—— (in press) 'Scenes from a marriage: the coupling of support, coping and gender within the context of chronic illness,' in J. Suls and K. Wallston (eds) *Social Psychological Foundations of Health and Illness*, Malden, MA: Blackwell Publishers.

Rose, G., Suls, J., Green, P., Lounsbury, P. and Gordon, E. (1996) 'Comparison of adjustment, activity, and tangible support in men and women patients and their spouses during the six months post-myocardial infarction,' *Annals of Behavioral Medicine* **18**: 264–272.

Sharkey, S.W., Brunette, D.D., Ruiz, E., Hession, W.T., Wysham, D.G. and Goldenberg, I.F. (1989) 'An analysis of time delays preceding thrombolysis for acute myocardial infarction,' *Journal of the American Medical Association* **262**: 3171–3174.

Shumaker, S.A. and Czajkowski, S.M. (1993) 'A review of health-related quality-of-life and psychosocial factors in women with cardiovascular disease,' *Annals of Behavioral Medicine* **15**: 149–155.

Shumaker, S.A. and Hill, D.R. (1991) 'Gender differences in social support and physical health,' *Health Psychology* **10**: 102–111.

Stone, P.H., Thompson, B., Anderson, H.V., Kronenberg, M.W., Gibson, R.S., Rogers, W.J., Diver, D.J., Theroux, P., Warnica, J.W., Nasmith, J.B., Kells, C., Kleiman, N., McCabe, C.H., Schactman, M., Knatterud, G.L. and Braunwald, E. (1996) 'Influence of race, sex, and age on management of unstable angina and non-Q-wave myocardial infarction,' *Journal of the American Medical Association* **275**: 1104–1112.

Suls, J., Green, P., Rose, G., Lounsbury, P. and Gordon, E. (1997) 'Hiding worries from one's spouse: associations between coping via protective buffering and distress in male post-myocardial infarction patients and their wives,' *Journal of Behavioral Medicine* **20**: 333–349.

Turi, Z.G., Stone, P.H., Muller, K.E., Parker, C., Rude, R.E., Raabe, D.E., Jaffe, A.S., Hartwell, T.D., Robertson, T.L. and Braunwald, E. (1986) 'Implications for acute intervention related to time of hospital arrival in acute myocardial infarction,' *American Journal of Cardiology* **58**: 203–209.

Tversky, A. and Kahneman, D. (1973) 'Availability: a heuristic for judging frequency and probability,' *Cognitive Psychology* **5**: 207–232.

Weaver, W.D., White, H.D. and Wilcox, R.G. (1996) 'Comparisons of characteristics and outcomes among women and men with acute myocardial infarction treated with thrombolytic therapy,' *Journal of the American Medical Association* **275**: 777–782.

Wethington, E., McLeod, J. and Kessler, R. (1987) 'The importance of life events for explaining sex differences in mental health,' in R.C. Barnett, L. Biener and G.K. Baruch (eds) *Gender and Stress*, New York: Free Press, pp. 144–155.

Young, R.F. and Kahana, E. (1993) 'Gender, recovery from late life heart attack and medical care,' *Women and Health* **20**: 11–31.

12 Culture and illness representation

Linda Ciofu Baumann[1]

As the intersections between diverse world cultures increase, the need for an appreciation of cultural influences on health behavior becomes more critical to our understanding of self-regulation processes. By failing to adequately acknowledge culture, health care practitioners as well as researchers decontextualize social problems and objectify them as individual problems. This approach to health and illness predominates in the Western world, despite evidence that most factors which affect health are outside the traditional sphere of medical care and reside in the lifestyles of persons within a community (Mechanic, 1995; McGinnis and Foege, 1993). This chapter provides a conceptual overview of self-regulation processes within a cultural context and explores how the interpretations of somatic experiences used to guide behavior vary among cultures.

Culture defined

Numerous definitions of culture exist, but they all imply a dynamic process (Andrews and Boyle, 1999; Leininger, 1991). Moreover, there is a general agreement that defining culture too narrowly or too broadly makes it lose much of its significance. Giger and Davidhizar (1999) provide a useful definition, identifying culture as a metacommunication system based on non-physical traits, such as values, beliefs, attitudes, customs, language, and behaviors that are shared by a group of people and passed down to generations through formal communication and imitation. Health beliefs and practices arise from normative or collective cultural values that interact with an individual's unique experiences, beliefs, and values that have been learned in and adapted to a particular context.

Cultural researchers have noted fundamental differences between illness beliefs held by egocentric cultures and those held by sociocentric cultures (Landrine and Klonoff, 2001). Egocentric cultures, largely those of white Europeans and North Americans, embrace the biomedical model of disease and illness and mind-body duality. Sociocentric cultures draw few distinctions between mind-body, religious, medical, spiritual, emotional, and social processes. Landrine and Klonoff (2001) compare health beliefs across seven sociocentric cultural groups and find strong similarities among these cultures in their holistic assumptions, definitions of health, causal attributions for illness, folk disorders, and use of indigenous healers. For example, these groups (which include various Latino, Asian, African American, and Native American cultures) view illness as a result of imbalance and disharmony that arises out of relationship conflicts, behavioral and moral transgressions, and negative emotions. Moreover, they share a view that illness manifests itself not only at the physical level, but at the psychological, social, and spiritual/moral levels as well. The fundamentally different world-views of illness held by egocentric and sociocentric cultures give rise to the prospects of significant clashes when members of these respective types of cultures attempt to understand and communicate with each other about illnesses and their treatment and prevention.

How is self-regulation theory relevant to the study of cultural beliefs?

Even though self-regulation models do take into account the social context of individual behavior, personal and internal processes are viewed as the primary determinants of behavior (Jackson *et al.*, 2000). For example, the common-sense model (Leventhal *et al.*, 1984) delineates the parallel yet highly interactive cognitive and affective processes that shape and direct illness-related behavior. This model also identifies the roles of abstract and concrete-perceptual processes in formulating cognitive representations of illnesses.

A basic assumption underlying self-regulation models is that the individual is a problem-solver, such as a 'common-sense' psychologist or biologist. The individual is actively involved in: (a) interpreting the meaning of somatic experiences; (b) deciding how to best respond to these experiences; and (c) evaluating the effectiveness of the response for achieving a desired outcome – for example, the relief of bothersome symptoms. Because an active problem-solver is involved in interpreting the meanings of somatic experiences of daily life, there is an intimate connection between self-regulation and the culture. The culture and the experiences of the individual are melded in their mental representations and health practices through the processing of information about the external and internal environments. The internal environment involves a continual flux of somatic experiences, many of which may be ambiguous in nature. These body sensations can be clarified in a variety of ways, including by taking action to modify the experience or to categorize it in order to establish meaning and implications. Categorization can be based on prior experience, social comparison, or through seeking advice. Culture plays a critical role in this evaluative process and provides the context of normative beliefs.

Folk illnesses are culturally constructed categories that may be in conflict with the biomedical paradigm. Folk illnesses can be identified and shared within cultural systems that span wide geographic regions and subgroups. In a sample of Latinos living in the US, Central America, and the Caribbean, beliefs about AIDS, diabetes, the common cold, *empacho*, and *mal de ojo* reflected strong, shared illness representations with little unique regional or ethnic variation (Weller and Baer, 2001). *Empacho*, or blocked intestines, results from an imbalance of hot and cold foods, causing food to get stuck in the gastrointestinal tract, leading to symptoms of bloating, cramps, and stomach ache. Older women treat the condition in children by massaging the stomach and back to dislodge the bolus of food and thus allow passage to the rectum. *Mal de ojo*, or 'evil eye,' is caused when a person, usually older, looks at a younger person in an admiring fashion. The eye contact can be deliberate or accidental. The symptoms of *mal de ojo* range from fever, nausea, and diarrhea to irritability and anxiety. The spell can be broken if the admirer touches the person while admiring them. Children are more susceptible to this condition, and many wear a bracelet with a seed (*ojo de venado*) or a bag of seeds pinned to their clothing (Purnell and Paulanka, 1998). Folk illnesses such as these reflect cultural constructions involving the integration of beliefs, actions, and social dynamics as guides to the self-regulation of somatic experiences.

Empirical approaches to exploring cultural models

The most influential work in understanding culture and health beliefs has been done by Arthur Kleinman *et al.* (1978) using situated discourse to elicit *explanatory models* or illness stories about how people interpret the somatic, psychological, and social experience of illness, as told within a 'culture system.' These researchers developed a distinct sub-field in medical anthropology (Farmer and Good, 1991) and provided a means for health care providers to incorporate cultural beliefs into clinical strategies for care and treatment. Explanatory models reflect social class, cultural beliefs, religious beliefs, and past experience with illness. Lay explanatory models of illness begin with an awareness of body sensations and feelings and are elicited by a series of questions:

1   What do you think caused your problem?
2   Why do you think it started when it did?
3   What does your sickness do to you? How does it work?
4   How severe is your sickness? Will it have a long or short duration?
5   What kind of treatment do you think you should receive?
6   What are the most important results you hope to receive from this treatment?
7   What are the chief problems your sickness has caused you?
8   What do you fear most about your sickness?

This approach has been used to identify explanatory models of illness within a variety of cultural groups and settings (e.g., Kelly, 1999; Pachter, 1994; Patel, 1995).

This approach is also useful for exploring differences between explanatory models held by distinctive social groups within a community. Blumhagen (1980) compared lay and expert explanatory models of hypertension in Americans who were mostly white, middle-aged men. For laypersons, the most important causal attribution for the disorder labeled 'hypertension' was chronic external stress that was associated with nervousness, anxiety and worry; the health care experts, meanwhile, said that the cause of hypertension was largely unknown and acknowledged that stress and anxiety might contribute to the disorder. Thus the illness representations of each group were partially distinct, but they did share some overlap.

Recent research guided by self-regulation theory has tended to rely more on quantitative rather than qualitative measures to evaluate and describe illness representation attributes (Meyer *et al.*, 1985; Turk *et al.*, 1986; Weinman *et al.*, 1996). These methods can be used to derive predictive models that deepen our understanding of individual beliefs and behaviors. However, they are less effective than the explanatory model assessments in expanding our understanding of the cultural influences on these beliefs and behaviors. Situated discourse provides qualitative data that can be interpreted to reflect the richness of the historical, social, and political context in which individual behavior takes place, especially in cultures or populations that are infrequently studied.

Are illness representations shared across cultures?

The dimensions of illness representations are fairly universal across large populations, although the cultural context defines the distinct features of the phenomena that comprise an illness representation: (a) a specific label or identity for the symptoms; (b) the anticipated causes of a condition; (c) the anticipated outcomes or consequences; (d) a timeline; and (e) the possibility of control. The explanatory model assessment, which focuses directly on these five attributes, appears to be applicable across cultures. This generic applicability suggests that all people share a need to understand the meaning of the signs or symptoms, cause, outcomes, control over, and timeline of an illness.

Cultures linked by common languages, traditional heritages, and sociopolitical experiences can share similar representations of illnesses. Latino cultures, defined by a language shared among populations of Latin America and the Caribbean (including indigenous groups), share common beliefs about health and illness. In particular, they share a hot/cold theory of disease that explains not only causes of disease and illness but also beliefs about treatment and cure that maintain equilibrium or balance. For example, diarrhea is a 'hot' condition that is treated with 'cold' foods, such as honey or dairy products. Another predominant cultural belief is *fatalismo*, or the belief that one has little control over one's fate (Flores, 2000). Perez-Stable (1987) found that Latinos, when compared to white subjects, were more likely to view cancer as fatal, to prefer not to know the diagnosis, and to believe that there was little one could do to prevent the disease.

In a review of studies conducted in sub-Saharan Africa, Patel (1995) found that beliefs about the spiritual causes of mental illness were shared by the widely diverse cultures of this region. On the other hand, data from the Cornell Medical Index administered to 102 Arab Americans showed significant differences in beliefs according to the country of origin. Many of the differences could be explained by the differences in the country of origin's level of modernization and the subjects' reasons for immigration (Reizian and Meleis, 1987).

Individual or cultural representations?

Garro (1988) states that 'Although there is no sharp distinction between an individual and a cultural model that can be made, researchers focus on one or the other' (p. 98). She used cultural consensus analysis to study Canadian Ojibway models of high blood pressure and showed that despite there being some diversity across the informants' beliefs about what caused high blood pressure, much of the variation in beliefs had its origin in the key concepts of a prototypical, cultural model. Illness representations have been found by others to have a prototypical structure, in that they tend to reflect the most representative case of a particular condition (Bishop and Converse, 1986). When an individual's experience is discrepant with the prototypical illness representation, he or she resolves this discrepancy by considering himself or herself to be an exception to the usual case, yet continues to believe, in general, in the prevailing cultural belief.

This tendency to resolve discrepancies between personal experiences and general cultural models by viewing one's condition as an exceptional case can be observed in US adults with hypertension. Although these patients with hypertension generally agree with the medical cultural model that high blood pressure has no reliable symptoms, they rely on the presence of symptoms to determine the presence and severity of disease. To understand hypertension within a context of prior experience of acute symptomatic illness, persons report that their own hypertension is a symptomatic condition even though they say that it is asymptomatic for others (Baumann and Leventhal, 1985; Meyer *et al.*, 1985).

Illness representations, such as using symptoms to alert an individual to the dangers of high blood pressure, are not necessarily accurate. The implications of inaccurate beliefs are that they may lead to actions which are detrimental to health. For example, patients with hypertension who believed that symptoms were indicators of high blood pressure tended to drop out of treatment, as compared to patients who had an asymptomatic representation of the disease. However, beliefs that are inconsistent with a biomedical model may have social consequences that impact health related behavior. For example, a study eliciting explanatory models of diabetes from patients and professional care givers found that Latino patients attributed economic and family problems as factors that caused diabetes and influenced the course of the disease (Luyas, 1991). In Latino culture, the family and the quality of social relationships are values that serve as a social buffer for coping with life stressors. Professional health care providers, in contrast, did not view economic and family problems as directly affecting the disease process.

Cultural influences on illness representations

Numerous studies have provided evidence of how culture influences the specific contents of illness representation attributes. In some cultures, representational contents may be rich and elaborate integrations of disease characteristics with self-knowledge and personal experiences. For example, Kagawa-Singer and Chung (1994) describe how Asian Pacific Islander psychotherapy clients talk about symptoms of illness by reporting a life story that may provide insight into why the symptoms may have occurred and what the external forces were at the time. These stories build upon variations in the social definition of the self and the need to maintain harmony in interpersonal relationships. As a consequence, there are large individual variations in causal attributions of a particular illness, although it often does not change what people do. In contrast, Western clients are more likely to report symptoms as a list that includes details of duration, frequency, and intensity. Additionally, they focus more on the internal or intrapsychic forces that may be responsible for the occurrence of symptoms.

American Indian and native Alaskan cultures are rich with symbolism. The presence of symbols in a community is a measure of the health and positive energies present. For example, many indigenous peoples of the world use the Sacred Tree as a symbol that represents life, cycles of time, the earth, and the universe. Some common meanings of the tree include protection, nourishment, growth, and wholeness. For many Indians, great respect is given to the phenomenon of dreams and to their importance – not only to the individual but also to the family and tribe. In such cultures, facts and objectivity do not provide a sufficient world-view of a problem and do not acknowledge the harmony and balance between the individual, families, communities, tribes, and peoples of the world (Fleming, 1992). Illness representations are likely to be rich in symbolism and contain concrete imagery that may not be comprehended by those outside these cultures. Moreover, objective, fact-oriented information may be less persuasive for these cultural groups than messages that integrate cultural symbols and understandings (Hagey, 1984).

In most cultures of the world where psychological concepts are less developed, somatization of distress is the norm (Mechanic, 1995). Because these
cultures do not recognize affective distress conditions, somatic experiences
of distress are attributed to illness and incorporated into the illness representation. The bi-level nature of representations (whereby processing occurs at
both an abstract and a concrete level) helps to explain this aspect of self-
regulation. Mechanic (1995) observed in China that neurasthenia was a
disease that appeared to be depression but the patients and providers who
treated these patients denied it was depression. He noted that a patient with
neurasthenia is not necessarily interested in treatment as much as the social
meaning of the condition that allows the person to withdraw from an intol-
erable life situation.

Cultural values and belief systems can also shape the contents of the
emotional representations associated with illness, and these effects can alter
symptom experiences, coping responses, and other aspects of illness self-
regulation. A compelling example is provided by Zborowsky's classic study
(1952) examining ethnic reactions to pain. While Jewish and Italian patients
responded to pain with emotion, Irish Americans were more stoic and
frequently denied the pain.

Shared social experiences continually shape and mold explanatory models
of illness within a culture. An example of how social and historical experiences within a culture influence illness representations is provided by a study
examining illness beliefs and the factors that influence delay in care seeking
among a sample of 296 Vietnamese women with breast cancer (Baumann *et
al.*, 1997). Most women attributed the cause of breast cancer to both
emotional (e.g., stress) and environmental (e.g., pollution and agent orange)
threats associated with war.

'To the extent that an explanatory model as a prevailing consciousness is
internalized by the broad masses, it becomes part of "common sense"' (Greer,
cited in Martin, 1987: 23). As an example of this process, Farmer (1994)
described the development of a cultural representation of AIDS in Haiti from
interviews done over a time-span of five years. Initially the stories lacked a
clear, widely shared model. As exposure to the illness grew and individuals
had personal contact or knew someone with AIDS, the collective representation developed and reflected the understanding that AIDS was a new disease
caused by a germ that is strongly associated with tuberculosis. Symptoms
include 'drying up', skin sores, and diarrhea. The causes of AIDS were
natural (e.g., 'God's illness') or unnatural and caused by sexual contact with
someone who willfully inflicts the disease or germ. The term for AIDS, *sida*,
evoked a fear of the consequences suffered by the poor at the hands of
corrupt governments that do nothing to improve their life conditions.

Epilepsy provides a good illustration of how culture influences illness
representations because of its association with stigma, especially in families
who suffer both financially and in their social interactions. Stigma theory
(Goffman, 1963) holds that epilepsy is a culturally devalued condition. Once

this negative label is applied to a person with seizures, that person then bears the brunt of societal reactions that lower the sufferer's self-esteem (Kleinman *et al.*, 1995): 'To understand that lived experience we also suggest that the suffering associated with epilepsy has to be viewed as occupying interpersonal space, a world of local social experience that connects moral status with bodily status, family with afflicted person, perhaps even social networks with neural networks' (p. 1328). When asked about their beliefs about epilepsy, Chinese subjects from poor interior regions of China reported more negative views of treatment than did North Americans. This difference can be explained by the differences in context. Chinese subjects saw that a person with epilepsy was not treated and continued to have seizures. However, North Americans lived in a context where patients with epilepsy were treated and remained seizure free (Kleinman *et al.*, 1995).

Cultural differences in explanatory models create many challenges for communities in terms of meeting the health needs of immigrants. The clash of cultures in health beliefs is powerfully described in a book by Anne Fadiman (1997). She tells the story of how a Hmong family who had recently immigrated to California interacted with the US health care system in the care of their epilectic child. The Hmong culture in Laos had had little experience of epilepsy. The Lee family consequently developed an explanatory model for their child's epilepsy in which they viewed Lia, the child with epilepsy, as sacred and called the problem 'the spirit catches you and you fall down.' The cause was soul loss, the result of being frightened by a slammed door. The parents believed that Lia did not need medication, but needed instead to be taken home to receive Hmong traditional medicine and animal sacrifice. In the context of the US, the condition was seen not as a blessing but as something to be extinguished through medical treatment.

Future directions

There is a need for a better understanding of the context in which an individual resides in order to guide the interpretation of self-regulation processes (Farmer and Good, 1991; Jackson *et al.*, 2000). This applies not only when considering the cultural context but also when eliciting illness representations in different settings within a culture. For example, Cheung *et al.* (1984) found that illness narratives in physicians' offices were different from those obtained in other settings.

Clark (1996) identifies four basic principles of cultural assessment. First, the culture must be viewed within the context and history in which it developed. Second, the underlying premises of behavior must be examined, such as hot/cold beliefs in disease causation that affect the choice of food believed to alleviate or exacerbate a condition. Third, the meaning and purpose of specific behaviors must be interpreted within the context of the culture. And finally, one must acknowledge individual variation in experiences and beliefs.

A critical theorist may question how lay representations serve either a social or a political end. By way of an example of how this might occur, the social condition of poverty may be transformed into a medical model of individual illness conditions such as diarrhea, stress, or tuberculosis. This transformation may serve the interests of those in power by promoting a societal focus on the treatment of the proximal symptoms of poverty (i.e., the illness conditions) rather than the overarching social causes, which in turn fosters the blaming of individuals for their poor health rather than efforts to deal with the social determinants (Farmer and Good, 1991). Landrine and Klonoff (2001) suggest that when understanding the cultural context of diverse cultural groups who have immigrated to the US, it is important to appreciate that health behaviors (e.g., diet, smoking, alcohol and substance use, use of medical services, acceptance of health information, etc.) are influenced by discrimination, mistrust of whites, and levels of acculturation.

Knowledge of a culture will impact on the design of educational interventions aimed at modifying health-related behavior. Lessons need to be linked to the daily life experiences of an individual and to be consistent with cultural norms and social conditions. Interventions must be holistic for treatment to be consistent and coherent and to make sense. Attempts to understand self-regulation in diverse cultures need to incorporate an understanding of the family and social environments, especially in sociocentric cultures. Such approaches to understanding beliefs and behaviors acknowledge that learning is both cognitive and experiential.

Education about illness and health behaviors needs to be concrete and sensory, for example by focusing on the taste, smell, and texture of the food and on the eating experience in order to modify dietary habits. This approach is theoretically consistent with the dual levels of information processing, abstract and concrete-perceptual, of an illness experience. A new food or a lower-fat method of preparing the food will need to be experienced in order for a person to both understand and feel the implications of this behavior change within the particular culture. Additionally, when providing nutrition information, it is crucial to use familiar regional and ethnic foods for the target audience because individuals with different racial/ethnic backgrounds have different food preferences and food preparation methods (Patterson *et al.*, 1995).

In summary, self-regulation mechanisms arise from both individual and collective experience. Data derived from explanatory models have shown the powerful effects of cultural categories, collective experiences, and social conditions on the experience of illness. Understanding an individual's self-concept and lifestyle patterns can have a profound affect on the quality of interactions with health care providers and enhance the effectiveness of self-regulation strategies that impact on health and illness experiences. Understanding how a person sees him- or herself in the world is essential for obtaining a complete understanding of factors that shape a person's illness experience.

Note

1 Correspondence should be addressed to Linda C. Baumann, 600 Highland Avenue, K6/342, University of Wisconsin-Madison, School of Nursing, Madison, WI 53792–2455, USA. E-mail: ljbauman@facstaff.wisc.edu

References

Andrews, M.M. and Boyle, J.S. (1999) '*Transcultural Concepts in Nursing Care*, 3rd edn, Philadelphia: Lippincott.

Baumann, L.J. and Leventhal, H. (1985) 'I can tell if my blood pressure is up: can't I? *Health Psychology* **4**: 203–218.

Baumann, L.C., Han, Y. and Love, R.R. (1997) 'Beliefs about breast cancer and care seeking in Vietnam,' *Clinical Excellence for Nurse Practitioners: The International Journal of NPACE* **5**: 301–311.

Bishop, G.D. and Converse, S.A. (1986) 'Illness representations: a prototype approach,' *Health Psychology* **5**: 95–114.

Blumhagen, D. (1980) 'Hyper-tension: a folk illness with a medical name,' *Culture, Medicine and Psychiatry* **4**: 197–227.

Chueng, F.M., Lau, B.K.W. and Wong, S. (1984) 'Paths to psychiatric care in Hong Kong,' *Culture, Medicine and Psychiatry* **8**: 207–228.

Clark, M.J. (1996) 'Care of the community or target group,' in M.J. Clark (ed.) *Nursing in The Community*, 2nd edn, Stamford, CT: Appleton & Lange, pp. 389–421.

Fadiman, A. (1997) *The Spirit Catches You and You Fall Down*, New York: Farrar, Straus & Giroux.

Farmer, P. (1994) 'AIDS-talk and the constitution of cultural models,' *Social Science and Medicine* **38**: 801–809.

Farmer, P. and Good, B.J. (1991) 'Illness representations in medical anthropology: a critical review and a case study of the representation of AIDS in Haiti,' in J.A. Skelton and R.T. Croyle (eds) *Mental Representation in Health and Illness*, New York: Springer-Verlag, pp. 132–162.

Fleming, C.M. (1992) 'American Indians and Alaska Natives: changing societies past and present,' in M.A. Orlandi (ed.) *Cultural Competence for Evaluators: A Guide for Alcohol and Other Drug Abuse Prevention Practitioners Working with Ethnic/Racial Communities*, Rockville, MD: US Department of Health and Human Services, pp. 147–171.

Flores, G. (2000) 'Culture and the patient-physician relationship: achieving cultural competency in health care,' *Journal of Pediatrics* **136**: 14–23.

Garro, L. (1988) 'Explaining high blood pressure: variation in knowledge about knowledge,' *American Ethnologist* **15**: 98–119.

Giger, J.N. and Davidhizar, R.E. (1999) *Transcultural Nursing: Assessment and Intervention*, 3rd edn, St Louis, MO: Mosby.

Goffman, I. (1963) *Stigma*, New York: Simon & Schuster.

Hagey, R. (1984) 'The phenomena, the explanations and the responses: metaphors surrounding diabetes in urban Canadian Indians,' *Social Science and Medicine* **18**: 265.

Jackson, T., Mackenzie, J. and Hobfoll, S.E. (2000) 'Communal aspects of self-regulation,' in M. Boekaerts, P.R. Pintrich and M. Zeidner (eds) *Handbook of Self-Regulation*, New York: Academic Press, pp. 275–300.

Kagawa-Singer, M. and Chung, R.C. (1994) 'A paradigm for culturally based care in ethnic minority populations,' *Journal of Community Psychology* **22**: 192–208.

Kelly, P. (1999) 'Isolation and stigma: the experience of patients with active tuberculosis,' *Journal of Community Health Nursing* **16**: 233–241.

Kleinman, R., Eisenberg, E. and Good, B.J. (1978) 'Culture, illness and care: clinical lessons from anthropologic and cross-cultural research,' *Annals of Internal Medicine* **88**: 251–258.

Kleinman, A., Wang, W., Li, S., Cheng, X., Dai, X., Li, K. and Kleinman, J. (1995) 'The social course of epilepsy: chronic illness as social experience in interior China,' *Social Science and Medicine* **40**: 1319–1330.

Landrine, H. and Klonoff, E.A. (2001) 'Cultural diversity and health psychology,' in A. Baum, T.A. Revensen and J.E. Singer (eds), *Handbook of Health Psychology*, Mahwah, NJ: Lawrence Erlbaum Associates, pp. 851–891.

Leininger, M. (1991) *Culture Care Diversity and Universality: A Theory of Nursing*, New York: National League for Nursing.

Leventhal, H., Nerenz, D.R. and Steele, D.J. (1984) 'Illness representations and coping with health threats,' in A. Baum, S.E. Taylor and J.E. Singer (eds) *Handbook of Psychology and Health*, vol. 4, Hillsdale, NJ: Lawrence Erlbaum Associates, pp. 219–252.

Luyas, G.T. (1991) 'An explanatory model of diabetes,' *Western Journal of Nursing Research* **13**: 681–693.

Martin, E. (1987) *The Woman in the Body: A Cultural Analysis of Reproduction*, Boston: Beacon Press.

McGinnis, J.M. and Foege, W.H. (1993) 'Actual causes of death in the United States,' *Journal of the American Medical Association* **270**: 2207–2212.

Mechanic, D. (1995) 'Sociological dimensions of illness behavior,' *Social Science and Medicine* **41**: 1207–1216.

Meyer, D., Leventhal, H. and Gutmann, M. (1985) 'Common-sense models of illness: the example of hypertension,' *Health Psychology* **4**: 115–135.

Pachter, L.M. (1994) 'Culture and clinical care: folk illness beliefs and behaviors and their implications for health care delivery,' *Journal of the American Medical Associaton* **271**: 690–694.

Patel, V. (1995) 'Explanatory models of mental illness in sub-Saharan Africa,' *Social Science and Medicine* **40**: 1291–1298.

Patterson, B.H., Harlan, L.C., Block, G. and Kahle, L. (1995) 'Food choices of whites, blacks, and hispanics: data from the 1987 national health interview survey,' *Nutrition and Cancer* **23**: 105–119.

Perez-Stable, E.J. (1987) 'Issues in Latino health care,' *Western Journal of Medicine* **146**: 213–218.

Purnell, L.D. and Paulanka, B.J. (1998) *Transcultural Health Care: A Culturally Competent Approach*, Philadelphia: F.A. Davis Company.

Reizian, A. and Meleis, A.I. (1987) 'Symptoms reported by Arab-American patients on the Cornell Medical Index (CMI),' *Western Journal of Nursing Research* **9**: 368–384.

Turk, D.C., Rudy, T.E. and Salovey, P. (1986) 'Implicit models of illness,' *Journal of Behavioral Medicine* **9**: 453–474.

Weinman, J., Petrie, K.J., Moss-Morris, R. and Horne, R. (1996) 'The Illness Perception Questionnaire: a new method for assessing the cognitive representations of illness,' *Psychology and Health* **11**: 431–445.

Weller, S.C. and Baer, R.D. (2001) 'Intra- and intercultural variation in the definition of five illnesses: AIDS, diabetes, the common cold, *empacho*, and *mal de ojo*,' *Cross-Cultural Research: The Journal of Comparative Social Science* **35**: 201–226.

Zborowsky, M. (1952) 'Cultural components in response to pain,' *Journal of Social Issues* **84**: 16–44.

Part V

Applications and interventions

13 Self-regulatory interventions for improving the management of chronic illness

Keith J. Petrie, Elizabeth Broadbent, and Geraldine Meechan[1]

The theory of self-regulation elaborated by Leventhal and colleagues (Leventhal *et al.*, 1997; Leventhal *et al.*, 1984) as well as others (Carver and Scheier, 1981) is in many ways ideally suited to understanding and improving patients' management of chronic illness. The theory, simply conceptualized, involves individuals monitoring their efforts and outcomes in managing tasks and using this information to regulate the process towards achieving desired goals. Self-regulation theory proposes that individuals will use strategies that are based on their understanding of the experience. The process is a dynamic one that changes in response to shifts in patients' perceptions. The theory starts with the premise that individuals are active problem-solvers who make sense of a threat to their health, such as physical symptoms or an illness, by developing their own cognitive representations of the threat which, in turn, determine how they respond.

The value of self-regulation theory to chronic disease lies in its dynamic nature. Chronic illnesses and their effects are rarely static, and patients need to integrate feedback on a constant basis in order to manage the illness successfully. Although the symptoms and effects of some chronic illnesses, such as multiple sclerosis or chronic lymphoidleukemia, change slowly over time, other illnesses, such as insulin-dependent diabetes and asthma, may change rapidly if not actively managed by the patient. For optimal management, the patient needs to be aware of the natural pace and course of the illness as well as the links between feedback and action.

The coping strategies adopted by the patient at an immediate level involve managing symptoms and treatment. Yet the demands of the illness may be even more complex, as it usually involves interacting effectively with health care providers and extracting suitable social support or information from others (Petrie, 2002). The psychological distress created by the impact of the illness also needs to be actively managed. For many patients, the physical effects of the illness may be severe and affect many aspects of their lives and identity. For others, prognosis may be poor or uncertain, in which case emotional functioning and personal relationships will be affected.

In this chapter we review a number of interventions that have applied or drawn on a self-regulatory framework in chronic illness populations. Studies were selected for the review if they fulfilled the following three criteria: (1) the intervention needed to be designed to improve the patients' understanding of their chronic illness; (2) the intervention had to aim to link coping or behavioural strategies to specific illness outcomes; and (3) the intervention needed to incorporate some appraisal or monitoring into the programme. The interventions are organized by type of chronic illness rather than by type of therapeutic approach.

We start with diabetes as an example of an illness for which the self-regulatory process is most explicit. Following this section we cover interventions for asthma, HIV, cancer and a set of other chronic illnesses. In the final section, a recent intervention for myocardial infarction (MI) patients is discussed in some detail. This intervention was explicitly developed to change patients' inaccurate and negative illness perceptions of their heart attack. In contrast to other interventions that typically deliver the same behavioural or cognitive intervention to each patient, this programme used an individualized approach in which the content of each patient's intervention was based on an assessment of their perceptions of their MI.

Diabetes mellitus

Successful management of diabetes requires the implementation of a classic self-regulatory process. Diabetic patients must monitor their symptoms and blood glucose levels in order to detect times when they are in danger of suffering from hypoglycaemia or hyperglycaemia. This information then forms the basis of self-treatment with insulin and informs the adjustment of diet – the goal being to regulate blood sugar levels. When the process is working well, changes in blood glucose status are accurately reflected in compensatory patient behaviour. However, difficulties with self-monitoring, ongoing self-treatment, or health behaviours can cause this self-regulatory system to break down. An additional problem is that good adherence does not directly correspond with good control. Although adherence leads to better control than non-adherence, there is still a lot of 'noise' in the feedback received by patients. Emotionally, this leads to considerable frustration over failing to achieve good control despite diligence in monitoring and treatment use.

A number of successful interventions have been developed to improve various aspects of the feedback system and thus the patient's management of diabetes. Research has demonstrated that patients' cognitive representations of diabetes play an important role in instituting a successful self-management process. A survey of 296 diabetic adults found that greater understanding of the condition and higher perceived control of diabetes were associated with greater engagement in diabetes-specific health behaviours (Watkins *et al.*, 2000). These representations were also associated with fewer negative feelings towards the disease and lower perceived interference with social and personal functioning. Similar results were found in a study of young people with Type 1 diabetes (Griva *et al.*, 2000). Higher self-efficacy beliefs, higher control perceptions and lower identity perceptions were associated with greater adherence to various lifestyle, monitoring and treatment behaviours. Along with lower consequence perceptions, these beliefs were also associated with better metabolic control.

Interventions that change mental representations offer a way to improve the self-management process. This is illustrated by an evaluation of an intervention that targeted the mental representations of patients with poorly controlled, insulin-dependent diabetes (Snoek *et al.*, 2001). The intervention focused on identifying and challenging negative thoughts as well as on introducing behavioural strategies such as cueing, rewards and stress management. Six months after the intervention, perceived barriers in diabetes self-care had significantly decreased in intervention patients. The intervention also resulted in increased self-care behaviours, including self-monitoring of blood glucose and adherence to diet and exercise recommendations, as well as improved mean glycaemic control.

Several interventions have been developed to improve the accuracy of patients' self-monitoring of blood glucose levels using home glucose-testing equipment and instructions for self-treatment (Muhlhauser *et al.*, 1987; Starostina *et al.*, 1994). Intervention effects have included improved metabolic control, fewer days of sick leave and reduced numbers of hospitalizations. However, patients typically perform glucose testing only a few times per day. At other times, patients must remain vigilant for other signs of hypoglycaemia or hyperglycaemia. If patients do not correctly read these physical sensations then it is possible to make potentially serious errors in self-management. The Blood Glucose Awareness Training programme (BGAT) aims to improve symptom monitoring and the accuracy of patients' blood glucose estimation (Gonder-Frederick and Cox, 1991). The intervention consists of seven weekly group sessions focusing on the recognition of symptoms associated with hypo-glycaemia and hyperglycaemia, inaccurate symptom beliefs and external influences on blood glucose levels. BGAT patients keep a diary recording internal cues (symptoms) and external cues (timing and amount of last insulin dose, food and exercise), estimates of blood glucose levels, and actual blood glucose readings. These diaries are reviewed at the weekly sessions. Studies have shown that BGAT not only improves blood glucose estimates and recognition of hypoglycaemic and hyperglycaemic episodes, it also results in improved metabolic control (Cox *et al.*, 1988; Cox *et al.*, 1989; Cox *et al.*, 1991).

As well as accurately monitoring symptoms and blood glucose levels, diabetic patients must engage in corrective medication, diet and exercise behaviours in order to keep glucose levels within a normal range. Results from studies that have aimed to improve self-care behaviours suggest that monitoring and medication behaviours are more successfully changed than diet and exercise behaviours (Halford *et al.*, 1997; Rubin *et al.*, 1991; Sawicki *et al.*, 1995; Wing *et al.*, 1988). One reason for the difficulties experienced when changing general dietary behaviours, such as eating more healthy food, may be that their effects on blood glucose are too delayed to provide effective feedback and so they are not reinforced. This possibility was suggested by findings from a study assessing an intervention that taught patients about diet, provided behavioural strategies to improve eating habits and appropriate exercise goals, and asked patients to monitor their blood glucose and diet (Wing *et al.*, 1988). At the end of treatment, patients showed improvements in weight, HbA and blood glucose compared to baseline; however, only weight reduction remained significant at a one-year follow-up. Further analyses revealed that dietary changes made by patients did not have an immediate effect on measured blood glucose levels. This absence of positive feedback failed to reinforce behavioural change.

In contrast, interventions that target behaviours with more immediate and identifiable outcomes have been very successful. This is demonstrated by a randomized, controlled trial of an intervention that was designed to control blood pressure levels in hypertensive Type 1 diabetics with overt nephropathology (Sawicki *et al.*, 1995). Patients in the intervention group were informed about hypertension, taught how to measure their own blood pressure and how to adjust their anti-hypertensive medication dose in response to blood pressure readings. Patients were also taught about non-pharmacological ways in which to reduce blood pressure, such as making appropriate changes to diet, exercise, alcohol intake and smoking, and using psychological techniques. At a five-year follow-up there were large and clinically significant differences between groups. The intervention group had lower rates of death and renal dialysis, less deteriorated retinopathy and renal disease, and lower blood pressure than the control group.

These studies have shown that interventions designed to improve aspects of the self-regulation process, including mental representations, self-monitoring and self-care behaviours, can improve the self-management of diabetes with clinically significant results. Improvements have been documented in self-monitoring, treatment adherence, metabolic control, weight reduction and reduced long-term complications. Interventions have been particularly successful at improving behaviours that have an immediate and measurable effect.

Asthma

Asthma is another chronic illness that requires patients to develop self-regulatory repertoires. Patients must regulate their lifestyle behaviours and medication use to prevent and alleviate respiratory symptoms. A number of interventions have successfully improved management of asthma using treatments that improve components of the self-regulatory processes involved in asthma care. Many of these programmes involve the teaching of better symptom monitoring and more effective self-management skills.

Interventions that have placed a strong emphasis on specific behavioural programmes and action plans have been particularly successful. An eight-session, asthma self-management programme taught patients how to use inhalers, peak flow meters and a journal to monitor self-care (Lucas *et al.*, 2001). Patients were taught how to identify and avoid asthma triggers, given information about controller and reliever drugs, and taught how to develop and modify an action plan with medical staff. Patients were contacted at regular intervals for follow-up sessions to reinforce these skills and assess progress. One year later, patients reported increases in asthma knowledge and self-efficacy, and reductions in smoking, night-wakings, days off work and visits to emergency departments. Patients also reported greater physical and social functioning, vitality and general health. A cost-benefit economic analysis showed that the programme led to a return on investment of 254 percent. Educational programmes that have placed less emphasis on changing behavioural strategies have been less successful in improving long-term outcomes (e.g., Abdulwadud, 1999).

A number of interventions have provided patients with specific rules for adjusting medication in response to peak flow measurements. One programme instructed patients to record peak flow measurements each morning and provided guidelines on how to alter medication in response to the readings (Lahdensuo *et al.*, 1996). Patients were also instructed in asthma physiology, medication, and in breathing and relaxation techniques. Compared to standard care patients, intervention group patients over the following year experienced fewer asthma incidents, such as unscheduled outpatient visits, days off work and courses of antibiotic or prednisone, and reported an improved quality of life. Analysis showed that patients were most likely to follow the guidelines for self-treatment in response to peak flow readings when their symptoms were consistent with the readings.

As these findings show, peak flow measurement is not the only source of information used by patients to monitor their illness. Patients naturally monitor their symptoms and incorporate this information into their decisions regarding management behaviour. One randomized, controlled trial compared asthma self-management using peak flow measurements with asthma self-management using symptom recognition (Turner *et al.*, 1998). Patients were given rules for altering medication in response to either spirometry readings or asthma symptoms, depending on the intervention group. All patients were educated in pathophysiology, medication, recognition of symptoms, trigger avoidance and patient–doctor communication. Patients in both groups experienced significant increases in forced expiration volume, peak expiratory flow and quality of life as well as decreased symptoms, improved airway responsiveness and fewer unscheduled doctor visits. Adherence to management plans was relatively poor in both groups (approximately 60 percent); although this rate represents an improvement when compared to standard care, adherence is an area that future interventions need to address.

These studies demonstrate that interventions can substantially improve asthma patients' functioning and reduce medical care costs. The research highlights the utility of developing specific action plans in psychosocial interventions for chronic illnesses.

HIV interventions

A diagnosis of HIV infection triggers a cascade of psychosocial issues for the patient. Individuals are typically asymptomatic during the initial stages of the illness, but progression sees decline in immunological function and the emergence of HIV-related symptoms (Chesney and Folkman, 1994). Although drug treatment is now available for HIV infection, the regimen requires strict adherence. Effective management of HIV infection therefore requires a self-regulatory process of symptom monitoring and medication management. The profound psychological impact of HIV infection has been well documented. Individuals with HIV infection face a variety of complex stressors, including multiple symptoms (Chesney and Folkman, 1994), discrimination (Bartlett and Finkbeiner, 1998) and loss of social support resources (Antoni *et al.*, 1991). In order to meet the challenge of the HIV epidemic, an extensive multidisciplinary effort has developed across the fields of public health, behavioural medicine, and community and health psychology (Chesney, 1993). Since the late 1980s an important focus for many researchers has become the implementation and evaluation of psychosocial interventions that provide coping strategies for HIV-infected individuals. These interventions incorporate strategies for reducing distress, encourage the use of active coping and aim to enhance self-efficacy.

An early self-regulatory intervention developed by Coates and colleagues (Coates *et al.*, 1989) was designed to reduce unsafe sex and improve immune function through the provision of education about HIV infection and stress management training. Sixty-four HIV-positive gay men were assigned randomly to either a stress management training group or a control group. The intervention group met for eight two-hour sessions and a one-day retreat and were taught systematic relaxation, health education (the execution of behavioural contracts covering diet, rest, alcohol and drug use, smoking, and exercise) and skills for stress management through group discussion, teaching and modelling. Intervention group participants subsequently reported fewer sexual partners post-intervention than did control participants, although group differences in immune function were not observed.

A subsequent group intervention, known as Coping Effectiveness Training (CET), was developed based on the cognitive theory of stress and coping. The key component of CET is the promotion of the match between appraisals and coping strategies. Patients are taught a meta-strategy that emphasises 'fitting' the coping strategy to characteristics of the stressful situation (Chesney and Folkman, 1994). This design fits elegantly with the self-regulation model in assuming that illness adaptation is driven by an individual's cognitive and emotional representations, by coping responses directed by these representations, and by appraisals of coping outcomes. CET comprises a training phase involving ten, two-hour weekly sessions and a day-long retreat. Following the training phase, bi-monthly meetings are held for the remainder of one year so that the effects of CET can be maintained. CET teaches the following strategies: appraisal of stressful situations; cognitive-behavioural approaches to problem-focused and emotion-focused coping; appraisal-coping fit; the use of social support; and self-efficacy and maintenance training. In the initial pilot study, conducted with forty HIV-infected and non-HIV infected men, CET was effective in improving coping, depression and positive morale (Chesney and Folkman, 1994). This initial study did not include the maintenance phase aimed at enhancing self-efficacy through the use of cognitive-behavioural strategies for coping across diverse stressful situations. A later CET trial, which included the maintenance phase, found significant increases in self-efficacy and reductions in distress compared to a waiting-list control group and an information group (Chesney *et al.*, 1996). The social support component of this intervention provides patients with skills to access networks in the wider community. The maintenance training is important as it allows for self-appraisal resulting in a potential update of their illness representation and revised coping efforts.

Some of the most prolific HIV intervention research has evolved within a psychoneuroimmunology framework. Along with psychological self-regulation, this work has investigated the impact of interventions on immune regulation. Over the past decade, Antoni and colleagues have developed a group cognitive-behavioural stress management (CBSM) intervention (Antoni *et al.*, 1991). CBSM encompasses multiple levels of support for patients and typically involves ten weekly sessions to address the psychosocial sequelae experienced by HIV-infected individuals. The programme aims to increase personal awareness by providing information on the sources of stress, the human stress response and on different coping strategies to deal with specific stressors. Progressive muscle relaxation and imagery techniques are incorporated to reduce anxiety. Cognitive restructuring is used to modify maladaptive appraisals. Coping-skills training, anger management techniques and assertion training are employed to enhance cognitive, behavioural and interpersonal coping skills. Overall, CBSM attempts to provide a supportive group dynamic and increase utilisation of social support networks (Antoni and Schneiderman, 2001). Study findings suggest that individuals experience improvement in cognitive coping strategies involving positive reframing and acceptance (Lutgendorf *et al.*, 1998), and also reduction in anxiety, anger, perceived stress and total mood disturbance (Antoni *et al.*, 2000). Positive reframing is an important strategy for improving self-regulation. By addressing and restructuring the existing beliefs an individual has, for example, about the consequences of their illness and the perception of uncontrollable burdens, a vital step is taken towards reaching cognitive and emotional integration.

Both CBSM and existential-experiential group interventions were found to be effective in reducing distress and depressive symptoms among HIV-infected gay men (Mulder *et al.*, 1994). Similarly, both a cognitive-behavioural group intervention and a support-group intervention resulted in significant reductions in somatisation, hostility and depression compared to a control condition (Kelly *et al.*, 1993). CBSM may act to regulate psychological distress and immune function in HIV-infected patients. As discussed below, this CBSM intervention has also been successfully used among women newly treated for breast cancer (Antoni *et al.*, 2001). The promising results from these studies involving different illness groups indicates the potential for using a similar intervention framework across diseases that share common characteristics. In the case of HIV and breast cancer, individuals have to deal with lifestyle changes, potential stigma and isolation, and the demands of treatment and ongoing medication.

Overall, successful intervention studies with HIV-infected patients have been those that focus on providing multiple levels of support. Helping patients understand their illness through the provision of accurate information corresponds to the idea that negative cognitions may guide their coping processes. Although coping skills training is typically promoted, CET's inclusion of 'fitting' the coping strategy to the stressful situation fits coherently into the self-regulatory process. Encouraging patients to access social support networks beyond the original support group environment is particularly important. Recognition that the patient's illness representations may differ dramatically from those held by members of their social network highlights the significance of encouraging patients to share information about their illness with a view to dispelling misconceptions others may have. Further exploration of the social and cultural environment is essential in order to advance our understanding of self-regulation in chronic illnesses such as HIV and to provide optimal intervention strategies for patients.

Cancer interventions

A wealth of research has focused on the psychosocial sequelae of cancer. Diagnosis of cancer is a frightening and difficult experience, as a person suddenly has to adjust to treatment, ongoing physical symptoms, emotional distress, a threat to personal identity and the possibility of death. For example, Glanz and Lerman (1992) reported that 80 per cent of women diagnosed with breast cancer experienced emotional distress and vulnerability. Few individuals are adequately prepared to handle all of these problems at once (Spiegel and Diamond, 2001). With these issues in mind, a broad range of interventions have been designed to teach individuals ways of coping with cancer and its accompanying emotional distress.

From a self-regulatory perspective, the cancer patient is regarded as an active seeker and processor of illness information. The process of self-regulation is therefore a dynamic one, as a patient's cognitive and emotional representations ultimately direct their selection and application of coping procedures used to meet the illness threat. Research has illustrated the relevance of the self-regulatory model as an integrative framework for understanding the cancer experience. Buick (1997) found that negative illness perceptions impacted on psychological morbidity for breast cancer patients. For example, those patients who had diminished beliefs that their breast cancer could be controlled or cured were more likely to experience psychological distress before radiation treatment and at a three-month follow-up. Self-regulatory interventions for cancer patients are designed to help patients develop adaptive representations and coping strategies over the illness continuum, enabling the patient to function optimally within the demands of their illness, treatment and accompanying emotional sequelae.

Psychosocial interventions for cancer patients tend to address three points in the disease timeline: diagnosis; immediately pre- or post-surgery or during adjuvant treatment following surgery; and metastatic disease and death (Andersen, 1992). These interventions can take the form of behavioural training, education and supportive therapy in both individual and group settings (Fawzy *et al.*, 2001). Reviews of the psychosocial intervention literature typically highlight a number of key studies that have informed and influenced ongoing research in this area. A number of these interventions can be considered within a self-regulatory framework and are discussed below.

An early intervention study by Telch and Telch (1986) randomly assigned patients with various cancer types to one of three conditions: group coping-skills instruction; support group therapy; and no-treatment control. Group coping-skills instruction emphasised teaching and the rehearsal of cognitive, behavioural and affective coping strategies. Patients were instructed in communication and assertion, relaxation, stress management, problem solving, feelings management and pleasant-activity planning. The intervention involved patients completing homework assignments, setting goals and self-monitoring their progress. In contrast, participants undergoing support group therapy had no preplanned agenda or set of structured exercises, although patients' feelings and concerns were openly discussed. Results indicated that patients in the coping-skills group showed more improvement than patients in the other two groups on a variety of measures, including affect, the ability to cope with medical procedures, communication skills and levels of cognitive distress. The success of this intervention strongly supports the efficacy of coping-skills training to enable cancer patients to adjust to their illness. In self-regulatory terms, the intervention encouraged active participation on behalf of the individual by linking beneficial coping techniques to common patient situations. This may have increased patients' perceptions of control, enabling them to avoid or reduce the negative consequences of their illness.

After reviewing the psychosocial intervention literature, Fawzy and colleagues developed an intervention model that incorporated what they identified as the effective components of previous intervention research (Fawzy *et al.*, 1990). A six-week group intervention was conducted with post-surgical malignant melanoma patients. The intervention consisted of four key components: health education; stress management techniques; enhancement of coping skills; and supportive group psychotherapy. Health education focused on improving patients' understanding of their illness by providing information specific to skin cancer, including risk factors and preventive measures. Stress management involved identifying sources of stress and personal reactions to stress, and learning management techniques. The coping skills component taught participants how to identify the problem, consider possible solutions, implement a strategy and appraise its success. Finally, supportive group psychotherapy was available throughout the intervention timeframe.

At the end of the six-week programme, intervention group participants showed some reduction in levels of psychological distress compared to control group participants. More definitive group differences were observed at a six-month follow-up, with intervention participants reporting lower levels of confusion, fatigue and depression, and higher levels of vigour. At a five year follow-up, intervention participants continued to exhibit lower levels of anxiety, depression and total mood disturbance, along with a decreased rate of recurrence and an increased rate of survival (Fawzy *et al.*, 1993). An assessment of coping and adjustment showed promising results, with intervention participants using active behavioural and active cognitive coping strategies significantly more often than control participants. These findings suggest the importance of providing multifaceted interventions for cancer patients. This comprehensive study provided patients with accurate information about melanoma, thereby addressing negative perceptions and increasing adherence. Stress management and coping-skills training gave patients clear strategies to draw upon when confronting the demands of their illness. The final essential component was ongoing patient self-monitoring, which reflects the feedback mechanism inherent in the self-regulation model.

A key intervention study involved the provision of cognitive-behavioural therapy for individual cancer patients (Greer *et al.*, 1992). The programme consisted of addressing the personal meaning of cancer for the individual and developing strategies directed at alleviating problems identified by the patient. Specific coping and behavioural strategies taught to patients included progressive muscle relaxation, using imagination and role play as a means of coping with stressors, encouraging emotional expression, and participation in activities designed to generate a sense of achievement. Four months post-intervention, patients receiving therapy had significantly lower levels of anxiety and distress than those in a control group.

Further research supports the efficacy of cognitive-behavioural-type interventions for cancer patients (Bottomley *et al.*, 1996). Cunningham *et al.* (1998) tested the effects on cancer patients of combined cognitive-behavioural therapy and supportive group therapy; a control group received only a home-study cognitive-behavioural package. The intervention was based on components of the programme developed by Spiegel *et al.* (1989) and also included self-help relaxation and meditation strategies, thought monitoring and changing, goal setting, and mental imaging. Although no significant effects were found on health outcomes, the authors state that some participants may have been discouraged by the demands of learning and practising self-regulation strategies.

Helgeson and colleagues compared the effectiveness of education-based and peer discussion-based group interventions among women with breast cancer. Participants were randomly assigned to one of four conditions: peer discussion; education; combined education; and peer discussion and control. The education-based programme provided participants with information about the disease, treatment and strategies for coping with their illness, whereas the peer discussion group focused on sharing experiences and expressing feelings. The study found positive effects on adjustment in the education group immediately after and at six months post-intervention; no participation benefits were found in the peer discussion group (Helgeson *et al.*, 1999).

Although interventions for cancer patients typically include support group therapy, the addition of self-regulation strategies such as relaxation, coping skills, goal setting and positive reframing provide direction for patients over the course of their illness. Recognising that patients have to deal with a multitude of challenges, effective interventions need to incorporate strategies which initiate self-monitoring over the course of the illness to allow appraisal of physical, emotional and spiritual progress.

Recent work by Antoni and colleagues investigated the effects of a ten-week group cognitive-behavioural stress management intervention among women newly treated for early-stage breast cancer. Participants met weekly for ten two-hour sessions and the intervention focused on learning to cope with the stressors of cancer- and treatment-related issues, and to optimise the use of social support networks. Patients undertook out-of-session assignments and monitored their stress responses. The intervention resulted in a reduction of moderate depression but did not affect other measures of emotional distress. The intervention also increased participants' reports that breast cancer had impacted positively on their lives (Antoni *et al.*, 2001).

Studies have provided considerable evidence that psychological interventions for cancer patients can improve their quality of life and reduce levels of distress through the teaching of techniques such as relaxation and coping skills. However, identifying which intervention components are the effective 'ingredients' is problematic. Although intervention work to date may raise more questions than answers, the self-regulatory perspective offers a powerful framework for further exploration of the most effective intervention methods for cancer patients.

Other illnesses

Self-regulatory interventions have also been successful among a number of other chronic illness groups. This type of intervention was used, for example, with patients in need of oral anti-coagulation medication who normally must undergo regular blood tests and clinic visits to monitor dose requirements. A randomized controlled trial investigated an extensive teaching and training programme that taught patients to self-regulate their treatment using home blood analyzers and provided rules for adjusting their own medication dose (Sawicki, 1999). Patients were also taught about the effects of diet and other medications on anti-coagulation control. The intervention resulted in improved anti-coagulation control compared to the results of standard treatment. It also resulted in improved quality-of-life scores, especially in the area of treatment satisfaction. Moreover, intervention patients reported decreases in illness-related distress and daily hassles. The cost savings resulting from improved self-regulation of anti-coagulation therapy are considerable.

Kate Lorig and her colleagues have extensively evaluated an arthritis self-management programme that addresses illness beliefs, teaches coping techniques and encourages individual experimentation with various self-management strategies (Lorig *et al.*, 1993). Over a four-year follow-up period, patients reported a 15–20 per cent reduction in pain compared to baseline. The same patients also made 40 per cent fewer physician visits and reported higher perceived self-efficacy. Patients receiving standard care over the same period made no such improvements. The most important mediator of improved health status over time was a change in the patient's self-efficacy beliefs – in particular, in their ability to control pain – rather than through the use of taught behaviours, indicating the ability of self-regulation interventions to improve health status by altering mental representations.

Lorig and her colleagues have adapted this intervention to form the Chronic Disease Self-Management Programme (Lorig *et al.*, 1999). A randomized, controlled trial tested the feasibility of conducting this programme with a combined group of patients with chronic lung disease, heart disease, stroke, and chronic arthritis. The intervention focused on enhancing self-efficacy and assisted patients in choosing self-management techniques. The programme also involved having patients set goals and identify effective feedback. After six months, intervention participants showed significant improvements in self-reported health behaviours and health status compared to standard care participants. They also had fewer hospitalizations and doctor visits. Importantly, both the arthritis and chronic illness programmes improved health status while cutting medical care costs.

These studies highlight the health and economic benefits that can be gained from using a self-regulation model as a basis for instructing patients in the management of their illness. These benefits are often gained from the patients' ability to monitor themselves and adjust their treatment far more frequently than is possible through reliance on management by health care providers. Furthermore, research shows that self-regulatory interventions often enhance the patients' control beliefs, treatment satisfaction, adherence and quality of life.

A self-regulatory intervention following myocardial infarction

Recent advances in the medical treatment of myocardial infarction (MI) have resulted in fewer patients dying during the acute stage. However, these gains contrast with the small progress achieved in understanding and improving the rehabilitation phase following MI. The problems that patients face in changing their lifestyle behaviours and returning to work can be more debilitating than the physical effects of the MI itself.

For many patients, the return to work is an important milestone in their recovery. However, a significant number of patients do not return to work following their MI although they are physically capable of doing so; vocational disability remains one of the important negative consequences of MI (Shanfield, 1990). It is estimated that in 40–50 percent of cases, the failure to return to work cannot be explained by limitations due to illness (Lewin, 1995), and existing cardiac rehabilitation programmes seem to have minimal impact on a patient's decision to return to work (Wenger and Froelicher, 1996). The fact that a significant proportion of patients fail to return to work and resume normal functioning represents a significant social and economic cost in terms of lost work hours, increased medical care use and diminished life satisfaction (Cay, 1995).

Research points to the fact that patients' beliefs about their illness are important determinants of behaviour during the recovery phase (Lewin, 1999; Petrie and Weinman, 1997; Weinman *et al.*, 2000). Studies have found that a patient's in-hospital expectations of their future work capacity are a strong predictor of an eventual return to work (Byrne, 1982; Maeland and Havik, 1987). An extreme form of negative health perceptions is seen in 'cardiac invalidism'. Here patients adopt an extremely passive, dependant and helpless role in the belief that any form of overly vigorous activity will bring on another MI (Riegel, 1993). A hypersensitivity to bodily symptoms means that normal sensations may be misconstrued as indicating over-exertion, cardiac damage or an impending fatal MI. This pattern often results in a cycle of inactivity and loss of physical condition which, in turn, supports these beliefs and leads to an overuse of medical services mainly for obtaining reassurances about symptoms (Maeland and Havik, 1989).

Research indicates that an MI patient's perceptions of illness, assessed a few days after the MI, have important effects on different aspects of recovery. Patients who believed that their MI would have more serious, long-lasting consequences were found to have greater levels of illness-related disability and were slower to return to work (Petrie *et al.*, 1996). Similarly, those patients who had weaker beliefs in the ability of their heart condition to be controlled or cured were less likely to attend cardiac rehabilitation (Cooper *et al.*, 1999; Petrie *et al.*, 1996). In these studies, illness representations were not closely related to medical indicators of MI severity and they were more predictive than medical factors of outcomes such as return to work.

Patients' and their spouses' beliefs about whether the heart attack was caused by stress, genetic factors, or poor health habits also seem to act as a clear starting point for deciding whether to change health behaviours. For many, a heart attack is seen as a clear warning of the consequences of smoking, poor diet and a sedentary lifestyle. However, other patients do not make these associations and see stress or family problems as the main reasons for their illness. Research indicates that patients and their spouses who believe that the MI was caused by poor health habits are more likely to make dietary changes six months post-MI (Weinman *et al.*, 2000).

These results suggest that if negative and maladaptive cognitions can be identified at an early stage following MI and an intervention instituted to foster more adaptive models and expectations, then improved levels of functioning and a return to work may be expected. A recent study investigated whether a brief, hospital-based intervention designed to change inaccurate and negative illness perceptions of MI would result in an earlier return to work, less long-term disability and improved cardiac rehabilitation attendance (Petrie *et al.*, 2002). The intervention, conducted by a psychologist several days after the patient's MI, followed an equivalent structure for all patients but its exact content was individualized according to the patient's responses on the Illness Perception Questionnaire – a scale that measures beliefs about the cause, expected timeline, consequences, symptoms and controllability of one's illness (Moss-Morris *et al.*, 2002). The first session consisted of a brief explanation of the physiology of MI using drawings to provide concrete images of the illness. This session also explored the patient's beliefs about the causes of the MI. Attention was given to addressing the common misconception that stress was singularly responsible for the MI and attempts were made to broaden the patient's causal model by including the importance of other factors such as poor diet, exercise and smoking. Expanding the patient's causal model in this manner provided more avenues for future personal control and disease management.

The second session built on the causes identified by the patient and focused on developing a plan for minimizing future risk by altering risk factors specific to the patient and increasing beliefs about personal control. Highly negative beliefs about consequences, particularly beliefs about needing to significantly reduce activities over the long-term, were challenged and a personalized recovery plan was developed. This plan included an explicit schedule for exercise, dietary change and a return to work tailor-made for the patient. The linking of beliefs about timeline and consequences was achieved by explaining that, as patients recovered from the illness, they could expect to return to work and resume normal activities.

In the third session, the patient's action plan was reviewed and symptoms of recovery were discussed. Symptoms that are a normal part of the recovery process were distinguished from symptoms that may be warning signs of a further MI. For example, symptoms that might be experienced during exercise, such as slight breathlessness while still being able to speak, were distinguished from symptoms that are not expected, such as severe chest pain. Concerns about medication were also explored. The need to take medication consistently and the hazards of relying on symptoms as guides for taking medication were also discussed in this final session, along with concerns about going home.

Results from a randomized, controlled trial showed that this intervention improved functional outcome following MI when compared to the effects of routine care received from rehabilitation nurses. The intervention induced significant, positive changes in patients' illness beliefs during their time in hospital. Intervention patients returned to work at a significantly faster rate and experienced significantly less angina symptoms than did control patients (Petrie *et al.*, 2002). This study suggests that illness perceptions may be successfully altered by brief cognitive-based interventions and provides further evidence that interventions based on the self-regulatory model have considerable potential to improve adjustment to chronic illness.

Conclusion

This review has examined how self-regulatory approaches have been applied to interventions for patients with chronic illness. Self-regulation principles have served as the basis for interventions for numerous chronic illness populations that have employed a variety of therapeutic approaches. Although the illnesses vary widely in their biological and psychological demands, self-regulatory models provide clinicians with a practical and workable blueprint on which to design an intervention. The view of the patient as an active participant in illness management contrasts with the passive role to which patients are often consigned by the medical treatment process. It is also a view that is compatible with the current Zeitgeist that favours a less paternalistic model of health care and a greater involvement of patients in decisions and management (Holman and Lorig, 2000).

The central role that is given to the patient's view of his/her illness provides clinicians intervening in chronic illness populations with several advantages. Perhaps most importantly, it provides both a target for intervention efforts and a marker for the effectiveness of the therapy. The importance of this advantage should not be understated, as most current interventions in the behavioural medicine area, such as cardiac rehabilitation and pain management programmes, are rarely theoretically based and often unclear about the type of behaviours or attitudes they are attempting to change. The smorgasbord of strategies that are used in these programs often reflect this lack of theoretical focus.

Several points are raised by the current review. First, interventions that are able to successfully incorporate short-term concrete feedback and tie these to action plans are more successful than those where feedback is either greatly delayed or nonexistent. This, of course, is a longstanding problem in therapeutic interventions but it highlights the importance of being imaginative when providing patients with proximal or immediate goals in order to maintain long-term behaviour change (Norman et al., 2000). The area of patient adherence to health psychology interventions is a new one, but it provides the opportunity to apply many of the techniques identified in other treatments in the health field (Burns and Nolen-Hoeksema, 1991).

Self-regulatory interventions have often targeted illnesses, such as diabetes and asthma, that require the patient to manage his or her medication or lifestyle behaviours in response to symptoms. In such illnesses, the results of behavioural change are often clearly evident both in terms of quality of life and biomedical markers. In other illnesses, such as cancer and HIV, the patient does not have the same amount of control through the self-management of symptoms. Interventions for these illnesses have tended to focus instead on distress management via psychological techniques, which are less able to provide immediate concrete feedback. It is therefore more difficult to develop self-regulatory interventions for these illnesses, as indicated by their relative lack of success. This highlights the need for researchers to study the fundamental qualities of different illnesses when designing interventions.

Another important shortcoming highlighted by the review is that more work is needed on identifying which clinical techniques are best employed to achieve change in illness populations. Often cognitive-behavioural techniques are borrowed from clinical psychology and applied in the health psychology area without information on how the intervention is best applied. Two important factors that ought to be considered are the timing of the intervention and the format in which it is best presented. For example, the illness perception intervention for MI patients is administered in-hospital immediately following the MI and thus allows for misperceptions and negative beliefs to be modified early on in the recovery process. Furthermore, individuals are often more amenable to interventions that encourage changes in behaviours immediately following a major illness or health threat (Weinstein, 1989). In other illnesses, however, interventions may be best implemented after the initial illness threat has been overcome and the patient is no longer overloaded with information or learning new illness-related behaviours. This aspect clearly needs further research.

Another issue that requires further research is whether the intervention should be applied in an individualized or small-group format. Although small groups can be more cost-effective in terms of clinician time, the importance of understanding the patient's illness beliefs and personalizing the intervention so that it fits the patient's circumstances and lifestyle means that an individualized approach may be more suitable for many patients.

The area of chronic illness intervention is likely to provide a great deal of future research as the need for more collaborative programmes incorporating the patient's view of their illness grows. The self-regulatory models developed by Leventhal and others have provided an excellent theoretical base on which to build the many future therapeutic interventions that will undoubtedly follow.

Note

1   Correspondence should be addressed to Keith J. Petrie, Health Psychology, Faculty of Medical and Health Sciences, University of Auckland, Private Bag 92019, Auckland, New Zealand. E-mail: kj.petrie@auckland.ac.nz

References

Abdulwadud, O., Abramson, M., Forbes, A., James, A. and Walters, E.H. (1999) 'Evaluation of a randomised controlled trial of adult education in a hospital setting', *Thorax* **54**: 493–500.

Andersen, B. (1992) 'Psychological interventions for cancer patients to enhance the quality of life', *Journal of Consulting and Clinical Psychology* **60**: 552–568.

Antoni, M.H. and Schneiderman, N. (2001) 'HIV and AIDS', in D.W. Johnston and M. Johnston (eds) *Health Psychology. Vol. 8: Comprehensive Clinical Psychology*, Oxford: Elsevier Science, pp. 237–276.

Antoni, M.H., Baggett, L., Ironson, G., LaPerriere, A., August, S., Klimas, N., Schneiderman, N. and Fletcher, M.A. (1991) 'Cognitive-behavioral stress management intervention buffers distress responses and immunologic changes following notification of HIV-1 seropositivity', *Journal of Consulting and Clinical Psychology* **59**: 906–915.

Antoni, M.H., Cruess, D.G., Cruess, S., Lutgendorf, S., Kumar, M., Ironson, G., Klimas, N., Fletcher, M.A. and Schneiderman, N. (2000) 'Cognitive-behavioral stress management intervention effects on anxiety, 24-hr urinary norepinephrine output, and T-cytotoxic/suppressor cells over time among symptomatic HIV-infected gay men', *Journal of Consulting and Clinical Psychology* **68**: 31–45.

Antoni, M.H., Lehman, J.M., Kilbourn, K.M., Boyers, A.E., Culver, J.L., Alferi, S.M., Yount, S., McGregor, B.A., Arena, P.L., Harris, S.D., Price, A.A. and Carver, C.S. (2001) 'Cognitive-behavioral stress management intervention decreases the prevalence of depression and enhances benefit finding among women under treatment for early-stage breast cancer', *Health Psychology* **20**: 20–32.

Bartlett, J.G. and Finkbeiner, A.K. (1998) *The Guide to Living with HIV Infection*, 4th edn, Baltimore: Johns Hopkins University Press.

Bottomley, A., Hunton, S., Roberts, G., Jones, L. and Bradley, C. (1996) 'A pilot study of cognitive behavioral therapy and social support group interventions for newly diagnosed cancer patients', *Journal of Psychosocial Oncology* **14**: 65–83.

Buick, D.L. (1997) 'Illness representations and breast cancer: coping with radiation and chemotherapy', in K.J. Petrie and J. Weinman (eds) *Perceptions of Health and Illness*, Amsterdam: Harwood Academic, pp. 379–410.

Burns, D.D. and Nolen-Hoeksema, S. (1991) 'Coping styles, homework compliance, and the effectiveness of cognitive-behavioral therapy', *Journal of Consulting and Clinical Psychology* **59**: 305–311.

Byrne, D.G. (1982) 'Psychological responses to illness and outcome after survived myocardial infarction: a long-term follow-up', *Journal of Psychosomatic Research* **26**: 105–112.

Carver, C.S. and Scheier, M.F. (1981) *Attention and Self-Regualtion: A Control-Theory Approach to Human Behavior*, New York: Springer-Verlag.

Cay, E.L. (1995) 'Goals of rehabilitation', in D. Jones and R. West (eds) *Cardiac Rehabilitation*, London: BMJ Books.

Chesney, M.A. (1993) 'Health psychology in the 21st century: acquired immunodeficiency syndrome as a harbinger of things to come', *Health Psychology* **12**: 259–268.

Chesney, M.A. and Folkman, S. (1994) 'Psychological impact of HIV disease and implications for intervention', *Psychiatric Clinics of North America* **17**: 163–182.

Chesney, M.A., Folkman, S. and Chambers, D. (1996) 'Coping effectiveness training for men living with HIV: preliminary findings', *International Journal of STDs and AIDS* **7**: 75–82.

Coates, T.J., McKusick, L., Kuno, R. and Stites, D.P. (1989) 'Stress reduction training changed number of sexual partners but not immune function in men with HIV', *American Journal of Public Health* **79**: 885–887.

Cooper, A., Lloyd, G., Weinman, J. and Jackson, G. (1999) 'Why do patients not attend cardiac rehabilitation: role of intentions and illness beliefs', *Heart and Lung* **82**: 234–236.

Cox, D.J., Carter, W.R., Gonder-Frederick, L., Clarke, W. and Pohl, S. (1988) 'Training awareness of blood glucose in IDDM patients', *Biofeedback and Self-Regulation* **13**: 201–217.

Cox, D.J., Gonder-Frederick, L., Julian, D., Carter, W.R. and Clarke, W. (1989) 'Effects and correlates of blood glucose awareness training among patients with IDDM', *Diabetes Care* **12**: 313–318.

Cox, D.J., Gonder-Frederick, L., Julian, D., Cryer, P., Lee, J.H., Richards, P.E. and Clarke, W. (1991) 'Intensive versus standard glucose awareness training (BGAT) with insulin-dependent diabetes: mechanisms and ancillary effects', *Psychosomatic Medicine* **53**: 453–462.

Cunningham, A.J., Edmonds, C.V.I., Jenkins, G.P., Pollack, H., Lockwood, G.A. and Warr, D. (1998) 'A randomized controlled trial of the effects of group psychological therapy on survival in women with metastatic breast cancer', *Psycho-Oncology* **7**: 508–517.

Fawzy, F.I., Fawzy, N.W. and Canada, A.L. (2001) 'Psychoeducational intervention programs for patients with cancer', in A. Baum and B.L. Andersen (eds) *Psychosocial Interventions for Cancer*, Washington, DC: American Psychological Association, pp. 235–268.

Fawzy, F.I., Cousins, N., Fawzy, N.W., Kemeny, M.E., Elashoff, R. and Morton, D. (1990) 'A structured psychiatric intervention for cancer patients: I. Changes over time in methods of coping and affective disturbance', *Archives of General Psychiatry* **47**: 720–725.

Fawzy, F.I., Fawzy, N., Hyun, C.S., Guthrie, E., Fahey, J.L. and Morton, D. (1993) 'Malignant melanoma: effects of an early structured psychiatric intervention, coping, and affective state on recurrence and survival six years later' *Archives of General Psychiatry* **50**: 681–689.

Glanz, K. and Lerman, C. (1992) 'Psychosocial impact of breast cancer: a critical review', *Annals of Behavioral Medicine* **14**: 204–212.

Gonder-Frederick, L. and Cox, D.J. (1991) 'Symptom perception, symptom beliefs, and blood glucose discrimination in the self-treatment of insulin dependent diabetes', in J.A. Skelton and R.T. Croyle (eds) *Mental Representations in Health and Illness*, New York: Springer-Verlag, pp. 220–246.

Greer, S., Moorey, S., Baruch, J.D.R., Watson, M., Robertson, B.M., Mason, A., Rowden, L., Law, M.G. and Bliss, J.M. (1992) 'Adjuvant psychological therapy for patients with cancer: a prospective randomised trial', *British Medical Journal* **304**: 675–680.

Griva, K., Myers, L.B. and Newman, S. (2000) 'Illness perceptions and self-efficacy beliefs in adolescents and young adults with insulin dependent diabetes mellitus', *Psychology and Health* **15**: 733–750.

Halford, W.K., Goodall, T.A. and Nicholson, I.M. (1997) 'Diet and diabetes (II): a controlled trial of problem solving to improve dietary self-management in patients with insulin dependent diabetes', *Psychology and Health* **12**: 231–238.

Helgeson, V.S., Cohen, S., Schulz, R. and Yasko, J. (1999) 'Education and peer discussion group interventions and adjustment to breast cancer', *Archives of General Psychiatry* **56**: 340–347.

Holman, H. and Lorig, K.R. (2000) 'Patients as partners in managing chronic illness', *British Medical Journal* **320**: 526–527.

Kelly, J.A., Murphy, D., Bahr, G., Kobb, J., Morgan, M., Kalichman, S., Stevenson, L., Brashfield, T., Bernstein, B. and St Lawrence, J.S. (1993) 'Factors associated with severity of depression and high-risk sexual behavior among persons diagnosed with human immunodeficiency virus (HIV) infection', *Health Psychology* **12**: 215–219.

Lahdensuo, A., Haahtals, T., Herrala, J., Kava, T., Kiviranta, K., Kuusisto, P., Pera-maki, E., Poussa, T., Saarelainen, S. and Svahn, T. (1996) 'Randomised comparison of guided self-management and traditional treatment of asthma over one year', *British Medical Journal* **312**: 748–752.

Leventhal, H., Nerenz, D.R. and Steele, D.J. (1984) 'Illness representations and coping with health threats', in A. Baum and J. Singer (eds) *A Handbook of Psychology and Health*, vol. 4, Hillsdale: NJ: Lawrence Erlbaum Associates, pp. 219–252.

Leventhal, H., Benyamini, Y., Brownlee, S., Diefenbach, M., Leventhal, E.A., Patrick-Miller, L. and Robitaille, C. (1997) 'Illness representations: theoretical foundations', in K.J. Petrie and J. Weinman (eds) *Perceptions of Health and Illness*, Amsterdam: Harwood Academic Press, pp. 19–46.

Lewin, R. (1995) 'Psychological factors in cardiac rehabilitation', in D. Jones and R. West (eds) *Cardiac Rehabilitation*, London: BMJ Books.

—— (1999) 'Return to work after MI, the roles of depression, health beliefs and rehabilitation', *International Journal of Cardiology* **72**: 49–51.

Lorig, K.R., Mazonson, P. and Holman, H.R. (1993) 'Evidence suggesting that health education for self-management in patients with chronic arthritis has sustained health benefits while reducing health care costs', *Arthritis and Rheumatism* **36**: 439–446.

Lorig, K.R., Sobel, D.S., Stewart, A.L., Brown, B.W., Bandura, A., Ritter, P., Gonzalez, V.M., Laurent, D.D. and Holman, H.R. (1999) 'Evidence suggesting that a chronic disease self-management program can improve health status while reducing hospitalization: a randomized trial', *Medical Care* **37**: 5–14.

Lucas, D.O., Zimmer, L.O., Paul, J.E., Jones, D., Slatko, G., Liao, W. and Lashley, J. (2001) 'Two-year results of the Asthma Self-Management Programme: long-term impact on health care services, costs, functional status and productivity', *Journal of Asthma* **38**: 321–330.

Lutgendorf, S.K., Antoni, M.H., Ironson, G., Starr, K., Costello, N., Zuckerman, M., Klimas, N., Fletcher, M.A. and Schneiderman, N. (1998) 'Changes in cognitive coping skills and social support during cognitive behavioral stress management intervention and distress outcomes in symptomatic human immunodeficiency virus (HIV)-seropositive gay men', *Psychosomatic Medicine* **60**: 204–214.

Maeland, J.G. and Havik, O.E. (1987) 'Psychological predictors for return to work after a myocardial infarction', *Journal of Psychosomatic Research* **31**: 471–481.

—— (1989) 'Use of health services after a myocardial infarction', *Scandinavian Journal of Social Medicine* **17**: 93–102.

Moss-Morris, R., Petrie, K.J., Weinman, J., Horne, R., Buick, D.L. and Cameron, L.D. (2002) 'Measuring cognitive representations of illness: a revision of the illness perception questionnaire', *Psychology and Health* **17**: 1–16.

Muhlhauser, I., Bruckner, I., Berger, M., Cheta, D., Jorgens, V., Ionescu-Tirgoviste, C., Scholz, V. and Mincu, I. (1987) 'Evaluation of an intensified insulin treatment and teaching programme as routine management of Type 1 (insulin-dependent) diabetes', *Diabetologia* **30**: 681–690.

Mulder, C.L., Emmelkamp, P.M.G., Antoni, M.H., Mulder, J.W., Sandfort, T.G.M. and de Vries, M.J. (1994) 'Cognitive-behavioral and experiential group psychotherapy for HIV-infected homosexual men: a comparative study', *Psychosomatic Medicine* **56**: 423–431.

Norman, P., Abraham, C. and Conner, M. (eds) (2000) *Understanding and Changing Health Behaviour: From Health Beliefs to Self-Regulation*, Amsterdam: Harwood Academic.

Petrie, K.J. (2002) 'Social support and recovery from disease and medical procedures', in N.J. Smelser and P.B. Baltes (eds) *International Encyclopaedia of the Social and Behavioural Sciences*, Oxford: Elsevier Science.

Petrie, K.J. and Weinman, J. (1997) 'Illness representations and recovery from myocardial infarction', in K.J. Petrie and J. Weinman (eds) *Perceptions of Health and Illness*, Amsterdam: Harwood Academic, pp. 441–462.

Petrie, K.J., Weinman, J., Sharpe, N. and Buckley, J. (1996) 'Role of patients' view of their illness in predicting return to work and functioning after myocardial infarction: longitudinal study', *British Medical Journal* **312**: 1191–1194.

Petrie, K.J., Cameron, L.D., Ellis, C.J., Buick, D.L. and Weinman, J. (2002) 'Changing illness perceptions following myocardial infarction: an early intervention randomized controlled trial', *Psychological Medicine* **64**: 580–586.

Riegel, B.J. (1993) 'Contributors to cardiac invalidism after acute myocardial infarction', *Coronary Artery Disease* **4**: 215–220.

Rubin, R.R., Peyrot, M. and Saudek, C.D. (1991) 'Differential effect of diabetes education on self-regulation and life-style behavior', *Diabetes Care* **14**: 335–338.

Sawicki, P.T. (1999) 'A structured teaching and self-management program for patients receiving oral anticoagulation: a randomized controlled trial', *Journal of the American Medical Association* **281**: 145–150.

Sawicki, P.T., Muhlhauser, I., Didjurgeit, U., Baumgartner, A., Bender, R. and Berger, M. (1995) 'Intensified antihypertensive therapy is associated with improved survival in Type 1 diabetic patients with nephropathy', *Journal of Hypertension* **13**: 933–938.

Shanfield, S.B. (1990) 'Return to work after an acute myocardial infarction: a review', *Heart and Lung* **19**: 109–117.

Snoek, F.J., Ven, N.C.W.v.d., Lubach, C.H.C., Chatrou, M., Adèr, H.J., Heine, R.J. and Jacobson, A.M. (2001) 'Effects of cognitive behavioural group training (CBGT) in adult patients with poorly controlled insulin-dependent (Type 1) diabetes: a pilot study', *Patient Education and Counselling* **45**: 143–148.

Spiegel, D. and Diamond, S. (2001) 'Psychosocial interventions in cancer: group therapy techniques', in A. Baum and B.L. Andersen (eds) *Psychosocial Interventions for Cancer*, Washington, DC: American Psychological Society, pp. 215–234.

Spiegel, D., Bloom, J., Kraemer, H. and Gottheil, E. (1989) 'Effect of psychosocial treatment on survival of patients with metastatic breast cancer', *Lancet* **2**: 888–891.

Starostina, E.G., Antsiferov, M., Galstyan, G.R., Trautner, C., Jorgens, V., Bott, U., Muhlhauser, I., Berger, M. and Dedov, I.I. (1994) 'Effectiveness and cost-benefit analysis of intensive treatment and teaching programmes for Type 1 (insulin-dependent) diabetes mellitus in Moscow: blood glucose versus urine glucose self-monitoring', *Diabetologia* **37**: 170–176.

Telch, C.F. and Telch, M.J. (1986) 'Group coping skills instruction and supportive group therapy for cancer patients: a comparison of strategies', *Journal of Consulting and Clinical Psychology* **54**: 802–808.

Turner, M.O., Taylor, D., Bennett, R. and Fitzgerald, J.M. (1998) 'A randomized trial comparing peak expiratory flow and symptom self-management plans for patients with asthma attending a primary care clinic', *American Journal of Respiratory Critical Care Medicine* **157**: 540–546.

Watkins, K.W., Connell, C.M., Fitzgerald, J.T., Klem, L., Hickey, T. and Ingerson-Dayton, B. (2000) 'Effects of adults self-regulation of diabetes on quality of life outcomes', *Diabetes Care* **23**: 1511–1515.

Weinman, J., Petrie, K.J., Sharpe, N. and Walker, S. (2000) 'Causal attributions in patients and spouses following a heart attack and subsequent lifestyle changes', *British Journal of Health Psychology* **5**: 263–273.

Weinstein, N.D. (1989) 'Optimistic biases about personal risks', *Science* **246**: 1232–1233.

Wenger, H.K. and Froelicher, E.S. (1996) *National Practice Guideline: Cardiac Rehabilitation*, Maryland: US Department of Health and Human Services.

Wing, R.R., Epstein, L.H, Nowalk, M.P. and Scott, N. (1988) 'Self-regulation in the treatment of Type II diabetes', *Behavior Therapy* **19**: 11–23.

14 Message frames and illness representations

Implications for interventions to promote and sustain healthy behavior

Alexander J. Rothman, Kristina M. Kelly, Andrew W. Hertel, and Peter Salovey[1]

Given the premise that people are motivated to maximize their health and well-being, one might expect that providing people with valuable information about their health would not be complicated. Yet, effectively communicating health information has proven deceptively difficult. People fail to recognize, understand, or retain health information; even when this information is remembered, it does not necessarily affect behavior (Salovey *et al.*, 1998).

In response to this state of affairs, it has been proposed that people differ in their readiness to modify their behavior, and consequently messages must be targeted to a person's informational needs (Prochaska *et al.*, 1992). However, the conceptual basis for identifying what information a particular person or group of people require is not well specified (Weinstein *et al.*, 1998). Even if messages could be designed to meet an individual's informational needs, the question remains as to how the information should be communicated. Who should communicate the information: for example, are peers a more credible source than parents? And how should the information be framed: for example, should the benefits of taking action or the costs of failing to take action be emphasized? Although all aspects of the communication process are important, in this chapter we focus on the latter question and examine how framing health appeals in terms of the costs or benefits of action can affect behavioral decisions.

The material in this chapter is organized around two themes. First, we review research on message framing and health behavior and evaluate the degree to which the empirical evidence available supports a theoretical framework outlined by Rothman and Salovey (1997). Second, we identify the next phase of research in this area and articulate how framed health appeals could be used to sustain ongoing behavioral practices. This approach to framing health promotion communications is grounded on the premise that to be effective, framed appeals must correspond to people's representations of the health behavior and thus investigators must be attentive to how these representations may change with repeated use of the behavior.

Preference reversals: an illustration of message framing

Information about health behaviors can focus on either the benefits of performing them or the costs of failing to perform them. For example, a brochure to promote skin cancer screening could adopt a gain-frame (i.e., emphasizing the benefits afforded by screening) or a loss-frame (i.e., focusing on the costs of failing to be screened).[2] According to the framing postulate of Prospect Theory (Tversky and Kahneman, 1981), how information is framed elicits systematic differences in people's preferences. Specifically, people act to avoid risks when considering the potential gains afforded by their decision (they are risk-averse in their preferences), but take risks when considering the potential losses afforded by their decision (they are risk-seeking in their preferences).

The empirical basis for this postulate rests primarily on people's responses to hypothetical scenarios framed in terms of gains or losses. For example, people are informed about an epidemic that is expected to affect 600 individuals and have to choose between two interventions to combat the disease (Tversky and Kahneman, 1981). Although each intervention affords the same expected utility, one offers a certain outcome, whereas the other offers an uncertain or risky outcome. In the gain-framed condition, the interventions are described in terms of the number of lives that would be *saved* (e.g., if Program A is adopted, 200 people will be saved; if Program B is adopted, there is a 1/3 probability that all 600 people will be saved, and a 2/3 probability that nobody will be saved). In the loss-framed condition, the interventions are presented in terms of the number of lives that would be *lost* (e.g., if Program C is adopted, 400 people will die; if Program D is adopted, there is a 1/3 probability that nobody will die, and a 2/3 probability that all 600 people will die). When presented with information about the number of lives that could be saved, most people prefer the program that offers a certain gain (i.e., Program A). Yet, when presented with information about the number of lives that could be lost, most people reject the program describing a certain loss in favor of the one that offers a risky outcome (i.e., Program D).

Why do preferences depend on how the programs are framed? Although the specific cognitive processes that underlie the impact of framed information on choice are not well specified, the differential response to gain- and loss-framed information is thought to reflect the shape of the value function that relates objective outcomes (e.g., losing 200 lives) to subjective values (e.g., the distress elicited by losing 200 lives). In the domain of losses, the value function is steep as people find even modest losses distressing (Taylor, 1991). Furthermore, the shape of the function is convex, such that increases in potential losses have a rapidly diminishing impact on the perceived value of the outcome. If the subjective cost of losing 600 lives is not appreciably greater than losing 400 lives, people accept the risk of a larger loss in order to try to avoid any losses. In the domain of gains, the shape of the value function is concave, and thus the satisfaction derived from any increase in potential gains is associated with relatively smaller increases in perceived value. However, in the domain of gains, the modest improvement in value leads people to be risk-averse rather than risk-seeking in their preferences (i.e., the increase in value associated with saving 600 rather than 400 lives is not worth the risk of saving no lives).

Some investigators have expressed concern about failures to replicate the preference reversal predicted by Prospect Theory (e.g., Fagley and Miller, 1990; Wang, 1996; for a meta-analytic review see Kuhberger *et al.*, 1999). Although people's preferences are contingent on whether a decision involves potential gains or losses, investigators have tended to ignore whether there is any variability in how people construe a framed outcome (but see Elliott and Archibald, 1989; Levin and Chapman, 1990). People's preferences for a certain or an uncertain outcome should depend on whether the outcome is perceived as unfavorable or favorable (Rothman *et al.*, 2000). For example, when asked to choose between two fitness programs that offer the potential to lose weight, people's preferences shifted depending on how they construed the opportunity to lose weight. People who perceived losing weight to be a desirable outcome preferred the program promising the certain weight loss, whereas those who perceived losing weight to be an undesirable outcome preferred the program offering an uncertain outcome. Participants' preferences for meal plans offering a certain or uncertain opportunity to gain weight similarly reflected the perceived desirability of weight gain. The difficulties investigators have had conceptually replicating the preference reversal specified by Prospect Theory may be due, in part, to variability in how outcomes are construed.

Applying message framing to health communications

Predictions regarding message-framing effects on decision-making are contingent on the status of two parameters: the relative desirability and (un)certainty of the potential outcomes. In tests of framing effects that involve hypothetical problems, these features are relatively easy to manipulate. First, gain- and loss-framed information is constructed by describing an outcome in relation to a particular reference point. Second, two response options are provided that differ systematically in the relative risk that an outcome is obtained – where risk is formally defined as the probability associated with obtaining a given outcome. The fact that framing can affect people's preferences systematically within the context of hypothetical scenarios is noteworthy, but what happens when it is applied to decision-making in more naturalistic situations, such as those involving personal health practices?

When message frames are integrated into health recommendations, operationalizing the underlying concepts of desirability and certainty can be complicated. First, decisions regarding a health behavior often do not involve a choice between two distinct options, but rather focus on whether or not to adopt a recommended course of action. For example, a woman must decide whether or not to schedule a mammogram. In these contexts, gain- and loss-framed information is operationalized as the benefits of engaging in the behavior and the costs of failing to engage in the behavior, respectively. Second, the risk associated with a given behavior is not defined in terms of the actual likelihood of a particular outcome. Instead, the relative risk posed by performing a behavior is conceptualized as the subjective perception that it will afford an unpleasant outcome. For example, choosing to perform a detection behavior could be perceived as risky, because by deciding to be screened for a potential health problem, one 'runs the risk' of receiving significant, unpleasant information.[3]

Given the complexity of translating a paradigm based on preferences within hypothetical scenarios to behavioral choices in response to health appeals, efforts to generate and test predictions regarding the relative impact of loss- and gain-framed appeals on health practices must be thoughtful. In particular, any predictions regarding the effects of message framing on health decision-making need to be grounded in the conceptual framework delineated by Prospect Theory (Rothman and Salovey, 1997). According to Prospect Theory, people are more willing to take risks when faced with loss-framed information, whereas they are more risk-averse in their preferences when faced with gain-framed information. Thus, the effect of a particular frame on people's willingness to perform a behavior is contingent on whether the option under consideration is perceived to reflect a risk-averse or risk-seeking course of action.

Consistent with the underlying tenets of Prospect Theory, a taxonomy of situations can be developed that affords predictions as to when gain- or loss-framed health appeals are maximally persuasive. When people are considering a behavior that they perceive involves some risk or uncertainty (e.g., it may detect a health problem), loss-framed appeals are more persuasive, but when people are considering a behavior that they perceive involves a relatively certain outcome (e.g., it prevents the onset of a health problem), gain-framed appeals are more persuasive. Moreover, the function served by a health behavior can operate as a reliable heuristic to predict which behaviors people tend to perceive as risky and which behaviors people tend to perceive as relatively certain or safe. Detection behaviors such as breast self-examination (BSE) or mammography serve to detect the presence of a health problem, and because they can inform people that they may be sick, initiating the behavior may be considered a risky decision. Although detection behaviors such as mammography provide critical long-term benefits, characterizing them as risky accurately captures people's subjective assessments of these behaviors (e.g., Lerman and Rimer, 1995; Mayer and Solomon, 1992; Meyerowitz and Chaiken, 1987). In contrast, prevention behaviors such as the regular use of sunscreen or condoms forestall the onset of an illness and maintain a person's current health status. In fact, these behaviors are risky only to the extent that one chooses *not* to take action. Taken together, this distinction suggests that loss-framed appeals would be more effective in promoting the use of detection behaviors but gain-framed appeals would be more effective in promoting the use of prevention behaviors (Rothman and Salovey, 1997).

Detection behaviors

Do loss-framed messages elicit greater interest in and use of detection behaviors? Our efforts to test this thesis have focused primarily on interventions to promote the use of screening mammography. According to current guidelines, women are encouraged to obtain mammograms annually after the age of 50. Mammograms, like most screening procedures, are designed to detect indicators of a health problem – in this case, abnormalities in breast tissue that could be cancerous. Because obtaining a mammogram involves the risk of discovering a health problem, a loss-framed appeal should be more effective than a gain-framed appeal in motivating women to have the procedure.

In an initial test of this prediction, women working at a telephone company who were not complying with prevailing mammography guidelines viewed a fifteen-minute videotape on breast cancer and mammography that emphasized either the costs of not being screened or the benefits of being screened. Women were then contacted a year later to ascertain who had obtained a mammogram. Although the two videos were rated equal in quality, women who viewed the loss-framed video were more likely to have subsequently obtained a mammogram than were women who viewed the gain-framed video (66.2 per cent compared to 51.5 per cent; Banks *et al.*, 1995). Similar findings have been obtained from an intervention directed at women recruited from community health clinics and public housing developments (Schneider *et al.*, 2001).

The finding that loss-framed appeals are more effective than gain-framed appeals when promoting screening mammography is consistent with the results obtained by other investigators who have tested the impact of message frame on people's interest in or use of a detection behavior. A loss-framed advantage has been obtained in studies involving BSE (Meyerowitz and Chaiken, 1987), mammography (Cox and Cox, 2001), HIV-testing (Kalichman and Coley, 1995), amniocentesis (Marteau, 1989), skin cancer examinations (Block and Keller, 1995; Rothman *et al.*, 1996), and blood-cholesterol screening (Maheswaran and Meyers-Levy, 1990).[4] Although three studies have reported a failure to find an advantage for either frame (Lalor and Hailey, 1990; Lauver and Rubin, 1990; Lerman *et al.*, 1992), two of them involved efforts to get women to take action following an abnormal screening test (Lauver and Rubin, 1990; Lerman *et al.*, 1992). As we discuss later in this chapter, how women respond to an abnormal test may create meaningful variability in how a screening test is construed, and thus mitigate any systematic effect of framing. Given the thesis that choosing to perform a detection behavior is construed as a risky option, the pattern of results across these studies is consistent with the prediction that people are more willing to take risks when faced with information about losses.

Prevention behaviors

Because prevention behaviors typically afford people the opportunity to maintain their health and minimize the risk of illness, gain-framed messages are predicted to elicit greater interest in and use of prevention behaviors. To date, only a few studies have tested the impact of gain- and loss-framed appeals on prevention behaviors, but of those that have been conducted a consistent advantage for gain-framed appeals has been found; for example, in studies on the use of condoms (Linville *et al.*, 1993), and sunscreen (Detweiler *et al.*, 1999; Rothman *et al.*, 1993).

The pair of studies that examined people's interest in the use of sunscreen has provided the most rigorous test of the effect of message frame on prevention behaviors. In an initial study, a sample of undergraduate men and women read either a gain- or a loss-framed pamphlet about skin cancer and sunscreen use (Rothman *et al.*, 1993, Experiment 2). After reading the pamphlet, participants were given the opportunity to request a free sample of sunscreen with a sun protection factor (SPF) of 2, 6, 8, or 15. Because sunscreen must have an SPF of 15 or higher to effectively prevent skin cancer, requests for sunscreen with an SPF of 15 were compared across conditions. Consistent with our predictions, students who read the gain-framed pamphlet were more likely to request an SPF of 15 than were those who read the loss-framed pamphlet. However, this effect was limited to the women who had enrolled in the study. Of the women who read a gain-framed pamphlet, 79 per cent requested sunscreen with an SPF of 15 as compared to 45 per cent who read the loss-framed pamphlet. For men, requests rates were 50 per cent and 47 per cent, respectively.

One reason why the gain-frame advantage might have been limited to women was that conducting the study during the winter in New England rendered the issue meaningful only to those people for whom skin care and protection is of chronic interest (i.e., women). In order to examine this thesis, a follow-up intervention was conducted during the summer on a public beach – a setting in which skin care and skin cancer should be of interest to everyone. People entering the beach were given either a gain- or loss-framed brochure about skin cancer (Detweiler *et al.*, 1999). After reading the brochure, participants received a coupon that they could exchange for a free sample of sunscreen from a 'distributor' several hundred yards down the beach. Consistent with our predictions, participants who read the gain-framed brochure were more likely to exchange their coupons for a free sample than were those who read the loss-framed brochure (71 per cent compared to 53 per cent, respectively). Moreover, the same pattern of results was obtained for men and women beach-goers.

Testing the distinction between detection and prevention

The empirical findings obtained across a broad range of studies have been consistent with the framework outlined by Rothman and Salovey (1997), yet any conclusions regarding the factors that determine the relative influence of gain- and loss-framed appeals are limited because comparisons are being drawn across studies and across health domains. The numerous differences between the health domains and health behaviors studied make it difficult to assert unequivocally that the influence of a framed appeal is contingent on the function of the behavior. Even within a single health domain, prevention and detection behaviors (e.g., the use of condoms and HIV testing) can differ on dimensions such as cost, familiarity, difficulty, frequency, and the need for trained personnel to perform the behavior. These substantial differences leave open the possibility of alternative explanations for the observed pattern of findings.

In order to confirm that the function of the health behavior determines the relative influence of gain- and loss-framed appeals, a series of studies was conducted that involved experimentally manipulating whether a single health behavior prevented or detected a health problem. In one study, college under-graduates received either a loss- or gain-framed pamphlet about a mouth rinse (Rothman *et al.*, 1999, Experiment 2). For half of the students, the mouth rinse was described as an effective means to prevent the build-up of plaque (i.e., a prevention behavior), whereas for the remaining students the mouth rinse was described as an effective means to detect the build-up of plaque (i.e., a detec-tion behavior). In both cases, the same behavior was described – one had to briefly gargle with a small amount of the mouth rinse. By manipulating both message frame and the function of the behavior within a single experiment, we were able to test for the predicted 'frame by behavior function' interaction. Consistent with predictions, the persuasiveness of the framed pamphlet was contingent on the function served by the mouth rinse. When the mouth rinse was described as a way to *prevent* the build-up of plaque, participants were more likely to request a free sample after having read the gain-framed rather than the loss-framed pamphlet (67 percent and 47 percent, respectively). However, when the mouth rinse was described as a way to *detect* the build-up of plaque, participants were more likely to request a free sample after having read the loss-framed as opposed to the gain-framed pamphlet (73 percent and 37 percent, respectively).

Taken together with the findings obtained in studies that focused solely on a prevention or a detection behavior, a compelling body of evidence has devel-oped to support the thesis that gain-framed messages are more effective when promoting a prevention behavior, whereas loss-framed messages are more effective when promoting a detection behavior. Yet, even in the face of this consistent set of findings, it is important to recognize that the distinction between prevention and detection behaviors rests on the premise that people perceive engaging in detection behaviors as posing some risk and engaging in prevention behaviors as posing little to no risk. The function of the behavior serves as a heuristic that investigators can use to anticipate how people construe a given behavior. To the extent that there is variability in how people construe a detection or a prevention behavior, the relative influence of gain- and loss-framed appeals is more complex. We now turn to studies that have begun to delineate how people's construal of a given behavior regulates the influences of framed appeals.

Unpacking the function of the behavior: the role of construals

Tests of the relative influence of gain- and loss-framed information have relied on the assumption that people perceive detection behaviors as risky and prevention behaviors as safe, and have treated any variability in these perceptions as error. Given that the demonstrated relationship between message frame and the function of the behavior has proven to be quite robust, it would appear that investigators have successfully targeted behaviors for which there has been considerable consensus in how they are construed. The observation that people predominantly perceive detection behaviors as posing a risk most likely reflects the fact that health professionals consistently describe the function of behaviors such as mammography as illness-detecting. Although it is possible for these behaviors to be re-framed as health-affirming behaviors – for example, a woman could get a mammogram in order to affirm that her breasts are healthy – the tendency to construe a detection behavior in terms of its ability to detect the presence rather than the absence of a problem is consistent with the finding that people have an easier time processing and reasoning about the presence rather than the absence of features (McGuire and McGuire, 1991).

Despite the prevailing tendency to perceive detection behaviors in terms of their ability to detect a health problem, there are at least two reasons why individuals might not perceive the decision to be screened as a risky choice. First, people who consistently follow a set of effective preventive behaviors, such as brushing and flossing their teeth, might feel that there is little risk of finding a health problem and thus not be concerned about having a screening examination. Second, although the screening tests currently available are designed to test for the presence of a health problem, advances in human genetics may lead to the development of tests that can identify factors that are health promoting. Given the tendency to construe detection behaviors in terms of what they are designed to detect, people may not perceive behaviors that screen for healthy attributes as risky (i.e., one no longer runs the risk of finding something wrong). Across both of these situations, to the extent that people perceive performing a detection behavior to be a safe, health-affirming practice, a gain-framed rather than a loss-framed appeal may prove to be more persuasive.

Only a few studies have examined how people's perceptions of a behavior moderate the influence of framed appeals, and they have all focused on perceptions of screening behaviors. In one study, Meyerowitz *et al.* (1991) assessed whether women perceived performing BSE to be a risky behavior prior to providing them with either a gain- or loss-framed brochure. They found that the loss-framed brochure was more effective, but only for those women who considered performing BSE to be risky. In fact, those women who did not perceive BSE to be a risky behavior were, if anything, more responsive to the gain-framed brochure. A similar pattern of results was obtained in a study designed to promote interest in skin cancer screening examinations (Rothman *et al.*, 1996). In this case, participants reported the likelihood that they might develop skin cancer prior to receiving either gain- or loss-framed information about skin cancer. A greater percentage of participants who received the loss-framed information was willing to schedule a screening examination (78 per cent) when compared to those who received the gain-framed information (57 per cent), but this effect was limited to people who perceived themselves to be at a relatively higher risk of developing skin cancer. People who perceived themselves to be at a relatively low risk of developing skin cancer were, if anything, more likely to schedule an examination if they had received the gain-framed as opposed to the loss-framed information (50 per cent and 44 per cent, respectively). Finally, Apanovitch *et al.* (in press) observed that women who strongly believed that they were not currently HIV positive – and thus had little to risk by being tested – were more likely to obtain an HIV test after having viewed a gain-framed appeal, whereas those who believed they could be HIV positive were slightly more likely to get tested after viewing a loss-framed appeal.

To date, only one study has attempted to manipulate how people construe the risk implications of a single screening behavior. Kelly and Rothman (in review) examined participants' willingness to schedule a screening examination that was presented as either a means to detect a health problem or a means to detect a health benefit. The perceived function of the screening examination was manipulated by adopting a version of the Thioamine Acelytase (TAA) paradigm (Croyle and Ditto, 1990). In this study, people were led to believe either that testing positive for TAA indicated a health benefit (i.e., it made people more resistant to a complex of pancreatic disorders) or that testing positive indicated a health problem (i.e., it made people more susceptible to a complex of pancreatic disorders). After receiving general information about TAA, participants were provided with a series of either gain- or loss-framed reasons to screen for TAA. At the close of the study, participants were provided an opportunity to schedule an appointment to be tested at the university health center. Consistent with prior research, the loss-framed pamphlet was predicted to be more effective when promoting a test designed to screen for a health problem. However, the gain-framed pamphlet was predicted to be more effective when promoting a test designed to screen for a health benefit. Among participants who reported having previously used the university health center, the effect of the message frame was shown to be contingent on the risk implications of the screening test. When TAA provided health benefits, a gain-framed pamphlet was more effective in getting people to schedule a test at the health center than was a loss-framed pamphlet (69 percent and 50 percent, respectively), but when TAA posed a health problem, participants were more likely to schedule a test when they had received a loss- rather than a gain-framed pamphlet (75 percent and 50 percent, respectively).[5]

The results from these studies provide converging evidence that it is the risk implications of a behavior that determine what type of message frame will most effectively motivate people to take action. Throughout our research, we have operationalized 'risk' as the perception that a procedure affords the possibility of learning undesirable information about one's health. The experimental design utilized by Kelly and Rothman (in review) provided an important opportunity to distinguish between this conceptualization of 'risk' and the objective likelihood or uncertainty of a given outcome. By systematically varying whether the test screened for a health problem or a health benefit, we were able to manipulate the risk posed by the test outcome while holding constant the uncertainty associated with it.

Although investigators have focused on differences in people's perceptions of screening behaviors, this line of analysis should extend to prevention behaviors as well. To the extent that adopting a prevention behavior is not perceived as a safe or certain option, gain-framed appeals should become less effective. Because the safety afforded by a prevention behavior is contingent on its ability to maintain one's health, the perceived effectiveness of the behavior may have an important influence on whether performing the behavior is considered a risky or safe proposition. Despite the fact that message frames can be used systematically to affect people's interest in and performance of health behaviors, our understanding of the processes that mediate this effect is strikingly limited. The increased attention investigators have begun to pay to how people construe the advocated behavior may improve their ability to specify the set of thoughts and/or feelings elicited by gain- and loss-framed appeals that, in turn, guide behavioral decisions. For example, Kelly and Rothman (in review) found that participants' feelings of concern about their health following the intervention mediated the effect that framing had on their willingness to schedule a screening test. Although this finding is consistent with the conceptual framework set forth by Rothman and Salovey (1997), additional empirical work is needed not only to replicate this finding but also to clarify more fully how gain- and loss-framed messages affect behavioral decision-making.

The dynamic relation between message frames and illness representations

The primary thesis that underlies research on message framing and health behavior is that how individuals construe a health behavior determines their response to framed appeals. Perhaps because Rothman and Salovey (1997) emphasized the utility of distinguishing between behaviors based on their function, investigators have treated people's representation of a behavior as a relatively stable and uniform construct. Although investigators have begun to document variability in how people construe a behavior, these efforts have been limited to cross-sectional comparisons between individuals. Little consideration has been given to how a person's representation of a behavior changes over time and how changes in construal might affect the use of message frames. In fact, the theoretical frameworks available offer little guidance regarding how message frames may be used to motivate ongoing behavioral practices. For example, what is the most effective way to promote regular screening mammography? Should women consistently receive a loss-framed appeal or should the message frame used shift in response to changes in how mammography is construed? If people's perceptions of a behavior determine their response to a framed appeal, predictions regarding the continued influence of gain- or loss-framed appeals will depend on the extent to which people's behavioral representations change over time.

We believe a more complex model of message framing is needed to specify the ongoing relationship between message frames and behavioral representations. By specifically raising this issue, we hope to encourage investigators – including ourselves – to consider and assess the effects of interventions beyond a one-time behavioral outcome. Given that the benefits afforded by most health practices require a sustained pattern of behavior, the practical value of understanding how people make decisions regarding ongoing behavioral practices is clear (for a broader analysis of this issue see Rothman, 2000).

If we hope to predict how people's representations of a health practice change, we first of all need to specify the factors that shape these representations. To date, empirical efforts have focused on documenting the consequences of people's illness representations and not the manner in which they develop (Leventhal *et al.*, 1997; but see Leventhal *et al.*, 1986). Consistent with broader theorizing regarding lay models of illness, how people construe a behavior is thought to be shaped in large part by how the behavior is characterized by professionals in the health care system (Cameron, 1997; Leventhal *et al.*, 1984). To the extent that detection behaviors are consistently described in terms of their ability to detect disease, thoughts about screening behaviors may automatically elicit images of illness and feelings of distress (Millar and Millar, 1995). People's personal experience with and beliefs about the relevant health issue should also inform how they construe the behavior (Pearlman *et al.*, 1997). For example, women may be more likely to construe screening mammography as an illness-detecting behavior if they have a family history of breast cancer and/or know other women who have been diagnosed with breast cancer. Because people's personalities shape the experiences and information they seek out, individual differences on dimensions such as dispositional optimism (Scheier and Carver, 1985), monitoring and blunting (Miller, 1995), or regulatory style (Higgins, 1998) may moderate the inferences that people draw about a behavior. Although each of the aforementioned factors is likely to be associated with people's perception of a health behavior, their personal experience with the behavior itself is likely to be the primary determinant of their construal. Direct behavioral experience has not only been shown to have a strong influence on people's attitudes (Fazio and Zanna, 1981), it is also the primary means by which people are exposed to health professionals' characterization of the behavior.

If people's perceptions of a health behavior are responsive to their behavioral experience, then the actions people take in response to a framed appeal may alter their construal of the behavior, and thus, in turn, their responsiveness to a subsequent framed appeal. To date, investigators have focused exclusively on how framed interventions affect a targeted behavior, with no attention having been paid to the elicited behavior's effect on any psychological (or behavioral) variable. In order to guide and encourage empirical work in this area, we have developed a conceptual framework that generates predictions regarding not only how people's actions shape their construal of the behavior but also how changes in construal affect the relative influence of gain- and loss-framed appeals. Because research on message framing has often focused on decisions regarding screening mammography, we have chosen to ground our theoretical discussion in this content area.

Imagine a group of women who have had a mammogram after viewing a loss-framed informational intervention. Consistent with prior research, we assume that prior to being screened they construe mammography as an illness-detecting procedure that poses some degree of psychological risk. Based on the outcome of the screening procedure, a woman typically will find herself in one of three situations: (a) the mammogram will be negative, revealing no indication of any health problem; (b) the mammogram will have raised suspicion of an abnormality that, ultimately, is determined to be a false positive; or (c) the mammogram will have detected an abnormality that, after biopsy, proves to be cancerous and requires some form of treatment. We propose that how a woman responds to each of these outcomes affects how she construes mammography and, thus, determines her response to framed appeals designed to promote further screening.

Consider first those women who receive an unambiguously clear screening. How might this experience affect their perceptions of mammography? Although investigators have spent considerable effort specifying the psychological consequences of receiving a positive or a false positive result (for a review see Lerman and Rimer, 1995), minimal consideration has been given to how women respond to the information that their breasts are healthy. We propose that women's affective and cognitive reactions to a clear screening can be used to distinguish between two broad classes of responses: one characterized by feelings of luck and the temporary relief from anxiety; and another characterized by feelings of reassurance and well-being.

The group of women who respond to the favorable news by feeling lucky and temporarily relieved are likely to interpret the screening outcome as a sign of the absence of disease. This emphasis on the absence of negative states – and the associated affective reactions it engenders – may reflect what Higgins (1998) has characterized as a prevention-focused self-regulatory style. With time, these initial feelings of relief are expected to dissipate as attention shifts from the recently completed screening to next year's procedure, eliciting new feelings of worry and concern about what might be found. For these women, the prospect of being screened remains a risky endeavor. Moreover, to the extent that they believe that the procedure inevitably will find a lump that proves to be cancerous, the experience of repeated negative screenings actually might lead the procedure to be seen as increasingly riskier – as women might infer their luck is bound to end. Given this construal of the behavior, we predict that a loss-framed appeal would consistently prove the most effective way to motivate these women to seek mammogram screening.

A second group of women is predicted to respond to a clear screening by feeling reassured by the news that they are in good health. In contrast to the first group, the reactions of these women would reflect a sensitivity to the presence of positive states, which is consistent with a promotion-focused self-regulatory style (Higgins, 1998). By conceptualizing the outcome as providing information about the presence of health rather than the absence of disease, these women may begin to modify how they have construed the screening procedure. To the extent that women begin to ascribe more favorable cognitive and affective associations to the process of screening mammography, the procedure may be seen as less of a risky endeavor and, in fact, over time it may be construed as an opportunity to affirm that one's breasts are healthy. At the point at which these women no longer construe mammography as an illness-detecting – or risky – behavior, the continued application of loss-framed appeals will prove ineffective. At this time, a shift to a gain-framed appeal would be predicted to be a more persuasive communication strategy.

Given that screening behaviors are consistently characterized in terms of their ability to detect disease, we would anticipate that the majority of women, at least initially, respond to a clear screening with feelings of relief and a reduction in concern. What remains to be determined are the factors that predispose women to reconceptualize the screening result as a reassuring and health-affirming outcome. We believe that some preliminary answers can be gleaned from research regarding predictors of elevated levels of concern and anxiety about breast cancer. Factors shown to predict feelings of concern about breast cancer – such as a family history of breast cancer and knowing women with breast cancer – are likely to decrease the chances that a woman would feel reassured following a clear screening. Although any transformation in how the screening procedure is construed should become more pronounced as the number of consecutive clear screenings increase, the rate at which perceptions of the behavior changes is likely to vary as a function of the characteristics listed above.

Taken together, the specifications of these two groups of women suggest that predictions regarding the relative impact of gain- and loss-framed appeals depend on how women respond to the behavioral outcome. Moreover, this perspective predicts that the number of women who respond more favorably to a gain-framed appeal about a screening behavior increases over time. How do these predictions fit with the consistent finding that loss-framed appeals are the most effective way to promote the use of screening mammography? It is possible that because prior intervention studies (Banks *et al.*, 1995; Schneider *et al.*, 2001) recruited only women who were not complying with prevailing screening guidelines, they may have unintentionally oversampled women who were less likely to have had a repeated series of clear mammograms and, thus, were more likely to perceive the behavior as a risky course of action. Consistent with this premise, women who use mammography irregularly (i.e., less than every two years) have been shown to have strikingly more negative attitudes toward the behavior than do women who get screened every one or two years (Rakowski *et al.*, 1997). However, the attitudinal measure used in this study did not specifically assess perceptions of the risk posed by the procedure.

We anticipate that the conceptual framework outlined with respect to how women may respond to a clear screening result can also be applied to women who have had to cope with an initially suspicious mammography finding as well as those who have completed treatment for breast cancer and have begun to monitor for a reoccurrence of cancer. Because researchers have consistently found that receiving an initially suspicious mammogram elicits elevated feelings of concern about the screening procedure (e.g., Lerman *et al.*, 1991), one might predict a loss-framed appeal would be the most effective way to encourage these women to return for a subsequent mammogram. However, any factors that elicit variability in how women respond to the initial screening outcome should affect the relative influence of gain- and loss-framed appeals. This might explain why an earlier study failed to obtain a message-framing effect on the screening behaviors of women who recently had a suspicious mammogram (Lerman *et al.*, 1992). In the case of women who have started to screen again following treatment, how they construe the screening procedure may depend on their response to the treatment. We expect that those women who complete treatment feeling confident and reassured about their health would be more likely to construe the test as a health-affirming procedure and, thus, be more responsive to a gain-framed appeal, whereas those who complete treatment anxious about the possibility of a relapse would be more likely to construe the test as an illness-detecting procedure and, thus, be more responsive to a loss-framed appeal.[6]

As indicated at the outset of this section, our predictions regarding the interplay between framing and changes in how a behavior is construed remain untested. They require investigators not only to monitor a pattern of behavioral outcomes over time but also to track how people's actions affect their representation of the behavior. The framework we have outlined provides a clear set of testable predictions regarding how the repeated application of gain- and loss-framed messages can be used to motivate people to maintain a healthy pattern of behavior. In stating that message frames need to match people's perceptions of the behavior, our approach provides a theoretically grounded way to tailor an intervention to characteristics of the target audience (Kreuter *et al.*, 1999). Although investigators have begun to entertain questions regarding the decision processes that discriminate between consistent and inconsistent behavioral practices (e.g., Sheeran *et al.*, 2001), a new generation of intervention studies needs to be designed and implemented that afford repeated intervention contacts and that allow for the inclusion of framed appeals that can be matched or mismatched to an individual's representation of the behavior.

Final observations

Research on message framing has provided a theoretically grounded approach to health communication and health decision-making. Yet it should be clear that framing in and of itself is not a 'magic bullet,' such that an emphasis on gains or losses always leads to an increase in healthy behavioral practices. Rather, the effectiveness of a framed message is moderated by characteristics of the message recipient, characteristics of the desired behavior, or both. It is the further elucidation of these moderators as well as the psychological mediators that underlie framing effects that represents the research agenda of the coming decade.

Notes

1   Correspondence should be addressed to Alexander J. Rothman, Department of Psychology, University of Minnesota, Twin Cities Campus, Elliott Hall, 75 East River Road, Minneapolis, Minnesota 55455, USA. E-mail: rothm001@tc.umn.edu
2   A further distinction can be made within the classes of gain- and loss-framed appeals. Gain-framed messages can emphasize obtaining positive outcomes or avoiding negative outcomes, whereas loss-framed messages can emphasize obtaining negative outcomes or avoiding positive outcomes. To date, investigators have found consistent effects across the two different operationalizations (Detweiler *et al.*, 1999).
3   Although this operationalization of risk would seem to be less precise than one grounded on the probability of a given outcome, it has become increasingly clearer that people's responses to the stated probability of an outcome depend on the subjective meaning assigned to the potential outcome (Rothman and Kiviniemi, 1999). Moreover, this emphasis allows one to disentangle the objective benefits afforded by a behavior from how people construe the behavior.
4   Loss-framed information about a blood cholesterol test was effective only when college undergraduates were informed that coronary heart disease was a problem for people under 25 years old (for a broader analysis of this finding see Rothman and Salovey, 1997).

5   The behavioral decisions made by participants who had not used university health services failed to reveal any interpretable pattern.

6   The proposed conceptual framework could also be applied to the repeated use of prevention behaviors. Although space limitations preclude a complete discussion of this analysis here, the primary assumption would be that changes in people's perceptions of the behavior would depend on whether they remained confident about its effectiveness. For example, people who get the flu despite having obtained a flu vaccination might differ in whether this experience leads them to question the efficacy of the precaution. We predict that those who maintain their confidence in the behavior – perhaps believing that they would have been worse off if they had not received the vaccination – would be more responsive to a gain-framed appeal, whereas those who begin to lose confidence in the behavior would be more responsive to a loss-framed appeal.

References

Apanovitch, A.M., McCarthy, D. and Salovey, P. (in press) 'Using message framing to motivate HIV-testing among low-income, ethnic minority women,' *Health Psychology*.

Banks, S.M., Salovey, P., Greener, S., Rothman, A.J., Moyer, A., Beauvais, J. and Eppel, E. (1995) 'The effects of message framing on mammography utilization,' *Health Psychology* **14**: 178–184.

Block, L.G. and Keller, P.A. (1995) 'When to accentuate the negative: the effects of perceived efficacy and message framing on intentions to perform a health-related behavior,' *Journal of Marketing Research* **32**: 192–203.

Cameron, L.D. (1997) 'Screening for cancer: illness perceptions and illness worry,' in K.J. Petrie and J.A. Weinman (eds) *Perceptions of Health and Illness: Current Research and Applications*, Amsterdam: Harwood Academic, pp. 291–322.

Cox, D. and Cox, A.D. (2001) 'Communicating the consequences of early detection: the role of evidence and framing,' *Journal of Marketing* **65**: 91–103.

Croyle, R.T. and Ditto, P.H. (1990) 'Illness cognition and behavior: an experimental approach,' *Journal of Behavioral Medicine* **13**: 31–52.

Detweiler, J.B., Bedell, B.T., Salovey, P., Pronin, E. and Rothman, A.J. (1999) 'Message framing and sun screen use: gain-framed messages motivate beach-goers,' *Health Psychology* **18**: 189–196.

Elliott, C.S. and Archibald, R.B. (1989) 'Subjective framing and attitudes towards risk,' *Journal of Economic Psychology* **10**: 321–328.

Fagley, N.S. and Miller P.M. (1990) 'The effect of framing on choice: interactions with risk-taking propensity, cognitive style, and sex,' *Personality and Social Psychology Bulletin* **16**: 496–510.

Fazio, R.H. and Zanna, M.P. (1981) 'Direct experience and attitude-behavior consistency,' in L. Berkowitz (ed.) *Advances in Experimental Social Psychology*, vol. 14, New York: Academic Press, pp. 161–202.

Higgins, E.T. (1998) 'Promotion and prevention: regulatory focus as a motivational principle,' in M.P. Zanna (ed.) *Advances in Experimental Social Psychology*, vol. 30, New York: Academic Press, pp. 1–46.

Kalichman, S.C. and Coley, B. (1995) 'Context framing to enhance HIV-antibody-testing messages targeted to African American women,' *Health Psychology* **14**: 247–254.

Kelly, K.M. and Rothman, A.J. (in review) 'Screening for health and illness: an analysis of how and when message frames impact behavioral decision-making.'

Kreuter, M.W., Strecher, V.J. and Glassman, B. (1999) 'One size does not fit all: the case for tailored print materials,' *Annals of Behavioral Medicine* **21**: 276–283.

Kuhberger, A., Schulte-Mecklenbeck, M. and Perner, J. (1999) 'The effects of framing, reflection, probability, and payoff on risk preference in choice tasks,' *Organizational Behavior and Human Decision Processes* **78**: 204–231.

Lalor, K.M. and Hailey, B.J. (1990) 'The effects of message framing and feelings of susceptibility to breast cancer on reported frequency of breast self-examination,' *International Quarterly of Community Health Education* **10**: 183–192.

Lauver, D. and Rubin, M. (1990) 'Message framing, dispositional optimism, and follow-up for abnormal Papanicolaou tests,' *Research in Nursing and Health* **13**: 199–207.

Lerman, C. and Rimer, B.K. (1995) 'Psychosocial impact of cancer screening,' in R.T. Croyle (ed.) *Psychosocial Effects of Screening for Disease Prevention and Detection*, Oxford: Oxford University Press, pp. 65–81.

Lerman, C., Trock, B., Rimer, B.K., Jepson, C., Brody, D. and Boyce, A. (1991) 'Psychological side effects of breast cancer screening,' *Health Psychology* **10**: 259–267.

Lerman, C., Ross, E., Boyce, A., Gorchov, P.M., McLauglin, R., Rimer, B. and Engstrom, P. (1992) 'The impact of mailing psychoeducational materials to women with abnormal mammograms,' *American Journal of Public Health* **82**: 729–730.

Leventhal, H., Nerenz, D.R. and Steele, D.J. (1984) 'Illness representations and coping with health threats,' in A. Baum, S.E. Taylor, and J.E. Singer (eds) *Handbook of Psychology and Health*, vol. 4, Hillsdale, NJ: Lawrence Erlbaum Associates, pp. 219–252.

Leventhal, H., Easterling, D.V., Coons, H.L., Luchterhand, C.M. and Love, R.R. (1986) 'Adaptations to chemotherapy treatments,' in B.L. Anderson (ed.) *Women with Cancer*, NY: Springer-Verlag, pp. 172–203.

Leventhal, H., Benyamini, Y., Brownlee, S., Diefenbach, M., Leventhal, E.A., Patrick-Miller, L. and Robitaille, C. (1997) 'Illness representations: theoretical foundations,' in K.J. Petrie and J.A. Weinman (eds) *Perceptions of Health and Illness: Current Research and Applications*, London: Harwood Academic, pp. 19–45.

Levin, I.P. and Chapman, D.P. (1990) 'Risk taking, frame of reference, and characterization of victim groups in AIDS treatment decisions,' *Journal of Experimental Social Psychology* **26**: 421–434.

Linville, P.W., Fischer, G.W. and Fischhoff, B. (1993) 'AIDS risk perceptions and decision biases,' in J.B. Pryor and G.D. Reeder (eds) *The Social Psychology of HIV Infection*, Hillsdale, NJ: Lawrence Erlbaum Associates, pp. 5–38.

Maheswaran, D. and Meyers-Levy, J. (1990) 'The influence of message framing and issue involvement,' *Journal of Marketing Research* **27**: 361–367.

Marteau, T.M. (1989) 'Framing of information: its influence upon decisions of doctors and patients,' *British Journal of Social Psychology* **28**: 89–94.

Mayer, J.A. and Solomon, L. (1992) 'Breast self-examination skill and frequency: a review,' *Annals of Behavioral Medicine* **14**: 189–196.

McGuire, W.J. and McGuire, C.V. (1991) 'The content, structure, and operation of thought systems,' in R.S. Wyer, Jr and T.K. Srull (eds) *Advances in Social Cognition*, vol. 4, Hillsdale, NJ: Lawrence Erlbaum Associates, pp. 1–78.

Meyerowitz, B.E. and Chaiken, S. (1987) 'The effect of message framing on breast self-examination attitudes, intentions, and behavior,' *Journal of Personality and Social Psychology* **52**: 500–510.

Meyerowitz, B.E., Wilson, D.K. and Chaiken, S. (1991) 'Loss-framed messages increase breast self-examination for women who perceive risk,' paper presented at the Annual Convention of the American Psychological Society, Washington, DC.

Millar, M.G. and Millar, K. (1995) 'Negative affective consequences of thinking about disease detection behaviors,' *Health Psychology* **14**: 141–146.

Miller, S.M. (1995) 'Monitoring versus blunting styles of coping with cancer influence the information patients want and need about their disease,' *Cancer* **74**: 167–177.

Pearlman, D.N., Rakowski, W., Clark, M.A., Ehrich, B., Rimer, B.K., Goldstein, M.G., Woolverton, H. and Dube, C.E. (1997) 'Why do women's attitudes toward mammography change over time? Implications for physician–patient communication,' *Cancer Epidemiology, Biomarkers and Prevention* **6**: 451–457.

Prochaska, J.O., DiClemente, C.C. and Norcross, J.C. (1992) 'In search of how people change: applications to addictive behaviors,' *American Psychologist* **47**: 1102–1114.

Rakowski, W., Clark, M.A., Pearlman, D.N., Ehrich, B., Rimer, B.K., Goldstein, M.G., Dube, C.E. and Woolverton, H. (1997) 'Integrating pros and cons for mammography and pap testing: extending the construct of decisional balance to two behaviors,' *Preventive Medicine* **26**: 664–673.

Rothman, A.J. (2000) 'Toward a theory-based analysis of behavioral maintenance,' *Health Psychology* **19**: 64–69.

Rothman, A.J. and Kiviniemi, M. (1999) '"Treating people with health information": an analysis and review of approaches to communicating health risk information,' *Journal of the National Cancer Institute Monographs* **25**: 44–51.

Rothman, A.J. and Salovey, P. (1997) 'Shaping perceptions to motivate healthy behavior: the role of message framing,' *Psychological Bulletin* **121**: 3–19.

Rothman, A.J., Martino, S.C. and Jeffery, R. (2000) 'Predicting preferences for certain or uncertain options: the importance of knowing whether an outcome is construed as a gain or a loss,' unpublished manuscript, University of Minnesota.

Rothman, A.J., Pronin, E. and Salovey, P. (1996) 'The influence of prior concern on the persuasiveness of loss-framed messages about skin cancer,' paper presented at the Annual Meeting of the Society of Experimental Social Psychology, Sturbridge, MA.

Rothman, A.J., Martino, S.C., Bedell, B.T., Detweiler, J.B. and Salovey, P. (1999) 'The systematic influence of gain- and loss-framed messages on interest in and use of different types of health behavior,' *Personality and Social Psychology Bulletin* **25**: 1355–1369.

Rothman, A.J., Salovey, P., Antone, C., Keough, K. and Martin, C.D. (1993) 'The influence of message framing on intentions to perform health behaviors,' *Journal of Experimental Social Psychology* **29**: 408–433.

Salovey, P., Rothman, A.J. and Rodin, J. (1998) 'Health behavior,' in D. Gilbert, S. Fiske and G. Lindzey (eds) *Handbook of Social Psychology*, 4th edn, vol. 2, New York: McGraw-Hill, pp. 633–683.

Scheier, M.F. and Carver, C.S. (1985) 'Optimism, coping, and health: assessment and implications of generalized outcome expectancies,' *Health Psychology* **4**: 219–247.

Schneider, T.R., Salovey, P., Apanovitch, A.M., Pizarro, J., McCarthy, D., Zullo, J. and Rothman, A.J. (2001) 'The effects of message framing and ethnic targeting on mammography use among low-income women,' *Health Psychology* **20**: 256–266.

Sheeran, P., Connor, M. and Norman, P. (2001) 'Can the theory of planned behavior explain patterns of health behavior change? *Health Psychology* **20**: 12–19.

Taylor, S.E. (1991) 'Asymmetrical effects of positive and negative events: the mobilization-minimization hypothesis,' *Psychological Bulletin* **110**: 67–85.

Tversky, A. and Kahneman, D. (1981) 'The framing of decisions and the rationality of choice,' *Science* **221**: 453–458.

Wang, X.T. (1996) 'Framing effects: dynamics and task domains,' *Organizational Behavior and Human Decision Processes* **68**: 145–157.

Weinstein, N.D., Rothman, A.J. and Sutton, S.R. (1998) 'Stage theories of health behavior' *Health Psychology* **17**: 290–299.

15 Self-regulation and decision-making about cancer screening

Ronald E. Myers[1]

Routine screening for certain types of cancer is recommended for older adults and other at-risk populations by public and private health organizations, professional medical societies, medical practitioners, and advocacy groups. Many members of at-risk populations do not routinely follow these recommendations, however. A recent nationwide survey completed in the US found that only 19 per cent of adults aged 50 years old and above had completed a fecal occult blood test in the preceding year, and only 32 per cent had ever had a sigmoidoscopy or colonoscopy within the previous five years. About one-third of women aged 40 years old and above had not had a mammogram to screen for breast cancer in the year prior to the survey (Holtzman *et al.*, 2000).

Research has shown that demographic, cognitive, affective, social, and health care system factors can help to explain cancer-screening utilization. However, there is no consensus in the field about what factors are consistent predictors of screening modality use. There are a number of reasons for this state of affairs. First, few prospective, theory-based studies designed to identify cancer screening predictors have been reported in the literature. In addition, although several explanatory frameworks (e.g., the Health Belief Model, the Theory of Reasoned Action, and self-regulation theories such as the common-sense model) have been used to guide data collection and analyses in cancer screening research studies, little work has been done to standardize and validate measures of explanatory constructs drawn from such models. As a result, common theory-based constructs have not been measured in a consistent fashion across studies of screening modality use.

Our understanding of why some people choose to use cancer screening modalities while others do not is also limited by the fact that researchers have not thoroughly examined the dynamic interplay of internal and external forces influencing personal decision-making about cancer screening. One reason that this area of inquiry has been neglected is that cancer screening has been viewed traditionally as a universal good. Reflecting this public health perspective, researchers have directed their energies largely toward the goal of identifying the most effective methods for persuading populations to take advantage of existing and new cancer screening modalities. The view that cancer screening is a preventive health behavior that everyone should adopt is being challenged by research that suggests there may be little benefit from screening and there is reason to be concerned about the 'downstream' effects (e.g., the risk of exposure to unnecessary follow-up procedures, the emotional burden of receiving an abnormal screening test result, and the financial costs of testing). Increasingly, cancer screening is being viewed as a matter of personal decision-making. Interest is growing in the use of explanatory models of the decision-making process (e.g., the Analytic Hierarchy Processing model) and the application of these models in the development of decision-making tools for facilitating informed choices concerning cancer screening.

In this chapter, major health behavior explanatory frameworks that have been applied to cancer screening are outlined, and findings related to predictors of cancer screening are highlighted. Self-regulation theory is described, and studies using this theory to explain cancer screening are outlined. The Preventive Health Model, a framework that integrates major constructs from preventive health behavior theories and self-regulation theory, is described. Cancer screening studies that have used the Preventive Health Model are reviewed. Decision-making is discussed from a self-regulation perspective. Here, attention is paid to the need to use theory-based models not only to illuminate the decision-making process, but also to develop methods that are effective in facilitating informed choice. An illustrative study of decision-making about prostate cancer screening is presented.

Preventive health behavior theories

Different theoretical frameworks have been advanced to explain preventive health behaviors such as cancer screening (Weinstein *et al.*, 1998). Most of these frameworks are based on a subjective expected utility perspective. That is, they posit that people are highly rational in decision-making about health behavior, inasmuch as people carefully consider the likelihood that certain health-related events will or will not occur as well as personal values related to the occurrence of these events. It is expected that these considerations will lead to reasoned judgments about whether or not to use preventive health modalities such as cancer screening tests (Edwards, 1954; Keeney and Raiffa, 1976; Miller and Star, 1967).

One of the most commonly cited preventive health behavior frameworks is the Health Belief Model (HBM). This model assumes that people are motivated by a desire to avoid illness and the belief that taking preventive action can help them attain that goal (Strecher and Rosenstock, 1997). According to the HBM, people carefully assess personal susceptibility to a given disease, the severity of the disease, the benefits and barriers of preventive behavior, and external cues to action before engaging in the behavior.

The HBM has been used to inform data collection and to direct intervention delivery in a number of studies on cancer screening (Burack and Liang, 1989; Burak and Meyer, 1997; Fox *et al.*, 2001; Friedman *et al.*, 1995; Han *et al.*, 2000; Taplin *et al.*, 1989; Taplin *et al.*, 1994; Wardle *et al.*, 2000; Yarbrough and Braden, 2001).

The Theory of Reasoned Action, and the later Theory of Planned Behavior, are based on the notions that intention drives behavior and that intention is determined by the extent to which the individual holds favorable attitudes toward the behavior (Ajzen and Fishbein, 1980; Fishbein and Ajzen, 1975; Montano *et al.*, 1997). These attitudes include whether or not one believes that engaging in the behavior will result in desired outcomes, whether or not one thinks that significant others support the behavior, and one's sense of control over behavioral performance. These frameworks have found application in several cancer prevention and control research studies (Barling and Moore, 1996; Montano and Taplin, 1991; Sheeran and Orbell, 2000; Taplin and Montano, 1993).

Most studies of cancer screening that have used these frameworks have involved the analysis of cross-sectional survey data related to the intention to screen or actual screening compliance or adherence. Studies of breast, cervical, and skin cancer screening that have reported cross-sectional or retrospective analysis results (Barling and Moore, 1996; Burack and Liang, 1989; Burak and Meyer, 1997; Fox *et al.*, 2001; Friedman *et al.*, 1995; Han *et al.*, 2000; Hodge *et al.*, 1996; McBride *et al.*, 1993; Montano and Taplin, 1991; Navarro *et al.*, 1998; Sheeran and Orbell, 2000; Taplin *et al.*, 1989; Taplin *et al.*, 1994; Taplin and Montano, 1993; Wardle *et al.*, 2000; Yarbrough and Braden, 2001) show that a range of factors (i.e., sociodemographic background, personal health status, previous experience with screening, perceived benefits and barriers related to screening, perceived susceptibility, worry, intention, and cues to action) may help to explain screening utilization. These types of studies are useful in identifying variables that are associated with past screening or the intention to screen, but, by definition, do not serve to identify actual 'predictors' of future screening decisions.

Self-regulation theory

According to the common-sense model (CSM) of illness self-regulation, each individual is imbued with a 'self-system' that serves to guide conscious actions intended to maintain or achieve valued physical, emotional, and social states or well-being (Leventhal and Cameron, 1987; Leventhal and Cleary, 1979). The self-system may be described as a psychosocial identity structure that manages important health problems that are encountered in everyday life. Important health problems include events or conditions that are perceived as threatening to one's capacity to function physically, cognitively, emotionally, or socially. The theory posits that individuals form cognitive and affective representations related to health problems and that these representations affect whether or not people choose to engage in given health behaviors (Brownlee *et al.*, 2000). Cognitive representations may be conceived as a more or less dispassionate awareness of or knowledge about the etiology of the health problem; one's susceptibility to disease; the severity and duration of the problem; and the effectiveness of available behavioral alternatives or coping strategies. Affective representations incorporate emotional reactions to these and other aspects of the health problem and behavioral alternatives. The active consideration of cognitive and affective representations may lead the individual to adopt or reject a given behavioral alternative (Carver and Scheier, 1999; Lazarus, 1966; Leventhal *et al.*, 1965; Leventhal *et al.*, 1967). Furthermore, the selection and implementation of an alternative is followed by outcome appraisal. Outcomes of health behaviors are evaluated in terms of consequences that were anticipated and those that were actually experienced (Hayes-Bautista, 1976; Leventhal *et al.*, 1980; Meyer *et al.*, 1985). Perceptions generated as a result of this process become part of the representational repertoire of the self-system (Ellsworth and Smith, 1998; Frijda, 1988) and serve to guide future action (Carver and Scheier, 1982; Powers, 1973).

The predictive potential of self-regulation theory has not been realized relative to cancer screening because there have been few prospective studies that have used self-regulation constructs in this area. In one investigation, conducted among women involved in a chemo-prevention trial, it was observed that side-effects occasioned by the use of tamoxifen triggered intrusive cancer-worries and an increased use of breast self-examination. The researchers hypothesized that symptoms served to activate affective concerns regarding risk and induced the use of a coping strategy (Cameron *et al.*, 1998). The experience of these symptoms signaled an increased awareness of the potential for developing breast cancer and simulated affective concerns relative to the disease, thereby enhancing the use of breast self-examination. Other findings from a prospective study of mammography utilization indicated that being older and having a moderate level of worry about developing breast cancer were predictors of preventive behavior (Diefenbach *et al.*, 1999). In this study, there was no single precipitating event, such as the experience of symptoms, that moved women to take preventive action. Instead, awareness that breast cancer risk increases with age may have been sufficient to confer a more acute sense of susceptibility and attendant worry.

Other self-regulation models of health behavior posit similar processes and identify additional factors that may determine behavioral decisions. For example, Bandura (1986) proposes that people's interactions with the environment are facilitated by an internal self-control system that sets behavioral goals, initiates goal-directed behavior, and monitors outcomes. The theory also assumes that individuals may be differentiated according to their personal expectations (i.e., anticipated outcomes of a given behavior), expectancies (i.e., values associated with behavioral outcomes), and sense of 'self-efficacy,' or belief in one's capacity to carry out a given behavior (Baranowski *et al.*, 1997). Research evidence suggests that individuals are more likely to engage in cancer screening if they view it as helpful in achieving favorable expectations and as something that is easy to do (Hodge *et al.*, 1996; McBride *et al.*, 1993; Navarro *et al.*, 1998).

The Preventive Health Model: an integrative framework

The Preventive Health Model (PHM) is an explanatory framework for preventive health behavior (e.g., tests used to detect early disease) that integrates aspects of major preventive health behavior theories with self-regulation theory. Psychosocial constructs included in the model are: personal background and experience (e.g., sociodemographic characteristics, medical history, past preventive behavior), cognitive and affective representations associated with disease, and social influence (Myers and Wolf, 1990; Vernon *et al.*, 1997). In terms of representations, the contents (e.g., knowledge and beliefs, emotional responses, perceived social support and influence) and the properties of salience and coherence are expected to influence behavior. Specifically, the extent to which a given health threat and preventive behavior are viewed as salient or important, and the degree to which they are considered to be coherent insofar as they are sensible, consistent with values and beliefs, and integrative with the individual's everyday life, are central elements of the PHM. These elements serve to condition behavioral intention to engage or not to engage in available coping strategies and, ultimately, influence decision-making relative to the selection of a given behavioral alternative. The PHM also takes into account external stimuli or contacts that serve as motivational cues.

The PHM has been used in a study to identify factors that predict adherence to colorectal cancer screening. This study was conducted among men and women who were 50 years old or more and were members of a managed care organization (Myers *et al.*, 1994). In the study, a PHM-based telephone survey was administered to 501 (78 percent) of 646 individuals in the sampling frame. Survey responders were subsequently sent a fecal occult blood test (FOBT) kit for use in screening. Survey respondents were randomly assigned to either a 'usual care' control group or an intervention group. The control group received a fecal occult blood test kit and a separate reminder to complete and return tests in the kit. The intervention group received these same contacts, along with an informational booklet and a brief educational counseling telephone call. The call was designed to allow the caller to review the content of the booklet with the study participant. Consistent with the PHM, the intervention was designed to ensure that patients received and understood standard information about screening and to reinforce the notion that screening is a salient and coherent behavior. Only 72 (29 percent) of the control group participants completed and returned screening tests, while 126 (50 percent) of the intervention group participants completed and returned theirs. Multivariate analyses showed that different features of cognitive representations predicted screening test use among men and women. For men, the perceived salience and coherence of screening together with self-efficacy were positive predictors of behavior. These factors remained statistically significant after controlling for the significant intervention effect. Among women, only age and self-efficacy were positively and significantly associated with screening. Findings from this study provide preliminary evidence of the potential importance of representational salience and coherence in influencing FOBT use by men, although such evidence is lacking for women.

The PHM has also been applied in a study of prostate cancer screening (Myers *et al.*, 1999). In this investigation, 548 men – African Americans aged 40–74 years old, with no history of prostate cancer, and who were patients served by the health service clinic at the University of Chicago – were targeted for the administration of a PHM-based telephone survey questionnaire. Of the 548 men, 413 (78 percent) completed the survey. Responders were then randomly assigned to either a minimal intervention group or an enhanced intervention group. Men in the minimal intervention group received a letter inviting them to make an appointment for a clinic visit and prostate cancer screening. Those who made an appointment received a telephone reminder. At the office, patients were informed about the pros and cons of screening. Enhanced intervention group men received the same contacts. In addition, they also received a tailor-made informational booklet with the invitation letter, and subsequently an educational counseling telephone call. In the enhanced intervention group, 51 per cent of the men had a screening exam, while only 29 percent of the men in the minimal intervention group visited the clinic and underwent screening. In addition to the intervention effect, being 50 years old or more and being married positively predicted screening exam use. In terms of cognitive representations, the belief that screening should be done in the absence of symptoms was a positive predictor. Intention was also positively related to screening.

In both of these studies, cancer screening was presented to the participants as a preventive health behavior to consider. Presumably, most study participants had not experienced symptoms or events significant enough to trigger substantial introspection or affective concerns related to having a cancer screening test. Therefore, we found that demographic and cognitive components of the PHM were the most important predictors of screening test use, whereas affective representations and social support and influence did not predict screening use. In circumstances where the individual is encouraged to carefully consider the pros and cons of cancer screening, affective factors may become more prominent in explaining behavior. Such is likely to be the case in future investigations, as informed decision-making about cancer screening is promoted as a societal value.

Fostering progress through the stages of decision-making

Given the shift in orientation away from the simple promotion of cancer screening and toward encouraging informed, value-consistent decision-making about cancer screening, there is a need to develop intervention tools for facilitating effective decision-making that can be easily used by patients and adapted for implementation in various clinical and social environments. These tools must incorporate strategies for connecting with patients' multidimensional self-systems (e.g., their cognitive and affective representations, social influence factors, etc.) and guiding patients through the decision-making process.

Evidence suggests that people pass through a series of stages as they consider whether or not to undergo an event such as cancer screening (Prochaska and DiClemente, 1984; Weinstein, 1988). Although the different theoretical models each identify somewhat different steps, there is a general consensus that these stages involve varying degrees of being aware of the behavior, considering the personal utility of behavioral strategies, decision-making about taking action, and maintaining behavioral change over time. Moreover, progression through these stages has been found to be predicted by the decisional balance of the 'pros' and 'cons' of engaging in the behavior (Prochaska, 1994). It is expected that the delivery of educational messages emphasizing stage-specific 'pros' rather than the 'cons' that resonate with individual cognitive and affective factors related to the behavior may move the person from being less to being more ready to consider taking action, and, ultimately, to making and acting on a personal decision. Prospective studies of screening mammography using stage models have reported that a person's sociodemographic characteristics, previous screening record, decisional balance score, and stage of readiness predict mammography utilization (Rakowski *et al.*, 1998; Rimer *et al.*, 2001; Stoddard *et al.*, 2002). In addition, a study of screening mammography found that breast cancer risk, perceived risk of developing breast cancer, fear of breast cancer, and worry about being diagnosed with breast cancer significantly discriminated women at different decisional stages of mammogram use (Clemow *et al.*, 2000). It is important to point out that although this research has provided useful information about what characteristics are associated with movement through decision-making stages or steps, it has provided relatively little insight into the dynamic nature of the decision-making process itself.

Decision-making as self-regulation

One of the most important aspects of the CSM is the recognition that both cognitive and affective representations of health problems and coping strategies operate to influence behavior. The manner in which these aspects of the self-system serve to catalyze decision-making, the circumstances under which the decision-making process is initiated, and the dynamic nature of the decision-making process itself need further explication.

Baumeister and Newman (1994), from a self-regulation perspective, argue that decision-making about a given health behavior is occasioned by situational stress arising from awareness of a proximal threat to one's health (e.g., a disease diagnosis) or information signaling a threat that is more distal (e.g., learning that one is at risk of developing a disease). Steps that lead to making a decision about a response include:

1   becoming aware of the nature and cause of the health threat
2   understanding that health decisions are commonly made under conditions of uncertainty
3   identifying alternative courses of action
4   weighing available alternatives in terms of personal values and potential impact on vulnerability
5   selecting and implementing an alternative that is both consistent with one's values and viewed as most likely to lead to the maintenance or achievement of well-being

In self-regulation terms, decision-making related to health problems involves the inspection of aspects of the problem that are recognized as relevant and important, and careful consideration of behavioral alternatives in light of potential gains and losses relative to instrumental goals and values (Janis, 1984; Janis and Mann, 1977). This process draws on cognitive and affective representation content, as well as on social influence and other factors identified by the PHM. Effective decision-making tools for cancer screening must be designed to encourage systematic consideration of representational content related to cancer and screening, along with an awareness that there is uncertainty about whether the decision reached is, in fact, the optimal choice.

Analytic Hierarchy Processing (AHP) is a decision-making approach for choosing behavior options under conditions of uncertainty. AHP techniques are designed with the assumption that people construct multi-attribute utility functions that relate the alternatives to factors (criteria) that will be affected by choosing one alternative over another, and then consider each alternative in probabilistic terms. That is, people assess the likelihood that one alternative will contribute to the achievement of a criterion and the likelihood that it will not and estimate a set of utility functions in quantitative terms. Furthermore, it is assumed that people base decision-making on completely rational assessments of computed chances or on differential time trade-offs that are connected to options and goals. This iterative process continues until the individual identifies the alternative that has the highest overall value or represents the best trade-off (Saaty, 1996; see also methods based on multi-attribute utility theory: Carter, 1992; Winkler, 1990). In effect, people make decisions based not only on the perceived effect that available alternatives could have on defined criteria but also in relation to features of the alternatives and criteria themselves. In addition, it is assumed that people compare criteria in hierarchical terms (i.e., determine which is of greater importance), in addition to relating the alternatives to the criteria. AHP methods allow for individual variation in knowledge about available alternatives, the thoroughness with which criteria are defined, and psychosocial attributes associated with decision alternatives and decision-making criteria (Dolan, 2000). These techniques serve to engage the individual in the process of considering the salience and coherence of screening, and, thereby, serve to crystallize behavioral preferences. A recent report indicates that the use of this approach can lessen decisional conflict related to decision-making about colorectal cancer screening (Dolan and Frisina, 2002).

Decision counseling and cancer screening

In the late 1990s, researchers in Philadelphia sought to obtain a more complete understanding of how men actually decide whether or not to have a prostate cancer screening examination. Of particular interest was the feasibility of using an AHP decision-making method to promote informed decision-making about screening. Another important aim of the study was to ascertain from study participants different types of cognitive, affective, and social factors that they believed were likely to influence their decision-making. The study was also designed to assess the impact of decision counseling on screening preference.

The research team identified 329 men who were aged between 50 and 69 years old, had no history of prostate cancer or benign prostatic hyperplasia, had not undergone a prostate ultrasound or biopsy, had been seen at a particular practice in the past two years, and had a current address in the Philadelphia area. Following a protocol approved by an Institutional Review Board, each man was sent an advance letter describing the study and indicating that he would be asked to complete a baseline survey questionnaire. The survey included PHM items on sociodemographic background, cognitive and affective representations related to prostate cancer screening, and social support and influence. A total of 103 men completed a survey by telephone. A written version of the survey instrument was sent to non-responders, and an additional 96 completed surveys were returned as a result. Thus, survey data were collected for 199 (63 per cent) of the original sample.

Inspection of the baseline survey data produced the following observations: 70 percent of the men were 50–59 years old; 21 percent of the men were African American, 75 percent were white, 4 percent were Asian or Pacific Islanders, and 1 per cent were Hispanic; almost three-quarters of the men were married; 7 percent had received less than twelve years of education, 23 percent were high school graduates, and 70 percent had received some post-secondary education; 9 percent of the men reported a family history of prostate cancer; and less than half (44 percent) had had a prostate cancer screening examination (i.e., both a digital rectal examination (DRE) and a prostate specific antigen (PSA) test) during the previous year.

Survey responders were randomly assigned to either a control group ($N = 99$) or an intervention group ($N = 100$). Men in the control group were sent a copy of the informational booklet. Intervention group men were also sent a copy of the booklet, but in addition they received a telephone call to arrange an office visit with a practice health educator for an AHP-based decision counseling session on prostate cancer screening. This session was designed to assist the participant in deciding whether or not to have a prostate cancer screening examination. Sixty men completed the decision-counseling session. Reasons for not completing the session included being unavailable during the study period ($N = 20$), refusal ($N = 9$), no longer being a patient in the practice ($N = 5$), serious illness ($N = 4$), and death ($N = 2$).

In the decision counseling session, the health educator prompted the patient to identify decision-making criteria by asking him to complete the following sentences: 'I want to have a prostate screening examination because ...'; and 'I don't want to have a prostate cancer screening examination because ...' In response to each sentence, the patient was permitted to provide as many open-ended responses as he felt applied. He was then asked to identify the three criteria that would be most likely to influence his decision as to whether or not he would have the screening, and to rank the selections in order of influence (first, second, third).

The majority of participants cited cognitive, affective, and social influence factors as the critical criteria for making decisions, with all three types of criteria as being important to the decision-making process. In terms of the criteria that favored screening, 80 per cent of the men identified positive cognitive criteria (i.e., the belief that screening would help to maintain or improve personal health and the belief that screening would increase length of life); 77 per cent cited positive affective criteria (i.e., the desire to find out if one had prostate cancer or might develop the disease in the future); and 63 per cent stated that a significant other (physician, family member, or friend) had encouraged them to undergo the screening. Criteria that argued against screening were identified much less frequently: 8 per cent of the men identified negative cognitive criteria (i.e., the belief that screening is inaccurate and that treatment for early disease is ineffective); 23 per cent cited negative affective criteria (i.e., the desire to avoid finding out if one had prostate cancer or might develop the disease in the future, and the desire to avoid undergoing diagnostic procedures in the event of an abnormal screening test result); and 2 per cent stated that a significant other had encouraged them to undergo the screening.

During the next phase of decision counseling, the health educator guided the patient through a process of making pair-wise comparisons of the selected criteria (first to second, second to third, and first to third), using a six-level scale to indicate a relative level of importance (i.e., overwhelmingly more important, very much more important, much more important, somewhat more important, a little bit more important, not at all important) for each comparison. The patient was then asked to compare the alternatives (the decision to have a screening examination versus the decision not to have the examination) indicating a relative level of influence for each criterion; these judgments were also made using a six-point scale (i.e., overwhelmingly more influential, very much more influential, much more influential, somewhat more influential, a little bit more influential, not at all influential). Finally, numeric values for all pair-wise comparisons were entered into a programmable hand-held calculator. The calculator then executed an algorithm, using the aforementioned measures of criteria importance and influence, to compute a decision preference score.

Among the sixty decision counseling session participants, the strength of preference for *having* a screening examination relative to *not having* an examination were distributed as follows: overwhelmingly more preferred (70 percent), very much more preferred (7 per cent), much more preferred (7 percent), somewhat more preferred (3 percent), a little bit more preferred (5 percent); 3 per cent of the men had no preference. Strength of preference for *not having* a screening examination relative to *having* an examination was distributed as follows: much more preferred (3 percent), and overwhelmingly more preferred (2 percent). At the conclusion of the decision counseling session, personal decision preference information was provided to the participants. Each man will be subject to a follow-up to ascertain whether or not he had prostate cancer screening subsequent to the decision counseling session.

Findings from this investigation show that participants, when encouraged to consider cancer screening in the context of a structured decision counseling session, spontaneously identified specific cognitive, affective, and social criteria as important determinants of their decision-making about prostate cancer screening. Moreover, the vast majority of participants identified positive cognitive, affective, and social criteria with very few participants citing negative criteria. At the end of the process, almost all participants were oriented towards having the screening procedure.

The AHP method proved to be feasible and acceptable. The men were not only able to articulate such representations, but were also able to weight them in terms of importance and compare one to another in terms of its potential impact on decision-making. This process yielded a measure of decision preference that seemed to make sense to the participants. Conceivably, the PHM measures of cognitive, affective, and social support and influence collected at baseline may be highly correlated with the criteria that were articulated by the men who participated in the decision counseling session. If there is a high correspondence between baseline survey representations and decision counseling critieria, it should be possible to use baseline survey measures to guide the decision counseling session and, thus, further facilitate informed decision-making. Survey data analyses are being performed to assess this relationship.

Conclusion

Until recently, cancer screening has been viewed by health professionals and the public as a 'uniform good,' an effective preventive health behavior that people should embrace (Welch, 2001). Reflecting this point of view, educational outreach programs traditionally have been designed to promote screening utilization, rather than to encourage critical thinking about whether or not to have a screening examination. However, this type of approach is now being questioned.

Concerns have been raised about prostate cancer screening in light of the lack of randomized trial data showing the benefit of screening for this disease (Canadian Task Force on the Periodic Health Examination, 1991; US Preventive Services Taskforce, 1996). In addition, the value of breast and colorectal cancer screening is also being questioned (Agency for Healthcare Research and Quality, 2002; Bond and Koretz, 2002; Olsen and Gotzsche, 2001). Debate about the pros and cons associated with cancer screening is no longer confined to academic forums, but has become part of the wider public dialogue (National Cancer Institute, 1997). Increasingly, health care professionals and lay individuals have begun to wonder whether or not cancer screening is a worthwhile health behavior (Walter and Covinsky, 2001).

To date, most of the behavioral research on cancer screening has sought to identify factors that are associated with or that predict screening modality use. Preventive health behavior models (e.g., the Health Belief Model and the Theory of Reasoned Action) and the CSM have been used to guide research in this area. Research has also focused on delineating the stages of readiness for decision-making that lead to the adoption of cancer screening and on developing more persuasive educational messages to encourage screening use. Recent concerns about cancer screening have drawn increased attention to the need for an alternative paradigm to guide research in this area, one that can generate greater understanding of how people decide whether or not to engage in cancer screening together with effective methods for facilitating informed decision-making. Self-regulation and decision-making approaches provide useful constructs that could serve to inform research in these areas.

The CSM assumes the existence of a multidimensional 'self-system' in each person which influences the perception of health threats, guides the selection of coping strategies, and shapes the appraisal of outcomes. Analytic Hierarchy Processing methods are compatible with the self-regulation perspective, in that they illuminate the process by which individuals weigh alternatives and, ultimately, select a course of action. These methods have the potential to extend the contributions of preventive health behavior and stage theories by generating greater understanding of how cognitive, affective, and social factors interact and serve to guide preventive health behaviors. To date, few studies have been reported on the use of self-regulation models to explain cancer screening. More research is needed.

The Preventive Health Model integrates preventive health behavior theory and self-regulation (CSM) constructs. This framework assumes that people use representations of health problems and behaviors to make health care decisions in everyday life. Evidence to support this view is provided by the results of the study of decision-making about prostate cancer screening reported in this chapter. It is reasonable to propose that the Preventive Health Model could be used to identify decision criteria prospectively. This information could then be used by health care practitioners in decision counseling to clarify patient knowledge and attitudes related to screening and to facilitate value-based, informed decision-making about screening and other health care issues. Such an approach could contribute substantially to achieving the elusive goal of shared decision-making (Barry, 2002).

Note

1   Correspondence concerning this chapter should be sent to Ronald E. Myers, Thomas Jefferson University, Department of Medicine, Division of Genetic and Preventive Medicine, Behavioral Epidemiology Section, 1100 Walnut Street, Suite 400, Philadelphia, PA 19107, USA. E-mail: ron.myers@mail.tju.edu

References

Agency for Healthcare Research and Quality (2002) 'Screening for breast cancer: recommendations and rationale,' http://www.ahrq.gov/clinic/3rduspsf/brestcancer/brcanrr.htm, 7 March.

Ajzen, I. and Fishbein, M. (1980) *Understanding Attitudes and Predicting Social Behavior*, Englewood Cliffs, NJ: Prentice-Hall.

Bandura, A. (1986) *Social Foundations of Thought and Action : A Social Cognitive Theory*, Englewood Cliffs, NJ: Prentice-Hall.

Baranowski, T., Perry, C. and Parcel, G. (1997) 'How individuals, environments, and health behavior interact: Social Cognitive Theory,' in M.L.F. Glanz and K. Rimer (eds) *Health Behavior and Health Education*, San Francisco: Jossey-Bass Publishers, pp. 153–178.

Barling, N.R. and Moore, S.M. (1996) 'Prediction of cervical cancer screening using the theory of reasoned action,' *Psychological Reports* **79**: 77–78.

Barry, M.J. (2002) 'Health decision aids to facilitate shared decision making in office practice,' *Annals of Internal Medicine* **136**: 127–135.

Baumeister, R.F. and Newman, R.S. (1994) 'Self-regulation of cognitive inference and decision processes,' *Personality and Social Psychology Bulletin* **20**: 3–19.

Bond, J. and Koretz, R. (2002) 'Colon cancer screening: science, recommendations, and doubts,' *Medical Crossfire* **49**: 31–40.

Brownlee, S., Leventhal, H. and Leventhal, E. (2000) 'Regulation, self-regulation and construction of the self in the maintenance of physical health,' in M. Boekaerts, P.R. Pintrich and M. Zeidner (eds) *Handbook of Self-Regulation*, San Diego, CA: Academic Press, pp. 369–416.

Burack, R.C. and Liang, J. (1989) 'The acceptance and completion of mammography by older black women,' *American Journal of Public Health* **79**: 721–726.

Burak, L.J. and Meyer, M. (1997) 'Using the Health Belief Model to examine and predict college women's cervical cancer screening beliefs and behavior,' *Health Care Women International* **18**: 251–262.

Cameron, L.D., Leventhal, H. and Love, R.R. (1998) 'Trait anxiety, symptom perceptions, and illness-related responses among women with breast cancer in remission during a tamoxifen clinical trial,' *Health Psychology* **17**: 459–469.

Canadian Task Force on the Periodic Health Examination (1991) 'Periodic health examination, 1991 update 3: secondary prevention of prostate cancer,' *Canadian Medical Association Journal* **145**: 413–428.

Carter, W.B. (1992) 'Psychology and decision making: modeling health behavior with multiattribute utility theory,' *Journal of Dental Education* **56**: 800–807.

Carver, C.S. and Scheier, M.F. (1982) 'Control theory: a useful conceptual framework for personality-social, clinical, and health psychology,' *Psychological Bulletin* **92**: 111–135.

—— (1999) 'Themes and issues in the self-regulation of behavior,' in R.S. Wyer (ed.) *Advances in Social Cognition*, vol. 12, Mahwah, NJ: Lawrence Erlbaum Associates, pp. 1–105.

Clemow, L., Costanza, M.E., Haddad, W.P., Luckmann, R., White, M.J., Klaus, D. and Stoddard, A.M. (2000) 'Underutilizers of mammography screening today: characteristics of women planning, undecided about, and not planning a mammogram,' *Annals of Behavioral Medicine* **22**: 80–88.

Diefenbach, M.A., Miller, S.M. and Daly, M.B. (1999) 'Specific worry about breast cancer predicts mammography use in women at risk for breast and ovarian cancer,' *Health Psychology* **18**: 532–536.

Dolan, J.G. (2000) 'A randomized controlled trial of the effects of an individualized patient decision making regarding cancer screening for the average risk patient,' *Medical Decision Making* **20**: 506.

Dolan, J.G. and Frisina, S. (2002) 'Randomized controlled trial of a patient decision aid for colorectal cancer screening,' *Medical Decision Making* **22**: 125–139.

Edwards, W. (1954) 'The theory of decision making,' *Psychological Bulletin* **51**: 380–417.

Ellsworth, E. and Smith, C. (1998) 'From appraisal to emotion: differences among unpleasant feelings,' *Motivation and Emotion* **12**: 271–302.

Fishbein, M. and Ajzen, I. (1975) *Belief, Attitude, Intention and Behavior: An Introduction to Theory and Research*, Reading, MA: Addison-Wesley.

Fox, S.A., Stein, J.A., Sockloskie, R.J. and Ory, M.G. (2001) 'Targeted mailed materials and the Medicare beneficiary: increasing mammogram screening among the elderly,' *American Journal of Public Health* **91**: 55–61.

Friedman, L.C., Webb, J.A., Bruce, S., Weinberg, A.D. and Cooper, H.P. (1995) 'Skin cancer prevention and early detection intentions and behavior,' *American Journal of Preventive Medicine* **11**: 59–65.

Frijda, N.H. (1988) 'The laws of emotion,' *American Psychologist* **43**: 349–358.

Han, Y., Williams, R.D. and Harrison, R.A. (2000) 'Breast cancer screening knowledge, attitudes, and practices among Korean American women,' *Oncology Nursing Forum* **27**: 1585–1591.

Hayes-Bautista, D.E. (1976) 'Modifying the treatment: patient compliance, patient control and medical care,' *Social Science and Medicine* **10**: 233–238.

Hodge, F.S., Fredericks, L. and Rodriguez, B. (1996) 'American Indian women's talking circle: a cervical cancer screening and prevention project,' *Cancer* **78**: 1592–1597.

Holtzman, D., Powell-Griner, E., Bolen, J.C. and Rhodes, L. (2000) 'State- and sex-specific prevalence of selected characteristics – Behavioral Risk Factor Surveillance System, 1996 and 1997,' *Morbidity and Mortality Weekly Report CDC Surveillance Summaries* **49**: 1–39.

Janis, I.L. (1984) 'The patient as decision maker,' in D. Gentry (ed.) *Handbook of Behavioral Medicine*, New York: Guilford Press, pp. 326–368.

Janis, I.L. and Mann, L. (1977) *Decision Making: A Psychological Analysis of Conflict, Choice, and Commitment*, New York: The Free Press.

Keeney, R. and Raiffa, H. (1976) *Decisions with Multiple Objectives: Preferences and Value Tradeoffs*, New York: Wiley.

Lazarus, R. (1966) *Psychological Stress and the Coping Process*, New York: McGraw-Hill.

Leventhal, H. and Cameron, L. (1987) 'Behavioral theories and the problem of compliance,' *Patient Education and Counseling* **10**: 117–138.

Leventhal, H. and Cleary, P.D. (1979) 'Behavioral modification of risk factors: technology or science,' in M.L. Pollack and D.H. Schmidt (eds) *Health Disease and Rehabilitation: State of the Art*, Boston: Houghton Mifflin.

Leventhal, H., Meyer, D. and Nerenz, D. (1980) 'The common-sense representation of illness danger,' in S. Rachman (ed.) *Medical Psychology*, vol. 2, New York: Pergamon Press, pp. 7–30.

Leventhal, H., Singer, R. and Jones, S. (1965) 'Effects of fear and specificity of recommendations in persuasive communications,' *Journal of Personality and Social Psychology* **2**: 20–29.

Leventhal, H., Watts, J.C. and Pagano, F. (1967) 'Effects of fear and instructions on how to cope with danger,' *Journal of Personality and Social Psychology* **6**: 313–321.

McBride, C.M., Curry, S.J., Taplin, S., Anderman, C. and Grothaus, L. (1993) 'Exploring environmental barriers to participation in mammography screening in an HMO,' *Cancer Epidemiology, Biomarkers, and Prevention* **2**: 599–605.

Meyer, D., Leventhal, H. and Gutmann, M. (1985) 'Common-sense models of illness: the example of hypertension,' *Health Psychology* **4**: 115–135.

Miller, D. and Star, M. (1967) *The Structure of Human Decisions*, Englewood Cliffs, NJ: Prentice-Hall.

Montano, D.E. and Taplin, S.H. (1991) 'A test of an expanded theory of reasoned action to predict mammography participation,' *Social Science and Medicine* **32**: 733–741.

Montano, D., Kasprzyk, D. and Taplin, S. (1997) 'The theory of reasoned action and the theory of planned behavior,' in M.L.F. Glanz and K. Rimer (eds) *Health Behavior and Health Education*, San Francisco: Jossey-Bass Publishers, pp. 85–112.

Myers, R. and Wolf, T. (1990) *Instrument Development for a Colorectal Cancer Screening Survey: Scientific Report 1988–1989*, Philadelphia, PA: Fox Chase Cancer Center.

Myers, R.E., Ross, E., Jepson, C., Wolf, T., Balshem, A., Millner, L. and Leventhal, H. (1994) 'Modeling adherence to colorectal cancer screening,' *Preventive Medicine* **23**: 142–151.

Myers, R.E., Chodak, G.W., Wolf, T.A., Burgh, D.Y., McGrory, G.T., Marcus, S.M., Diehl, J.A. and Williams, M. (1999) 'Adherence by African American men to prostate cancer education and early detection,' *Cancer* **86**: 88–104.

National Cancer Institute (1997) *The Public's Perception of Medical and Cancer Research*, Bethesda, MD: National Cancer Institute, Office of Cancer Communications.

Navarro, A.M., Senn, K.L., McNicholas, L.J., Kaplan, R.M., Roppe, B. and Campo, M.C. (1998) '*Por La Vida* model intervention enhances use of cancer screening tests among Latinas,' *American Journal of Preventive Medicine* **15**: 32–41.

Olsen, O. and Gotzsche, P.C. (2001) 'Cochrane review on screening for breast cancer with mammography,' *Lancet* **358**: 1340–1342.

Powers, W.T. (1973) 'Feedback: beyond behaviorism,' *Science* **179**: 351–356.

Prochaska, J.O. (1994) 'Strong and weak principles for progressing from precontemplation to action on the basis of twelve problem behaviors,' *Health Psychology* **1**: 47–51.

Prochaska, J. and DiClemente, C. (1984) *The transtheoretical approach: crossing the traditional boundaries of therapy*, Homewood, IL: Dow Jones-Irwin.

Rakowski, W., Ehrich, B., Goldstein, M.G., Rimer, B.K., Pearlman, D.N., Clark, M.A., Velicer, W.F. and Woolverton, H., III (1998) 'Increasing mammography among women aged 40–74 by use of a stage-matched, tailored intervention,' *Preventive Medicine* **27**: 748–756.

Rimer, B.K., Halabi, S., Sugg Skinner, C., Kaplan, E.B., Crawford, Y., Samsa, G.P., Strigo, T.S. and Lipkus, I.M. (2001) 'The short-term impact of tailored mammography decision-making interventions,' *Patient Education and Counseling* **43**: 269–285.

Saaty, T.L. (1996) *The Analytic Hierarchy Process*, Pittsburgh, PA: RWS Publications.

Sheeran, P. and Orbell, S. (2000) 'Using implementation intentions to increase attendance for cervical cancer screening,' *Health Psychology* **19**: 283–289.

Stoddard, A.M., Fox, S.A., Costanza, M.E., Lane, D.S., Andersen, M.R., Urban, N., Lipkus, I. and Rimer, B.K. (2002) 'Effectiveness of telephone counseling for mammography: results from five randomized trials,' *Preventive Medicine* **34**: 90–99.

Strecher, V. and Rosenstock, I. (1997) 'The health belief model,' in M.L.F. Glanz and K. Rimer (eds) *Health Behavior and Health Education*, San Francisco: Jossey-Bass Publishers, pp. 41–59.

Taplin, S.H. and Montano, D.E. (1993) 'Attitudes, age, and participation in mammographic screening: a prospective analysis,' *Journal of the American Board of Family Practice* **6**: 13–23.

Taplin, S., Anderman, C. and Grothaus, L. (1989) 'Breast cancer risk and participation in mammographic screening,' *American Journal of Public Health* **79**: 1494–1498.

Taplin, S.H., Anderman, C., Grothaus, L., Curry, S. and Montano, D. (1994) 'Using physician correspondence and postcard reminders to promote mammography use,' *American Journal of Public Health* **84**: 571–574.

US Preventive Services Taskforce (1996) *Guide to Clinical Preventive Services*, 2nd edn, Baltimore, MD: Williams & Wilkins.

Vernon, S.W., Myers, R.E. and Tilley, B.C. (1997) 'Development and validation of an instrument to measure factors related to colorectal cancer screening adherence,' *Cancer Epidemiology, Biomarkers, and Prevention* **6**: 825–832.

Walter, L.C. and Covinsky, K.E. (2001) 'Cancer screening in elderly patients: a framework for individualized decision making,' *Journal of the American Medical Association* **285**: 2750–2756.

Wardle, J., Sutton, S., Williamson, S., Taylor, T., McCaffery, K., Cuzick, J., Hart, A. and Atkin, W. (2000) 'Psychosocial influences on older adults' interest in partici- pating in bowel cancer screening,' *Preventive Medicine* **31**: 323–334.

Weinstein, N.D. (1988) 'The precaution adoption process,' *Health Psychology* **7**: 355–386.

Weinstein, N.D., Rothman, A.J. and Sutton, S.R. (1998) 'Stage theories of health behavior: conceptual and methodological issues,' *Health Psychology* **17**: 290–299.

Welch, H.G. (2001) 'Informed choice in cancer screening,' *Journal of the American Medical Association* **285**: 2776–2778.

Winkler, R.L. (1990) 'Decision modeling and rational choice: AHP and utility theory,' *Management Science* **36**: 247–248.

Yarbrough, S.S. and Braden, C.J. (2001) 'Utility of health belief model as a guide for explaining or predicting breast cancer screening behaviors,' *Journal of Advanced Nursing* **33**: 677–688.

16 Self-regulation and genetic testing

Theory, practical considerations, and interventions

Michael A. Diefenbach and Natalie Hamrick[1]

Advances in molecular genetics over the past decade mean that it is now possible for individuals to be tested for their genetic susceptibility to developing specific cancers. It is estimated that mutations in the *BRCA1* and *BRCA2* breast cancer susceptibility genes account for up to 10 per cent of breast cancer cases in the US (Claus *et al.*, 1996). The lifetime risk of developing breast cancer among women with a *BRCA1* or *BRCA2* mutation is estimated to range between 45–80 per cent and between 15–60 per cent for ovarian cancer (Easton, Ford, Bishop, and The Breast Cancer Linkage Consortium, 1995; Ford *et al.*, 1994; Ford *et al.*, 1998; Struewing *et al.*, 1997). For colon cancer, the risk figures are much lower: 3–10 per cent of individuals with germline mutations of the APC colorectal cancer susceptibility gene develop colorectal cancer (Bjork *et al.*, 2001; Jagelman *et al.*, 1988; Spiegelman *et al.*, 1994). The possibility of genetic testing has given individuals previously unimaginable choices to learn about their risk of developing certain diseases. Such choices, however, are never without risk or costs that extend beyond the financial and time commitments that are required for a genetic testing protocol. Rather, they include psychological (i.e., cognitive and affective) and social-relationship risks that might impact on the entire family.

The purpose of this chapter is four-fold. First, we will argue that self-regulation theory offers a comprehensive framework to identify and to address relevant variables that influence decision-making for and coping with a decision to undergo genetic testing. Second, we will briefly review the psychological research of the past decade on issues surrounding genetic testing for breast cancer susceptibility. Third, we will critically evaluate intervention efforts designed to assist individuals in the genetic testing context. Finally, we will conclude by considering some directions for future research.

Self-regulation and genetic testing

The genetic testing procedure is a multi-step process that starts with the realization that one is at risk of developing cancer, which is often prompted by a cancer diagnosis, either one's own or that of a relative. Specifically, the steps involved in genetic testing begin with a person's interest in learning more about genetic testing and end with the provision of blood for testing and the receipt of the test results. Genetic counseling, with all its various components (i.e., education and counseling to help first with making the decision to test and then with coping with, both before and after, the receipt of the results), is usually part of a comprehensive risk-assessment program. At each of these steps, self-regulation theory can inform the researcher and the clinician about underlying psychological processes and aid in the development of counseling protocols. There are three central features of the common-sense model (CSM) of self-regulation that make it uniquely suited for application to the genetic testing situation.

The first central feature of the CSM comprises the five attributes of the threat or illness representations (Leventhal, 1970). The *identity* attribute defines and labels the threat. This identification process is usually triggered by an internal symptom, but it can also be set into motion by information from an external source, such as risk information given by a health care provider. A person's cancer risk perception can originate from a lump that is found during self-care, or stem from the processing of information that a relative has been diagnosed with cancer. The use of an *identity label* often determines subsequent attributes, such as *timeline* or duration, *consequences*, *cause*, and *controllability* (Lau *et al.*, 1989). Each attribute adds another piece of information to the definition of the unknown stimulus or situation and can contribute in its own way to perceptions of cancer risk and cancer-related worry. The *timeline* or duration addresses the perceived temporal progression of the stimulus. In the case of cancer, timeline is represented by the individual's beliefs about when and if cancer will occur and how long it will stay, including recurrences. The *consequence* attribute defines the stimulus in terms of the potential impact of the illness on the individual's overall quality of life (i.e., one's ability to continue a desired way of life) and life expectancy (i.e., whether it is a minor, major, or life-threatening illness). In the case of cancer, individuals invariably perceive the consequences as having the potential to alter one's quality of life and one's life expectancy. The *cause* attribute categorizes the stimulus in terms of the potential factors that might have led to the stimulus in the first place (e.g., family history, exposure to toxins), and *controllability* answers the question of whether or not there is anything that can be done about it. It is important to note that the attributes of illness representations are highly individualized, anchored in the person's concrete-perceptual realities, and they may not be consistent with medical knowledge. For example, individuals can wrongly assume that an illness with a potential genetic cause is not preventable and not treatable (Marteau and Senior, 1997). As a consequence of this individualization and its anchoring in a person's perceptual reality, the model suggests that beliefs about the disease (e.g., cancer) and associated expectations (e.g., vulnerability beliefs) are extremely difficult to change.

The second central feature is the parallel processing of cognitive and emotional stimuli. As described, the individual needs to process probabilistic information about the likelihood of developing the disease and comprehend information related to its cause(s) and controllability. In addition, the individual will respond emotionally to the potential threat of a life-altering disease by considering many causes and varying degrees of controllability. Thus, the parallel framework accounts for both cognitive and emotional processing pathways, their potential interaction, and their influence on behavior.

The third central feature of self-regulation theory is the iterative nature of evaluation and decision-making that influence behavior. Health behaviors and responses to health threats can be triggered as a result of a cognitive evaluation of the threat, the emotional impact of the threat, an interaction of the two, or motivations to achieve personal goals (e.g., screening to prevent disease). If the individual is confident that a particular health behavior or coping strategy will allow progress toward the achievement of the goal, it will be selected. If, however, the behavior or coping strategy's efficacy and availability are questionable, it is less likely to be utilized. For example, an individual learns of a sibling's recent cancer diagnosis. This information will be integrated with the individual's existing representations and beliefs and will most likely result in a heightened perception of cancer risk and cancer-related worries and fears. The result of such information processing will be an evaluation of one's available coping options. One such option would be to consider genetic testing to reduce the uncertainty about one's risk of developing cancer. The final stage in this self-regulation sequence is the appraisal process in which the chosen health behavior or coping response is evaluated for its effectiveness. If the coping response is successful, then no further change in behavior is necessary and no changes in threat representations will follow. If the coping response is not successful, however, then the individual will engage in a different response and will revise existing threat representations. In the case of genetic testing, after the individual has received intensive counseling she has to decide whether genetic testing is feasible, is psychologically right for her, and will yield the desired information about her future disease risk.

The process of genetic testing from a self-regulation perspective

One of the underlying principles of self-regulation theory is that individuals are seen as active problem-solvers. As active problem-solvers, individuals have to make sense of the often complicated information they receive while learning about genetic testing. Self-regulation theory suggests that individuals process such information through a filter of existing disease and threat-relevant beliefs and expectations. The case of genetic testing is particularly complex (and intriguing) because it provides multiple ways in which the individual's own beliefs and expectations, as well as worries and anxieties, can interact with the information. The result of such processing then determines health-relevant behaviors, such as cancer detection and prevention behaviors.

When examining illness representations as they pertain to genetic testing, it becomes clear that such representations are intricately linked with representations about cancer. As described in greater detail below, motivations to undergo testing can stem from a desire to obtain clarity about risk status, an increased sense of susceptibility to cancer, or worry about cancer. Thus, it is not only necessary to assess testing-specific representations but also cancer-relevant representations. In the case of breast cancer, for example, the identity representation clearly links genetic testing to the specific genes (*BRCA1/2*) that are responsible for a heightened susceptibility to cancer. With regard to the timeline attribute, individuals might exhibit expectations that they will definitely develop breast cancer if they receive a positive test result. When contemplating genetic testing for breast cancer the individual is likely to subscribe to a genetic, hereditary disease model. However, this may not be the only causal model an individual possesses. Alternative models might include causal beliefs about harmful environmental or dietary factors.

The consequence attribute in the case of genetic testing for *BRCA1/2* mutations is complicated by four possible test outcomes (Daly, 1999). A *true positive* result represents the identification of an alteration in a known cancer-predisposing gene. Conversely, a *true negative* result indicates that a person is not a carrier of a known cancer-predisposing gene that has been positively identified in another family member. *Indeterminate* status implies that a person is not a carrier of a known cancer-predisposing gene, and that the carrier status of other family members is either negative or unknown. The fourth possible outcome is an *inconclusive* test result. In this case, the person who was tested is a carrier of an alteration in a gene that currently has no known significance or is a carrier of a variant of a gene of uncertain significance. The individual needs to understand that a true negative test result will not preclude the diagnosis of cancer in the future. Conversely, a true positive test result is not a death sentence either. Finally, the indeterminate and inconclusive test results require the individual to exhibit a high level of tolerance for ambiguity, the ability to adhere to regular screening regimens, and to cope with potential feelings of anxiety.

Taken together, individuals enter the genetic testing situation with their own sets of beliefs, expectations, and emotional responses about genes, cancer, and the ability of modern medicine to provide a cure for the disease. These representations need to be assessed and integrated into discussions about the genetic testing procedure, about the implications of testing results on future prevention behaviors, and its importance for other family members.

Widening the circle: family and outside influences on the decision to
undergo genetic testing

To be eligible for genetic testing, an individual must fulfill three broad categories of eligibility: (1) the individual must meet the criteria for hereditary breast/ovarian cancer syndrome; (2) the candidate must have a high likelihood of being a mutation carrier based on personal and familial characteristics; and (3) the person needs to display the psychosocial readiness to receive the results of genetic testing (Daly, 1999). To meaningfully interpret test results, members of two or even three generations of a family are sometimes asked to undergo genetic testing. Thus, genetic testing is a family process. Usually one member of the family initiates the process of genetic testing by acting as the 'messenger of the news' (DudokdeWit *et al.*, 1997) and by persuading relevant family members to pursue testing. This is not an easy task for the 'messenger' as the information can potentially heighten perceptions of risk, cancer-related worries and fears, and prompt feelings of denial. The 'messenger' might also exert pressure on first-degree relatives to undergo testing because the relatives' genetic information is needed to complete the family pedigree. The first person in a family to undergo genetic testing has been termed the 'first utilizer' (DudokdeWit *et al.*, 1997). First testing by a family member can prompt other members to undergo testing as well. As more hereditary information is revealed to at-risk family members, the nature of the result can heighten or decrease the perceived risk of developing cancer and also the levels of cancer-related distress. As a pedigree is nearing completion, a family member can learn about his or her genetic carrier status even if the person has not been tested or has been unwilling to be tested. This is the case if a first-degree relative is 'sandwiched' between two generations who are both willing to be tested and who will reveal their test results. Results from genetic testing for cancer susceptibility therefore rarely remain private to one individual within a family. Thus, the decision to undergo genetic testing is by necessity a decision that involves not just one person but rather the whole family. As family members may hold conflicting representations of cancer – such as its consequences (e.g., death, pain, or disfigurement), cause, time frame, associated symptomatic indicators of risk, and means of prevention – many opportunities exist for conflict.

Psychological empirical research in the area of genetic testing for *BRCA1/2*

Now that we have laid the foundations for constructing a self-regulation approach to genetic testing, let us turn now to a discussion of the current genetic testing literature. Although research exists on genetic testing for other cancers, the literature concerning *BRCA1/2* is the most extensive. Despite the fact that genetic testing has been available for a little less than a decade, a number of studies have addressed patients' interest in and response to genetic testing. Research in this area can be roughly divided into three chronological phases. The first phase examined general interest among at-risk individuals and the general population (Lerman *et al.*, 1991; Struewing *et al.*, 1995; Lerman *et al.*, 1994a; Lerman *et al.*, 1994b; Lerman *et al.*, 1996). The second phase was concerned with the psychological impact of genetic testing (Lerman *et al.*, 1996; Croyle *et al.*, 1997; Lerman *et al.*, 1998; Lodder *et al.*, 2001; Coyne *et al.*, 2002; and Schwartz *et al.*, 2002). During the last phase, researchers turned their attention to examining the predictors of genetic testing uptake among various populations (Capelli *et al.*, 1999; Capelli *et al.*, 2001; Durfy *et al.*, 1999; Lipkus *et al.*, 1999; Kash *et al.*, 2000; Schwartz *et al.*, 2000; Yeomans-Kinney *et al.*, 2001). We will review each phase in turn.

Phase I: interest in genetic testing

When testing for *BRCA1* became a possibility, researchers first examined whether or not individuals were interested in undergoing tests to determine one's genetic susceptibility to developing cancer. Research by Lerman and colleagues demonstrated that interest in genetic testing was generally high, especially among breast cancer survivors and first-degree relatives (Struewing *et al.*, 1995; Lerman *et al.*, 1994a; Lerman *et al.*, 1994b). The CSM would suggest that interest was influenced by specific testing- and disease-related beliefs and outcome expectations, as well as by heightened worry about the disease. This interest in genetic testing was translated into action by women's willingness to donate blood for testing. However, only 57 percent of those tested opted to receive their results (Lerman *et al.*, 1998). Cancer-related stress and moderate depressive symptoms were suggested as possible barriers to participants' willingness to receive their test results.

Phase II: psychological outcomes of genetic testing for BRCA1/2

Of the six studies assessing the psychological outcomes of genetic testing, most studies report moderately elevated, sub-clinical to low-clinical levels of distress (Coyne *et al.*, 2002; Croyle *et al.*, 1997; Lerman *et al.*, 1995; Lerman *et al.*, 1996; Lerman *et al.*, 1998; Lodder *et al.*, 2001; Schwartz *et al.*, 2002). The main finding across these studies is a reduction of distress from before testing to one to six months after testing among individuals who received a true negative test result (Croyle *et al.*, 1997; Lodder *et al.*, 2001; Schwartz *et al.*, 2002). This, in line with self-regulation theory, would suggest that cancer-related worry and distress may have been a motivating factor behind individual test decisions. For individuals with a true positive test result, distress levels remained elevated at pre-testing levels (Croyle *et al.*, 1997; Lodder *et al.*, 2001; Schwartz *et al.*, 2002). Among those who reported high levels of stress before testing, deciding not to obtain one's test result after being tested resulted in higher rates of clinical depression one month posttest, compared to the group of individuals who were actual gene mutation carriers (Lerman *et al.*, 1998). Self-regulation theory provides at least two possible explanations for these results. First, patients may have found less solace in 'not knowing' their results than they had anticipated. Ruminating over thoughts about an inherent cancer risk may have led to higher levels of cancer worry and depression. An alternative explanation is that the cognitive effort involved in suppressing one's thoughts about cancer risk was too great, that the existing worry could not be contained and that it therefore manifested itself in increased depressive symptomatology.

Coyne *et al.* (2002) have critically evaluated this literature and concluded that many studies overstate the psychological impact of genetic testing on participants. They argue that many of the studies lack an adequate comparison group in which psychological distress is assessed. Such comparison groups should consist of individuals without a family history of cancer or of individuals who are not interested in genetic testing. Without such a comparison group, the association between genetic testing and distress remains tenuous. They further contend that a number of studies inflate the amount of psychiatric morbidity (i.e., clinical depression) found in their sample by lowering the cut-off-score for psychiatric diagnosis below any validated or clinically meaningful value. Their criticism is not, however, inconsistent with the recognition that the differences in distress and depressed affect among sub-groups of women at risk of developing breast cancer (e.g., the higher levels of distress and depression among participants who choose not to obtain their test results) are important to acknowledge. Their comments suggest that elaborate, individually focused psychological or pharmacological interventions might not be the appropriate way in which to address non-pathological levels of emotional distress that result from being part of a family where genetic risk is an issue. Offering information and counseling directed at illness representation attributes (e.g., cause, consequences), teaching the skills needed to share such information with others, and practicing conflict negotiation may prove to be a more effective approach to distress reduction. This is an ongoing controversy in the literature that can only be resolved by conducting additional, careful research. Methods to assess distress in participants need to be re-evaluated and alternative non-psychiatric terms (e.g., depressive affect, anxiety levels compared to clinical depression) are needed for describing and classifying participants.

Phase III: predictors of testing uptake

To date, seven studies have examined the psychological factors involved in predicting the uptake of *BRCA1/2* testing (Lipkus *et al.*, 1999; Durfy *et al.*, 1999; Kash *et al.*, 2000; Schwartz *et al.*, 2000; Yeomans-Kinney *et al.*, 2001; Cappelli *et al.*, 1999; Cappelli *et al.*, 2001). Across these studies three variables were consistently associated with a person's willingness to undergo genetic testing. In line with self-regulation predictions, these variables were:

having a family history of breast cancer; exhibiting increased levels of perceived risk of developing breast cancer; and having increased levels of cancer worry. The influence of these variables was consistently found across different study populations, including ethnic groups (i.e., African American at-risk groups; Yeomans-Kinney *et al.*, 2001; Durfy *et al.*, 1999) or different backgrounds (Ashkenazi Jewish women and lesbian/bisexual women; Durfy *et al.*, 1999).

In addition to these three variables, researchers found that certain demographic and personality factors were related to a genetic testing decision. Yeomans-Kinney *et al.* (2001) reported that younger age and lower levels of ambiguity tolerance were related to a positive genetic testing decision. A particular style of information seeking and information processing, monitoring, was also predictive of a positive genetic testing decision (Tercyak *et al.*, 2001; Miller *et al.*, 2001b), as was a higher level of spirituality (Schwartz *et al.*, 2000). From a self-regulation perspective, low ambiguity tolerance is likely to be associated with higher levels of negative affect and thus genetic testing might be perceived as a means of avoiding negative emotions and reducing ambiguity. This would also result in the formation of more complete, individualized cancer representations and the adoption of actions that are believed or experienced to be disease protective (e.g., adhering to a self-monitoring regimen, implementing diet changes, and adaptation of an exercise program). The finding that higher levels of spirituality were associated with a positive testing decision might be related to causal beliefs that a 'higher power' is ultimately responsible for health and disease, thus potentially positive test results are less threatening.

When asked, study participants cited a variety of beliefs about, and motivations behind, their testing decisions. Women expected that the genetic testing outcome would motivate them to adhere to a program of increased breast cancer surveillance (Durfy *et al.*, 1999; Yeomans-Kinney *et al.*, 2001; Clark *et al.*, 2000); help them make a decision regarding whether or not to have prophylactic surgery (Clark *et al.*, 2000, Yeomans-Kinney *et al.*, 2001; Durfy *et al.*, 1999) and also with important life decisions, such as having children (Yeomans-Kinney *et al.*, 2001; Cappelli *et al.*, 1999); and help their family decide whether or not to undergo testing (Yeomans-Kinney *et al.*, 2001; Cappelli *et al.*, 1999; Clark *et al.*, 2000). Some women also expressed the altruistic attitude of wanting to help science by participating in genetic testing research protocols (Clark *et al.*, 2000). In addition, women expressed beliefs about the barriers to testing, such as an increased worry about the effect of a positive screening result on female offspring or relatives (Yeomans-Kinney *et al.*, 2001; Cappelli *et al.*, 2001); the high cost and lack of availability of the test (Durfy *et al.*, 1999; Yeomans-Kinney *et al.*, 2001); and having a fatalistic attitude (e.g., 'If it's in the genes there is nothing that can be done, so why find out about it?'; Cappelli *et al.*, 2001).

To summarize, the reviewed studies suggest that despite some reservations, individuals are interested in genetic testing as a tool for facilitating life and health care decisions. Individuals come to these decisions by integrating information provided by genetic counselors, physicians, the media, and other sources with their own representations about genetic testing and breast cancer. Although existing research has shed light on some of the clinical, social, and psychological variables associated with genetic testing uptake, more research is needed that focuses on the interplay of affect and cognition, as emotions are clearly important influences in the process and may infuse information processing and decision-making. We also need to pay more attention to the potential moderators and mediators of testing uptake. For example, monitors or high information seekers have a tendency to seek out and scan for disease-related information (Miller *et al.*, 2001a). However, we do not know what type of information is preferred by monitors. Are monitors more concerned with information that points to possible causal associations, or do they prefer information that points to future consequences? Which kind of information has the most significant emotional impact? Answers to such questions are necessary if one wants to design effective educational and informational intervention sessions.

Recommendations for counseling protocols for genetic testing

We first review the minimum requirements for counseling protocols as set forth by the National Society of Genetic Counselors (1997) and the Task Force on Informed Consent as part of the Cancer Genetics Studies Consortium (CGSC). The recommendations for genetic testing for cancer susceptibility developed by the National Society of Genetic Counselors (1997) follows the model used for prenatal and pediatric counseling. In 1997, the Task Force published a consensus document recommending that participants planning to undergo genetic testing should receive ongoing education and counseling (Geller *et al.*, 1997). Specifically, the recommendations emphasize the importance of jargon-free education, paying deference to cultural differences, and in general using a client-centered approach to counseling. The report puts particular emphasis on using a shared decision-making approach, during which the participant's values and goals with regard to genetic testing are elicited and discussed in light of the provider's values and goals. Furthermore, the report recommends individualizing the information disclosure session, taking into account the participant's specific psychological and familial circumstances.

Botkin *et al.* (1996) published a model protocol for BRCA1/2 genetic testing among a large Utah family group (K2082). The protocol is based on recommendations for genetic counseling for BRCA1/2 (Biesecker *et al.*, 1993) and Huntingdon's disease (Quaid, 1992). The hallmark of this protocol is the frequent interaction of potential participants with genetic counselors. At-risk individuals are contacted by letter to elicit their interest in study participation. Recruitment follows the model that parents will be included and tested prior to testing their children. This strategy avoids de facto testing of parents, because detection of a mutation in a child means that the parent would be carrying the mutation as well. If participants show interest, they are given more information over the telephone and in an informed consent document. A session with a genetic counselor then follows, which also includes psychological screening by a family counselor. During the pre-testing counseling session participants are educated about genes, the associated cancer risk if a mutation is present, the efficacy of the DNA analyses, and the screening and prevention options available to them. A separate consent form for genetic testing is then signed if the participant wishes to undergo such a test. Next, a family therapist assesses the psychological functioning of the participant with respect to signs of depression and anxiety and explores the impact genetic testing results might have on the individual. It should be noted that the inclusion of a family therapist is not a standard of care, but a specific feature of the discussed protocol.

During the disclosure session the genetic testing results are revealed in the presence of both the genetic counselor and the family therapist. Cancer screening, prevention, and psychological issues are discussed as they arise. Special attention is given to feelings of depression, anxiety, loss, or guilt. A follow-up letter with an individualized summary of the information discussed during the disclosure session is sent to each participant. Participants are encouraged to contact the counselors and therapists with any concerns or problems they may have experienced following the disclosure session. This counseling protocol model has been widely adapted and expanded. One feature that has been added to the protocol is a pre-disclosure session which is accompanied by the receipt of a separate informed consent document for disclosure. The pre-disclosure session reinforces the main messages of the first genetic counseling session, and the informed consent document gives the participant the opportunity to refuse receipt of the test results.

After reviewing the literature, Marteau and Croyle (1998) suggest that adverse psychological reactions appear to be less common when testing is provided within a testing program that provides clear information and emotional support both before and after testing. Specifically, they argue that pre-decision counseling should provide clear and simple information concerning the advantages and disadvantages of testing, as well as the meaning of any possible result. Furthermore, the test results should be explained and support offered not only to the person being tested, but also to their relatives. From a self-regulation perspective, we would add that the individuals' representations about the meaning and process of testing, as well as their emotional responses to testing, should be elicited and addressed in the counseling program.

Genetic testing interventions and self-regulation

Although counseling interventions have been established in most academic institutions that offer genetic testing, few attempts have been made to evaluate the efficacy of such programs in a methodologically rigorous clinical trial (Croyle and Lerman, 1999). One exception is a study by Lerman and colleagues (Lerman *et al.*, 1997) that evaluated the effects of an education session and an education-plus-counseling session on women with a low to moderate risk of developing breast cancer, as compared to a waiting-list control condition. The education and counseling sessions followed standards set forth by the National Association of Genetic Counseling and incorporated behavioral variables that have been found to influence decision-making. Those in the education condition received information on the benefits, limitations, and risks of BRCA1 testing, assessed the options for screening and prevention, and discussed personal risk factors. For the counseling component, this information was personalized by addressing the individual's family history and discussing the psychological ramifications of genetic testing. The authors hypothesized that among those receiving the education sessions, testing knowledge would increase and the perceived risk of being a mutation carrier would decline, as compared to the control condition. In addition, it was predicted that those in the counseling condition would be left with fewer perceived benefits and more perceived costs of testing, with the result being a decreased willingness among the participants to undergo testing or to donate blood.

Data analyses revealed that both conditions were equally effective in enhancing genetic testing-related knowledge compared to the control group. As predicted, the personalized counseling approach was successful in decreasing perceived benefits and increasing perceived costs of testing. Neither approach, however, reduced intentions to undergo genetic testing or changed risk perceptions about breast cancer.

A self-regulation perspective might shed further light on these results. The educational component was designed to convey medical facts and technical information, but it did not address underlying beliefs or expectations surrounding genetic testing. Even the enhanced education session that included personalized counseling had little content addressing personal beliefs, expectations, and worries. Rather, the sessions addressed such topics as the experience of cancer within the family; the anticipated impact of positive or negative results on adjustment; coping; and the functional status of self and others. Beliefs about personal susceptibility and vulnerability are often deeply held based on individual experiences. As these results suggest, such beliefs are unlikely to be changed by educational sessions that convey medical and technical facts. To be successful in this regard, self-regulation theory suggests that the foundations of these exaggerated beliefs need to be explored. What is the cause of such a belief? Is it rooted in a particular traumatic experience (e.g., witnessing the death of a loved one)? How is it connected to the affect system? In other words, what are the emotional concomitants of this prior experience? Once the relationships among beliefs and affect have been established, the counseling process can then address any misconceptions and fears through common counseling approaches such as cognitive restructuring and stress management techniques.

The Family Risk Assessment Program at Fox Chase Cancer Center, a comprehensive counseling program for women at risk of developing breast and ovarian cancer, has recently undertaken a study to incorporate a cognitive and affective processing (CAP) counseling component into the genetic counseling process. The CAP intervention is based on the Cognitive-Social Health Information Processing (C-SHIP) theoretical framework, which has recently been developed by Miller and colleagues (Miller *et al.*, 1996; Miller *et al.*, 2001a; Miller and Diefenbach, 1998). In line with self-regulation theory, the C-SHIP postulates that cognitive-affective processing of cancer-relevant information takes place in cognitive-affective mediating units, which determine subsequent behavior. The mediating units encode and process cancer-relevant information, such as expectancies, beliefs, affects, values and goals, and self-regulatory strategies. The CAP intervention encourages intensive processing of the cognitive and affective responses to the information that is presented by the genetic counselor. The ultimate goal of the CAP sessions is to prepare the individual cognitively and emotionally to undergo genetic testing that is psychologically appropriate for her. In addition, the CAP prepares the individual to better cope with a positive or negative test result.

On a cognitive level, the counseling process ascertains the motivation for testing and investigates the person's representations about the testing process, addressing specific causal beliefs and consequence expectations about testing. During this process the counselor attempts to modify beliefs that could be the source of continued distress and maladaptive coping responses. For example, if an individual believes that she 'will definitely develop breast cancer' and that 'nothing can be done about it,' the counselor will attempt to correct these misconceptions by clarifying and emphasizing the role of genes in the development of breast cancer. For example, the counselor might point out that 'Just because you look like your mother/aunt (who had breast cancer) doesn't mean that you have the BRCA1/2 gene: as far as anyone knows, there is no relationship between that gene and the fact that you and your relative have both got black hair and green eyes.' In addition, the counselor will go over the breast cancer incidence statistics and will emphasize the different detection and prevention methods that the individual may choose from.

In addition to clarifying misconceptions, the counselor will address possible emotional reactions to the genetic testing information. This is achieved by actively 'pre-living' the likely consequences of receiving certain test results. Specifically, the participant pre-lives, under the guidance of the counselor, the receipt of a true positive and a true negative test result. During the pre-living process all aspects of result notification are addressed, including the moment of first learning about the results (e.g., 'Imagine that you sit in this room and you just hear from your doctor that you are/are not the carrier of a *BRCA1/2*mutation. What would your first response be? How would you feel? Would you be sad, anxious, angry? Describe what you would feel, think, or do'). Next, the individual is asked to imagine the sharing of the result information. To whom in her family would she reveal the test result, how would she do it, and what would her emotional responses be? During the end of the CAP intervention, the counselor assists the participant in formulating a decision plan that is psychologically and medically appropriate. Such a plan also includes strategies for informing her family of the results, monitoring future risk, and adhering to preventive and screening options. By taking the participant's cognitive representations and emotional reactions into account during the pre-living process, the individual will be better able to make a testing decision and be prepared to adjust to the genetic testing outcome. In addition, exploring an individual's representations and expectations will further help select the most appropriate coping strategies, as well as determine optimal prevention and screening options.

Conclusions

This chapter was designed to provide an overview of the various psychosocial issues related to genetic testing from a self-regulation perspective. It is hoped that the reader has been convinced that the CSM provides an excellent framework in which to examine the cognitive and highly charged emotional issues that surround genetic testing. Using this framework puts the individual's belief system and associated affective responses at the center of a complex information processing sequence that eventually determines decisions and actions. The individual is therefore seen not as a passive receiver of information but as an active information processor who integrates new information with past experiences, beliefs, and expectations. In the same vein, the CSM treats affects not as byproducts of cognitive processes but as constructs that are capable of driving behavior. An example of just how powerful these beliefs and expectations can be may be seen in some women's persistent and exaggerated sense of being vulnerable to breast cancer. From a self-regulatory perspective, we see a woman's sense of vulnerability not as a single isolated variable but as a complex construct that has connections to the cognitive and affective system. Further research is required, especially qualitative investigations, to explore what 'lies behind' women's answers to questions about their perceived chances of developing breast cancer. These findings then need to be integrated into the CSM framework. Furthermore, we need to pay attention to potential mediating and moderating factors and their influence on the self-regulation process. Dispositions such as optimism and preferences such as information seeking can influence the information processing sequence. It is necessary to investigate the individual and situational conditions under which such constructs operate and how they interact with self-regulation variables and eventually affect behavior.

An understanding of how individuals process information is only one side of the equation. It is also necessary to find better ways in which to present information that is personally relevant, understood, and retained. Research on tailoring such information has yielded important results in this respect, but more work is needed to address the timing, quantity, and frequency of information presentation. There is a space for the CSM here as well. Understanding an individual's pre-existing ideas concerning cancer's timeline, consequences, cause, and controllability has an obvious importance in the determination of the timing, quantity, and frequency of information presentation during the intervention. Clearing up misconstruals and reinforcing correct beliefs as appropriate sets the stage for the participant to make an informed decision regarding genetic testing. It should be reiterated that pre-existing beliefs, expectations, and emotional responses about genes, cancer, and the ability of modern medicine to provide a cure for the disease also have the potential to act as filters for ignoring some information, as well as structuring the interpretation of the information to which the individual attends. Thus, representations need to be assessed and integrated into discussions about the genetic testing procedure, the implications of test results on future prevention behaviors, and the importance of the results for other family members.

To summarize, we feel that self-regulation theory provides researchers and clinicians the tools with which to obtain a more complete understanding of the steps involved in the genetic testing process. Not only does it enable one to understand the motivation behind an individual's decision to undergo testing, it also provides a framework for predicting decision-making, adjustment, and the selection of screening and prevention behaviors.

Note

1   Preparation of this manuscript was supported in part by grants from the National Cancer Institute, CA6136-04 and CA06927, which supports the Behavioral Core Research Facility at Fox Chase Cancer Center; the Commonwealth of Pennsylvania PADOH ME-98155; and the Department of Defense DAMD 17-01-1-0006. We are indebted to Suzanne M. Miller Ph.D. for her comments and to Cecily Knauer and Mary Ann Ryan for their technical assistance. Correspondence concerning this chapter should be addressed to Michael A. Diefenbach PhD., Division of Population Science, Fox Chase Cancer Center, 510 Township Line Road 3rd Fl., Cheltenham, Pennsylvania 19012, USA. E-mail: ma_diefenbach@fccc.edu

References

Biesecker, B.B., Boehnke, M., Calzone, K., Markel, D.S., Garber, J.E., Collins, F.S. and Weber B.L. (1993) 'Genetic counseling for families with inherited susceptibility to breast and ovarian cancer,' *Journal of the American Medical Association* **269**: 1970–1974.

Bjork, J., Akerbrant, H., Iselius, L., Bergman, A., Engwall, Y., Wahlstrom, J., Martinsson, T., Nordling, M. and Hultcrantz, R. (2001) 'Periampullary adenomas and adenocarcinomas in familial adenomatous polyposis: cumulative risks and *APC* gene mutations,' *Gastroenterology* **121**: 1127–1135.

Botkin, J.R., Croyle, R.T., Smith, K.R., Baty, B.J., Lerman, C., Goldgar, D.E., Ward, J.M., Flick, B.J. and Nash, J.E. (1996) 'A model protocol for evaluating the behavioral and psychological effects of BRCA1 testing,' *Journal of the National Cancer Institute* **88**: 872–882.

Cappelli, M., Surh, L., Humphreys, L., Verma, S., Logan, D., Hunter, A. and Allanson, J. (1999) 'Psychological and social determinants of women's decisions to undergo genetic counseling and testing for breast cancer,' *Clinical Genetics* **55**: 419–430.

Cappelli, M., Surh, L., Walker, M., Korneluk, Y., Humphreys, L., Verma, S., Hunter, A., Allanson, J. and Logan, D. (2001) 'Psychological and social predictors of decisions about genetic testing for breast cancer in high-risk women,' *Psychology, Health and Medicine* **6**: 321–333.

Clark, S., Bluman, L.G., Borstelmann, N., Regan, K., Winer, E.P., Rimer, B.K. and Skinner, C.S. (2000) 'Patient motivation, satisfaction, and coping in genetic counseling and testing for BRCA1 and BRCA2,' *Journal of Genetic Counseling* **9**: 219–235.

Claus, E.B., Schildkraut, J.M., Thompson, W.D. and Risch, N.J. (1996) 'The genetic attributable risk of breast and ovarian cancer,' *Cancer (Phila.)* **77**: 2318–2324.

Coyne, J.C., Kruus, L., Kagee, A., Thompson, R. and Palmer, S. (2002) 'Benign mental health consequences of screening for mutations of *BRCA1/BRCA2,*' *American Journal of Medical Genetics* **107**: 346–347.

Croyle, R.T. and Lerman, C. (1999) 'Risk communication in genetic testing for cancer susceptibility,' *Journal of the National Cancer Institute Monographs No. 25*, pp. 59–66.

Croyle, R.T., Smith, H.R., Botkin, J.R., Baty, B. and Nash, J. (1997) 'Psychological responses to BRCA1 mutation testing: preliminary findings,' *Health Psychology* **16**: 63–72.

Daly, M. (1999) 'NCCN practice guidelines: genetics/familial high-risk cancer screening,' *Oncology* **13**: 161–183.

DudokdeWit, A.C., Tibben, A., Frets, P.G., Meijers-Heijboer, E.J., Devilee, P., Klijn, J.G.M., Oosterwijk, J.C. and Niermeijer, M.F. (1997) 'BRCA1 in the family: a case description of the psychological implications,' *American Journal of Medical Genetics* **71**: 63–71.

Durfy, S.J., Bowen, D.J., McTiernan, A., Sporleder, J. and Burke, W. (1999) 'Attitudes and interest in genetic testing for breast and ovarian cancer susceptibility in diverse groups of women in Western Washington,' *Cancer Epidemiology, Biomarkers and Prevention* **8**: 369–375.

Easton, D.F., Ford, D., Bishop, T. and the Breast Cancer Linkage Consortium. (1995) 'Breast and ovarian cancer incidence in BRCA1-mutation carriers,' *American Journal of Human Genetics* **56**: 265–271.

Ford, D., Easton, D.F., Bishop, D.T., Narod, S.A., Goldgar, D.E. and the Breast Cancer Linkage Consortium. (1994) 'Risks of cancer in BRCA1-mutation carriers,' *Lancet* **343**: 692–695.

Ford, D., Easton, D.F., Stratton, M., Narod, S., Goldgar, D., Devilee, P., Bishop, D.T., Weber, B., Lenoir, G., Chang-Claude, J., Sobol, H., Teare, M.D., Struewing,

J., Arason, A., Scherneck, S., Peto, J., Rebbeck, T.R., Tonin, P., Neuhausen, S., Barkardottir, R., Eyfjord, J., Lynch, H., Ponder, B.A., Gayther, S.A., Zelada-Hedman, M. and the Breast Cancer Linkage Consortium (1998) 'Genetic heterogeneity and penetrance analysis of the BRCA1 and BRCA2 genes in breast cancer families,' *American Journal of Human Genetics* **62**: 676–689.

Geller, G., Botkin, J.R., Green, M.J., Press, N., Biesecker, B.B., Wilfond, B., Grana, G., Daly, M.B., Schneider, K. and Kahn, M.J.E. (1997) 'Genetic testing for susceptibility to adult-onset cancer: the process and content of informed consent,' *Journal of the American Medical Association* **277**: 1467–1474.

Jagelman, D.G., DeCosse, J.J. and Bussey, H.J. (1988) 'Upper respiratory cancer in familial adenomatous polyposis,' *Lancet* **1**(8595): 1149–1151.

Kash, K.M., Ortega-Verdejo, K., Dabney, M.K., Holland, J.C., Miller, D.G. and Osborne, M.P. (2000) 'Psychosocial aspects of cancer genetics: women at high risk for breast and ovarian cancer,' *Seminars in Surgical Oncology* **18**: 333–338.

Lau, R.R., Bernard, T.M. and Hartman, K.A. (1989) 'Further explorations of common-sense representations of common illnesses,' *Health Psychology* **8**: 195–219.

Lerman, C., Audrain, J. and Croyle, R. (1994a) 'DNA testing for heritable breast cancer risks: lessons from traditional genetic counseling,' *Annals of Behavioral Medicine* **16**: 327–333.

Lerman, C., Rimer, B.K. and Engstrom, P.F. (1991) 'Cancer risk notification: psychosocial and ethical implications,' *Journal of Clinical Oncology* **9**: 1275–1282.

Lerman C., Daly, M., Masny, A. and Balshem, A. (1994b) 'Attitudes about genetic testing for breast-ovarian cancer susceptibility,' *Journal of Clinical Oncology* **12**: 843–850.

Lerman, C., Biesecker, B., Benkendorf, J.L., Kerner, J., Gomez-Caminero, A., Huges, C. and Reed, M.M. (1997) 'Controlled trial of pretest education approaches to enhance informed decision-making for BRCA1 gene testing,' *Journal of the National Cancer Institute* **89**: 148–157.

Lerman, C., Lustbader, E., Rimer, B., Daly, M., Miller, S., Sands, C. and Balshem, A. (1995) 'Effects of individualized breast cancer risk counseling: a randomized trial,' *Journal of the National Cancer Institute* **87**: 286–292.

Lerman, C., Hughes, C., Lemon, S.J., Main, D., Snyder, C., Durham, C., Narod, S. and Lunch, H.T. (1998) 'What you don't know can hurt you: adverse psychologic effects in members of *BRCA1*-linked and *BRCA2*-linked families who decline genetic testing,' *Journal of Clinical Oncology* **16**: 1650–1654.

Lerman, C., Narod, S., Schulman, K., Hughes, C., Gomez-Caminero, A., Bonney, G., Gold, K., Trock, B., Main, D., Lynch, J., Fulmore, C., Snyder, C., Lemon, S.J., Conway, T., Tonin, P., Lenior, G. and Lynch, H. (1996) 'BRCA1 testing in families with hereditary breast-ovarian cancer: a prospective study of patient decision-making and outcomes,' *Journal of the American Medical Association* **275**: 1885–1892.

Leventhal, H. (1970) 'Findings and theory in the study of fear communications,' in L. Berkowitz (ed.) *Advances in Experimental Social Psychology*, vol. 5, New York: Academic Press, pp. 120–186.

Lipkus, I.M., Iden D., Terrenoire, J. and Feaganes, J.R. (1999) 'Relationships among breast cancer concern, risk perceptions, and interest in genetic testing for breast cancer susceptibility among African-American women with and without a family history of breast cancer,' *Cancer Epidemiology, Biomarkers and Prevention* **8**: 533–539.

Lodder, L., Frets, P.G., Trijsburg, R.W., Meijers-Heijboer, E.J., Klijn, J.G.M., Duivenvoorden, H.J., Tibben, A., Wagner, A., van der Meer, C.A., van den Ouweland, A.M.W. and Niermeijer, M.F. (2001) 'Psychological impact of receiving a *BRCA1/BRCA2* test result,' *American Journal of Medical Genetics* **98**: 15–24.

Marteau, T.M. and Croyle, R.T. (1998) 'Psychological responses to genetic testing,' *British Medical Journal* **316**: 693–696.

Marteau, T.M. and Senior, V. (1997) 'Illness representations after the human genome project: the perceived role of genes in causing illness,' in K.J. Petrie and J.A. Weinman (eds) *Perceptions of Illness and Treatment*, Amsterdam: Harwood Academic, pp. 241–266.

Miller, S.M. and Diefenbach, M.A. (1998) 'C-SHIP: a cognitive-social health information processing approach to cancer,' in D. Krantz (ed.) *Perspectives in Behavioral Medicine*, Mahwah, NJ: Lawrence Erlbaum Associates, pp. 219–244

Miller, S.M., Shoda, Y. and Hurley, K. (1996) 'Applying cognitive-social theory to health-protective behavior: breast self-examination in cancer screening,' *Psychological Bulletin* **119**: 70–94.

Miller, S.M., Fang, C.Y., Diefenbach, M.A. and Bales, C.B. (2001a) 'Tailoring psychosocial interventions to the individual's health information processing style: the influence of monitoring versus blunting in cancer risk and disease,' in A. Baum and B. Anderson (eds) *Psychosocial Interventions and Cancer*, Washington, DC: American Psychological Association, pp. 343–362.

Miller, S.M., Driscoll, J.L., Rodoletz, M., Sherman, K.A., Daly, M.B., Diefenbach, M.A., Buzaglo, J.S., Godwin, A.K. and Babb, J.S. (2001b) 'Coping style correlates of participation in genetic testing for inherited breast and ovarian cancer risk,' poster session presented at A Decade of ELSI Research Conference, Bethesda, MD.

National Society of Genetic Counselors. (1997) 'Predisposition genetic testing for late-onset disorders in adults: a position paper of the National Society of Genetic Counselors,' *Journal of the American Medical Association* **278**: 1217–1220.

Quaid, K.A. (1992) 'Presymptomatic testing for Huntington's disease: recommendations for counseling,' *Journal of Genetic Counseling* **1**: 277–302.

Schwartz, M.D., Hughes, C., Roth, J., Main, D., Peshkin, B.N., Isaacs, C., Kavanagh, C. and Lerman, C. (2000) 'Spiritual faith and genetic testing decisions among high-risk breast cancer probands,' *Cancer Epidemiology, Biomarkers and Prevention* **9**: 381–385.

Schwartz, M.D., Peshkin, B.N., Hughes, C., Main, D., Isaacs, C. and Lerman, C. (2002) 'Impact of *BRCA1/BRCA2* mutation testing on psychologic distress in a clinic-based sample,' *Journal of Clinical Oncology* **20**: 514–520.

Spiegelman, A.D., Talbot, I.C., Penna, C., Nugent, K.P., Phillips, R.K., Costelli, C. and DeCosse, J.J. (1994) 'Evidence for adenoma-carcinoma sequence in the duodenum of patients with familial adenomatous polyposis: the Leeds Castle Polyposis Group (Upper Gastrointestinal Committee),' *Journal of Clinical Pathology* **47**: 709–710.

Struewing, J.P., Hartge, P., Wacholder, S., Baker, S.M., Berlin, M., McAdams, M., Timmerman, M.M., Brody, L.C. and Tucker, M.A. (1997) 'The risk of cancer associated with specific mutations of BRCA1 and BRCA2 among Ashkenazi Jews,' *New England Journal of Medicine* **336**: 1401–1408.

Struewing, J.P., Lerman, C., Kase, R.G., Giambarresi, T.R. and Tucker, M.A. (1995) 'Anticipated uptake and impact of genetic testing in hereditary breast and ovarian cancer families,' *Cancer Epidemiology, Biomarkers and Prevention* **4**: 169–173.

Tercyak, K.P., Lerman, C., Peshkin, B.N., Hughes, C., Main, D., Isaacs, C. and Schwartz, M.D. (2001) 'Effects of coping style and BRCA1 and BRCA2 test results on anxiety among women participating in genetic counseling and testing for breast and ovarian cancer risk,' *Health Psychology* **20**: 217–222.

Yeomans-Kinney, A., Croyle, R.T., Dudley, W.N., Bailey, C.A., Pelias, M.K. and Neuhausen, S.L. (2001) 'Knowledge, attitudes, and interest in breast-ovarian cancer gene testing: a survey of a large African-American kindred with a BRCA1 mutation,' *Preventive Medicine* **33**: 543–551.

Index

abstract, conceptual processes 2–3, 158, 184, 248–9, 316, 325
activities of daily living 43
Addison's disease (AD): spouse/carer perceptions 209–11
adherence to treatment 28, 141–2, 261
adjustment to stressful events 30–2, 67, 175–6
affect 22–3, 184–199; approach systems 22–3, 158–9; avoidance systems 22–3, 158–9; discrepancy reduction 22; negative 22–3, 157–77, 184–99; positive 22–3, 196–7; regulating systems and goals 194, 223; role of confidence and doubt 23–5; role of effort 25; role of giving up 25
aging and self-regulation 51, 54–5, 80, 149, 223
AHP see Analytic Hierarchy Processing
AIDS and adjustment 29, 248
Analytic Hierarchy Processing (AHP) 11, 304–7
anxiety 23, 157–77, 317; and cognition 158–9; Common Sense Model (CSM) 158–9; coping responses 129–30, 165–8; illness–related responses 165–8; illness representations 159–60; influences on concrete processing 163; influences on information processing 161–3; influences on perception and attention 160–1; interventions 173–6; physiological processes 158–9, 170; in response to health threats 169–73; and self-regulation 173–6; self–regulation theory 158–9; and sustained health habits 167–8; and symptom reporting 170–1; trait 84, 169–74

arthritis see osteoarthritis, rheumatoid arthritis
asthma 102–4, 141; interventions 175, 260–2, 272
avoidance 76, 129, 132, 185
behavioural avoidance system (BAS) 157–9, 165, 169, 171, 177
Beliefs about Medicines Questionnaire (BMQ) 103, 139–42
blood glucose awareness training 259
BMQ see Beliefs about Medicines Questionnaire
bone density screening 187
breast cancer: and anxiety 53–4, 172; and genetic testing 162, 170, 172, 248, 304, 307–27
breast self-examination (BSE) 281–2, 286, 300
cancer 108–12; coping with 32, 172; interventions 33–5, 264–7, 322–6; role of hope and purpose 33–6; and self-concept 195; worry 48, 162, 319, 321
cancer screening 8, 297–309; Analytic Hierarchy Processing (AHP) 304–5; decision making 297–309; interventions 303–4, 322–6; preventive health behaviour theories 298–9; Preventive Health Model (PHM) 301–2; self-regulation 297–309; see also breast self–examination, colorectal cancer screening, mammography, prostate cancer screening, skin cancer screening
cardiac disease: activity patterns after hospitalisation 229–233; adaptation to 220–36; belief systems 9; emotional support 234; gender differences 223–4, gender linked traits

235; gender stereotypes 220–36; health care setting 220–36; interventions 173–4, 233–4; medical self–referral 222; psychological adjustment to 27–8; self–regulation 220–36; symptom levels after hospitalisation 231–2; symptom perceptions 164, 222–8; treatment delay and gender 222–3; treatment seeking 223–8; Type A personality 223–4

cardiac invalidism 232, 269

cardiovascular disorders 112

causal beliefs 20–1, 49–52, 100, 159, 243, 245; in cardiac disease 112–13, 164, 270; carer perceptions 210–12, 214, 215; in chronic obstructive pulmonary disorder 104; in functional somatic syndromes 124–6; in genetic testing 315, 321; and treatment perceptions 145

CET see Coping Effectiveness Training Intervention

CFS see chronic fatigue syndrome

Chronic Disease Self-Management Programme 268

chronic fatigue syndrome (CFS) 119–20, 12–8, 130–1; spouse / carer perceptions 209–11

chronic illness: behavioural perspective 99–102; carer perceptions 56, 131, 207–17; Common Sense Model (CSM) 101–2; coping 101–2, 196; core concept 98–9; family context 207–8; management of 257–73; patient outcomes 214–16; perceptions of professional care 212–14; perceptions of spouse 208–12; representations of 97–114; self-regulatory interventions 257–73; see also Addison's disease (AD), AIDS and adjustment, asthma, cancer, cardiac disease, cardiovascular disorders, chronic fatigue syndrome (CFS), chronic obstructive pulmonary disease (COPD), diabetes mellitus, HIV, myocardial infarction (MI), neurological disorders, osteoarthritis, rheumatoid arthritis

chronic obstructive pulmonary disease (COPD) 104

chronic pain 123–5

chronic pelvic pain 120, 122

cognitive-affective units of illness representations 75, 77, 325

cognitive appraisal in psychological stress 67

cognitive behavioural stress management intervention 34–5, 263–4, 267

cognitive behaviour therapy 266–7

colorectal cancer screening 301–2, 314

Common Sense Model (CSM) 4–5, 7–8, 20–2, 42–60, 184, 221, 241; anxiety and cognition 157–9; and cancer screening 299–301, 303; and chronic illness 101–2; and functional somatic syndromes (FSS) 121–32; future directions 58–60; and genetic testing 315; history of 43–6; and medication use 139, 144–7; process rules 58; representations 48–53; and the self 58–9

competence beliefs 5

complementary therapies 144, 149

concerns beliefs and medication 139–44

concrete, experiential processes 2–3, 158, 184, 248–9, 316, 325

confidence 23–5, 28; in health and illness behaviour 17–36

congruence in carer–patient beliefs 208–15

conscious versus non–conscious processes 2–3

consequences beliefs 20–1, 49–52, 100, 159, 245; carer perceptions 210–12; in chronic obstructive pulmonary disorder 104; in functional somatic syndromes 125–7; in genetic testing 315, 317; in myocardial infarction 269, and treatment perceptions 145

control/cure beliefs 20–1, 49–52, 100, 245, 265; in cardiac disease 112–13; carer perceptions 210–12; in chronic obstructive pulmonary disorder 104; in functional somatic syndromes 126; in genetic testing 315; and treatment perceptions 145; see also locus of control

COPD see chronic obstructive pulmonary disease

coping 67–73, 76–89, 234; accommodative 80; anxiety and 165–8, 171; assimilative 80; avoidant 76; carer influence on 208–12, 214; cognitive representations 52–3, 127–8, 208; cognitive representations in chronic fatigue syndrome (CFS) 128; cognitive representations in functional somatic syndrome (FSS) 127; emotion–focused 44–6, 67, 84, 166, 175, 215; as a predictor of health outcomes 113; problem–focused 44–7, 67, 78, 84, 165–6, 215; repressive style 76; styles 84; vigilant 76

Coping Effectiveness Training Intervention (CET) 262–4

coping skills training 259, 261–9

coronary artery bypass surgery 27

coronary heart disease (CHD) see cardiac disease, cardiovascular disorders, myocardial infarction

cultural beliefs and self–regulation theory 52, 57, 243–4

cultural differences in medical treatment use 150, 247, 249

culture: assessment of 249–50; definition of 242–3; and illness representations 242–50; and personality 88–9

cybernetic control theory 43, 66–8

decision making: Analytic Hierarchy Processing (AHP) 304–5; cancer screening 297–309; self-regulatory perspectives 7–8

defensive denial 184–99, 215; affect regulation 191–2; and avoidance 185; behavioural costs 192–3; definition 185; self–regulation model 184; self-system influences 194–5

defensive processing 3, 161–3, 190–1, 195–6; in diabetes mellitus 196; interventions 258–60

depression 23, 27, 32, 33, 196, 215, 234, 248

detection behaviour 281–5; see also breast self-examination, mammography, prostate cancer screening, skin cancer screening

diabetes 85, 170, 196, 213, 258–60, 272

dispositional optimism see optimism

doctors and medical knowledge 212–14

doubt 23–5

emotion-focused interventions 173–6

emotion regulation 2, 10, 34, 184–99; and anxiety 129–30, 157–77, 166–7

emotional constraint/suppression 172, 174, 234

emotional disclosure techniques 175

emotional intelligence 82–3

emotional representations 104, 129, 147, 159, 248

emotional response tendencies 84

empacho 244

epilepsy beliefs 249

expectancies 5, 25, 77; control-related 78–9; generalised 25; global 79; in personality 77–9; role of thoughts 24–5

expectancy–based theories 25

expectancy–value theories 33

explanatory models of illness 100, 244–5, 247

extraversion 70

false consensus bias 188

family influences on illness 207–8

fear 44–8, 129, 132, 157, 175, 185; fear–drive model 44–5

feedback loops 1, 18–19, 66–7, 220–1; discrepancy–enlarging 18–19; discrepancy–reducing 18–19, 22

FFM see Five Factor Model

fibrocystic disease 190

fibromyalgia 86, 119–20, 122–3, 126–7

Five Factor Model (FFM) 68–71, 84–86

folk illnesses 114, 244

functional somatic syndromes (FSS): aetiology 121; cognitive representations 122–8; common functional syndromes 120; emotional representations 129–30; illness representations 130–2; interactional model 121; representational beliefs 119–32; role of socio-cultural factors in 131–2; see also chronic fatigue syndrome (CFS), chronic fibromyalgia, chronic pain, chronic pelvic pain, hyperventilation syndrome, irritable bowel syndrome, multiple chemical sensitivity, non-cardiac chest pain, premenstrual syndrome, somatization, temporomandibular joint disfunction, tension headache

gain frames for health messages 279–92

gender stereotypes 222–36

genetic testing 8, 314–27; for BRCA1/2 162, 170, 172, 248, 304, 317–327; in cancer 314–27; Common Sense Model (CSM) 315; counselling protocols 315, 322–23; eligibility 318; illness representations 317; interventions 323–6; predictors of testing uptake 320–2; psychological outcomes 320–322; role of family 318; self-regulation 314–27

giving-up 28–33, 171; limited disengagement 29; partial disengagement 29

goals: and affect regulation 194; anti-goals 19; approach 19, 80; avoidance 19, 80; cognitive representations of 5; coherence 4, 8; constructs in personality and health 67, 74, 79–80, 87–88; disengagement 29–33, 171; emotion-focused 2; and feedback processes 17–19; in health and illness behaviour 17–36; hierarchical organisation of 2, 19–22, 26, 68; and hope 28–31, 33–5; level of abstraction 19–20; non–conscious 3; parallel processing of 2; Power's hierarchy 20–1; problem–focused 2; and purpose 33–5; re-engagement 30–1; self-presentation 80–1; social-cognitive view 79–82; survival 4, 8

HBM see Health Belief Model

health action process approach 7

health behaviour 5, 167–8, 187, 192–3, 250, 283–5; attitudinal models 57; Fear-Drive Model 44–5; goals 2, 26; and illness representations 211, 278–92; interventions 278–92; message framing 278–92; parallel–processing model 44–5; role of discrepancy enlargement goals 19; role of discrepancy reduction goals 19; see also prevention behaviour

Health Behaviour Goal Model 2, 5

Health Belief Model (HBM) 7; in cancer screening 298

health threats: bogus 188–9; control-systems approach 220–1; defensive responses 194–7; emotion-focused coping 165; information 189–91; minimisation of 186–8; multiple process model 220–1; problem–focused coping 165–6; responses to 157–77; role of anxiety 157–77; role of cognition 157–177; self–regulation of 169, 184–99, 220–2; social comparisons 56, 188–9; trait anxiety 169–71

heart disease see cardiac disease, myocardial infarction

heart transplant surgery: role of positive expectations 28

HIV: interventions 262–4; medication use 142–4, 146; prevention 82; response to diagnosis 186; testing 286

hope 28–31, 33–5

hot/cold theory of disease 245–6, 249

hypertension 187–8, 246, 260; feedback 19; identity of illness threat 49; symptoms 19, 50–1

hyperventilation syndrome 119–20, 123

hypochondriasis and goal cognition 79–80

identity beliefs 20–1, 48–52, 100, 159, 245; in cardiac disease 112–13; carer perceptions 210–12; in chronic obstructive pulmonary disorder 104; in functional somatic syndromes 122–4, 127; in genetic testing 315, 317; and treatment perceptions 145

if-then profiles 53–4, 75, 87

Illness Perceptions Questionnaire (IPQ) 102–3, 105, 111–13, 210, 216, 270

Illness Perceptions Questionnaire Revised (IPQ–R) 102

illness representations 20–1, 48–52, 58–60, 195, 242–50, 258–9, 315; across cultures 131, 242–50; age–illness rule 51; anthropological studies 52–3, 242–50; anxiety influences 159–63; of carers 207–17; chronic illness 93–114; coherence 301–2, 145; content domains 50–2; cultural influences on 131, 242–50; functional somatic syndromes (FSS) 130–2; health behaviour 278–92; of health care providers 212–14; prevalence rule 51; stress-illness rule 51; symmetry rule 50; and treatment 138–50

individual differences approach to personality 68–71, 76–84, 86

intelligence 81–83, 87; emotional 83; social 82; somatic and visceral 83

interpersonal skills 82

interventions 8–9, 33–5, 59–60, 198, 233–4; chronic illness 33–5, 257–73; emotion–focused 173–6; emotional disclosure techniques 175; genetic counselling 323–6; mental simulation 175–6; objective processing strategies 174

IPQ see Illness Perceptions
   Questionnaire
IPQ–R see Illness Perceptions
   Questionnaire (Revised)
irritable bowel syndrome 119–20, 122–4,
   128–9
locus of control 78
loss frames in health messages 279–92
mal de ojo 244
mammography 281–2, 288–92, 303
marital stress 232
medical care seeking 54–6, 163, 165, 175,
   213–14, 220–36, 269; rule of
   conservation 54
medical treatments and self-regulation
   46–8
medication adherence 141–4, 268;
   barriers to use 138; common–sense
   representations 140–4; demographic
   variables 149–50; personal sensitivity
   to 149; resilience to 149
melanoma and coping 236, 266
mental simulation techniques 25, 175–6
message framing 278–92; application to
   health communications 280–2;
   detection behaviours 282–7;
   preference reversals 279–80;
   prevention behaviours 283–7;
   Prospect Theory 279–81; role of
   construals 285–7
MI see myocardial infarction
minimization of health threats 186–8
molera caida 52
monitoring-blunting 76–8, 288
multiple chemical sensitivity 119–20
myocardial infarction (MI): causal
   attributions 164; interventions 174,
   269–72; and marital stress 232;
   perceptions of spouse 208, 211–12,
   214; recovery from 211–12; social
   support 228–9; treatment delay and
   gender 222–3
necessity beliefs and medication 139–44
negative affect 22–3, 157–77, 184–99
negative affectivity 172, 174; see also
   neuroticism, trait anxiety
neurological disorders 104–8
neuroticism 70, 73, 169, 171; see also
   negative affect, trait anxiety
non-adherenceto treatment 142–4
non-cardiac chest pain 120, 123, 126
noxious medical treatments and self-
   regulation 46–8

openness to experience 71
optimism 27–8, 34; dispositional 27–8,
   79, 264
osteoarthritis: coping 213, 215, 268;
   interventions 268
pain 46–8, 129, 174, 268; chronic 120,
   122–5
Parallel Processing Model 44–6
personality, 68–89; attention to threat
   76–7; and competencies 81–2;
   dispositional perspective 68, 85;
   expectancies 77–9; Five Factor
   Model (FFM) 68–71, 84–86; goal
   constructs 17–19, 74, 87–8; goals
   79–82; in health and disease 66–89;
   individual differences 68–9, 76–7; and
   intelligence 81–3;
   personality–stressor–illness
   relationship 71–3; process
   perspectives 74; processing approach
   68, 85; research models 69–70; and
   response tendencies 84; and risk
   behaviour 81; self/identity constructs
   74; self–relevance 77; social–cognitive
   approaches 74–76, 81–82, 84–86;
   social-cognitive model 75; traits 68–9
pessimism 27–8
pessimistic explanatory style 77
PHM see Preventive Health Model
positive expectations 28
post-traumatic growth 175
Power's hierarchy of goals 20–1
precaution adoption process 7
precautionary behaviour see prevention
   behaviour
premenstrual syndrome 120, 123
prevalence beliefs 188–9
prevention behaviour 167–8, 186–93,
   283–5
Preventive Health Model (PHM) 4, 11,
   301–2
problem maximization and minimization
   209–11
problem-solving 43–4: goals of 43–4
Prospect Theory 11, 279–81
prostate cancer screening 305–8
provider–patient communications 82,
   170–1
psychosocial interventions 33–5
purpose: sense of 33–5
qualitative methods 49, 100–1, 244–5
quality-of-processing hypothesis 190
reassurance from medical staff 174

regrets: management of 32–3
repressive coping style 76
response tendencies in personality 84
rheumatoid arthritis 123, 126
risk behaviours 188–9; and
    self–presentation goals 80–1
risk perceptions 48, 149, 164, 186–8,
    192–3, 316, 321
schizophrenia: perceptions of 215
screening 285–7; cancer 297–309
self 5, 43–4, 53–4, 58–9, 130–1, 194–7,
    299
self-constructs 74,77
self-control 75, 167–8, 193
self-efficacy 5, 78–9, 191
self-guides 77, 195
sexually transmitted diseases 192
skin cancer screening 286
smoking 187–8, 195
smoking cessation 178, 186–7
social-cognitive approaches to
    personality and health 74–86
social comparison 24, 188–9
social influences on health 6, 54–8,
    131–2, 207–17, 224, 227, 318
social intelligence 82–3
social skills 82
social support 35, 72, 82, 172, 208, 209,
    214–17, 228–9, 263; gender
    differences in 228–33, 234
somatic and visceral intelligence 83
somatization 79, 119–37, 236, 248
somatoform disorders see
    hypochondriasis, somatization
spouses, influences on coping 208–12
stage theories of health behaviour 7;
    health action process approach 7;
    precaution adoption process 7;
    transtheoretical model 7;
statistical accounts of personality 71–3,
    75, 85–6
stereotypes: gender 222–36; old age 236
stress 67–73, 78–9, 84; behaviour-
    focused research 67; cognitive
    appraisal 67; emotion–focused coping
    67; and illness appraisals 51–2, 164–5;
    problem-focused coping 67; stress-
    focused research 67
stress-coping models 2–3, 67–73, 101

stress-management interventions 34–5,
    173, 175–6, 262, 266
stressed power motivation 70
subjective utility models 7; Health Belief
    Model (HBM) 7; Theory of Planned
    Behaviour (TPB)7; Theory of
    Reasoned Action (TRA) 7
suicide and disengagement 31
sunscreen use 281, 283
support group therapy 35, 265
support groups 131
symmetry rule 50–1
symptoms 9; Common Sense Model
    (CSM) 58; interpretations of 19, 49,
    51, 122–4, 127, 145, 164, 170, 214,
    223, 235, 247, 271; and life regrets 33;
    medically unexplained 119;
    monitoring 47–8, 258–61; self-
    regulation responses 48, 68
temporomandibular joint disfunction
    120
tension headache 120
Theory of Planned Behaviour 7, 57, 299;
    in cancer screening 299
Theory of Reasoned Action (TRA) 7,
    57; in cancer screening 299
timeline beliefs 20–1, 49–52, 100, 187,
    245, 265; in cardiac disease 112–13;
    carer perceptions 210–12; in chronic
    obstructive pulmonary disorder 104;
    in functional somatic syndrome
    125–6; in genetic testing 315; and
    treatment perceptions 145
TOTE unit 1, 43, 57
TPB see Theory of Planned Behaviour
TRA see Theory of Reasoned Action
trait anxiety 84, 169–74
trait hostility 70
transtheoretical model 7, 303
treatment beliefs 139–49; cognitive and
    emotional representations 147; as
    health threat 146–7; perceptions of
    138–50; self-regulation 138–50; self-
    regulation model 147
Type A personality 70, 223–4
unmitigated communion orientation 235
validity perceptions of information
    189–91

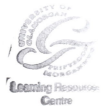